Skeletal Muscle Structure, Function, & Plasticity

Second Edition

The Physiological Basis of Rehabilitation

Skeletal Muscle Structure, Function, & Plasticity

Second Edition

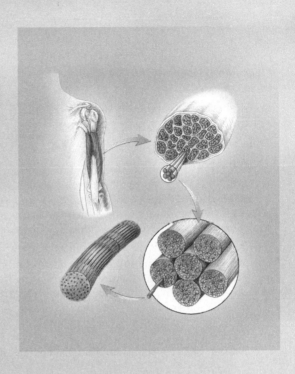

The Physiological Basis of Rehabilitation

Richard L. Lieber, PhD

Professor of Orthopaedics and Bioengineering
Departments of Orthopaedics and Bioengineering
Biomedical Sciences Graduate Program
University of California, San Diego
and V.A. Medical Center

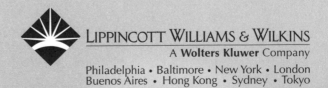

LIPPINCOTT WILLIAMS & WILKINS
A **Wolters Kluwer** Company

Philadelphia • Baltimore • New York • London
Buenos Aires • Hong Kong • Sydney • Tokyo

Editor: Tim Julet
Managing Editor: David Payne
Marketing Manager: Debbie Hartman
Production Editor: Jennifer Ajello
Designer: Risa Clow
Compositor: Graphic World
Printer: Maple-Vail

Printed in the United States of America

First Edition, 1992

Coventry University

Library of Congress Cataloging-in-Publication Data is available

ISBN 0-7817-30619-X

To purchase additional copies of this book, call our customer service department at **(800) 638-3030** or fax orders to **(301) 824-7390**. International customers should call **(301) 714-2324**.

Visit Lippincott Williams & Wilkins on the Internet: *http://www.LWW.com.* Lippincott Williams & Wilkins customer service representatives are available from 8:30 am to 6:00 pm, EST.

05
2 3 4 5 6 7 8 9 10

To my mother, Janet Stone Lieber, who gave me her brains and her humor.
Mom, I thank God that I learned this precious lesson just before your untimely death.

Preface

Understanding such universal phenomenon as movement or strength requires an understanding of the neuromuscular system. Since muscle represents about 3/4 of the body mass, a healthy muscular system is associated with healthy cardiovascular, pulmonary, and endocrine systems. Conversely, disorders of the neuromuscular system have dramatic effects on daily activities and independence. Unfortunately, there is currently no text available that presents evidence-based muscle basic science and plasticity in a simple, unified manner. Therefore, the purpose of this book is to provide useful information for understanding strength and movement, by describing the structure, function, and plasticity of the neuromuscular system.

The second edition of this book is actually a new book. Based on the thoughtful and critical feedback from students, I have endeavored to revise all of the experimental examples to use the newly available data that permit a focus on the human musculoskeletal system. In addition, I have added thought-provoking "boxes" that pose questions and provide answers that are clinically relevant if not a bit controversial. Finally, at several points, "Therapist's Comments" provide feedback and perspective from a noted academic physical therapist, Dr. Gary Chleboun (Ohio University). Taken together, my goal is to make this book more relevant, more rigorous, and more interactive than the previous edition.

As with the first edition, this book is conceptually divided into two parts: Part 1 (Chapters 1–3) represents the foundations of basic science. Part 2 (Chapters 4–6) represents illustrations of these basic science concepts by illustrating the adaptive capacity of muscle.

● Chapter 1 begins with an integrated presentation of muscle development and anatomy. The significance of these anatomical features is discussed in later book chapters.

● Chapter 2 (the longest chapter) describes both the mechanical and physiological properties of skeletal muscle. The elegance of structure-function relationships in the neuromuscular system is emphasized. Again, the significance of these properties is foreshadowed as it relates to the practice of physical therapy.

● Chapter 3 describes the way in which muscles, tendons, and joints interact to produce movement, using Chapters 1 and 2 as a conceptual base. The key to this chapter is to understand that the whole muscle-tendon-joint system does not simply represent the sum of the parts.

● Chapter 4 presents various ways of increasing muscle use and their effects: chronic electrical stimulation, passive stretch, voluntary exercise, surgical transfer, etc. By looking at the detailed muscle response to these interventions, you will begin to understand the response of muscle to almost any type of increased use and will be able to strategize regarding optimal methods for strengthening muscle.

● Chapter 5 continues our discussion of plasticity in the context of decreased-use models: immobilization, spinal cord injury, denervation, and weightlessness. Again, you will learn the way in which a muscle adapts when the level of use is decreased. You will also learn why some muscles are not vulnerable to the atrophy experienced by others.

● Chapter 6 ends the book with a description of muscle's cellular and physiological response to injury as well as some exciting experimental treatments of muscle disease. Since injury can arise in the form of trauma, intense exercise, laceration, or injection of local anesthetic, a rationale for avoiding such injuries is also presented.

Based on this broad presentation, the rehabilitation professional can focus his/her attention on the scientific basis for muscle treatment. Throughout the text, intervention strategies and traditional thinking are critically evaluated in light of the data presented. Many of the world's most outstanding experiments are presented and interpreted in a way that provides unifying principles to the understanding of skeletal muscle structure, function, and plasticity.

Acknowledgments

Special thanks to my colleagues who have read various chapters and provided helpful criticism in this as well as the first edition: Frank Booth, Bruce Carlson, Reggie Edgerton, Brenda Eisenberg, Bob Gregor, Roland Roy, and Tricia Silva. Of course, no scientist is an island and thus I acknowledge the support and leadership of my scientific collaborators: Reid Abrams, David Amiel, Wayne Akeson, Ron Baskin, Mike Botte, Gary Chleboun, Dale Daniel, Reggie Edgerton, Jan Fridén, Richard Gelberman, Bob Gregor, Alan Hargens, Ken Kaufman, Gordon Lutz, Odile Mathieu-Costello, Roland Roy, Allen Ryan, David Sutherland, Lars-Eric Thornell, and Yin Yeh. In the same way, I have benefited from the interaction with current and former laboratory students and staff: Marcia Beckman, Field Blevins, Jenny Boakes, Shannon Bremner, Cindy Brown, Tom Burkholder, Clark Campbell, Jennifer Davis, Brendan Donoghue, Babak Fazeli, Tom Ferro, Mark Jacobson, Amir Jamali, Yasuo Kawakami, Jeanne Kelly, Björn-Ove Ljung, Greg Loren, Margot Leonard, Michael Mai, Dev Mishra, Randy Mohler, Tina Patel, Eva Pontén, Rajnik Raab, Michel Sam, Tony Sanzone, Sameer Shah, Tricia Silva, Mary Schmitz, Scott Shoemaker, Christy Trestik-Farnsworth, Thalia Woodburn, Al Tsai, Nancy Wudek, and Abbe Zaro. Thank you to colleagues who generously provided access to unpublished material in order to enhance this text: Jon Covault, Reggie Edgerton, Jan Fridén, Tetsuo Fukanaga, Bob Gregor, Yasuo Kawakami, Paavo Komi, and Roland Roy. I very much appreciate the thoughtful feedback from Dr. Gary Chleboun, who scoured the entire book to create the "Therapist's Comments" sections. I am indebted to medical artist Rebecca Chamberlain who enthusiastically and cheerfully created many of the beautiful illustrations contained herein, learning more about muscle than I'm sure she ever wanted to know! In addition to scientific support, I am deeply indebted to Dina Clark, Jennifer Davis, and Yvonne Hall for the tremendous administrative assistance and the moral support needed to complete this two-year project.

I would also like to specifically acknowledge my close friend Jan Fridén, who has become my "brother-in-science" during the last 15 years and Allen Ryan who has acted as my trusted confidante, running partner, and mentor for almost 20 years.

Thanks also to the editorial staff at Lippincott Williams & Wilkins—John Butler who originally supported the idea of this text, Linda Napora, who taught me the meaning of editing in the first edition, and Ulita Lushnycky who provided the encouragement and guidance that I needed in just the right way at just the right time in order to create this second edition.

Finally, I would like to express my love to my sister, Susan Clark-Laughlin, for her never-ending support and love, and to my girls, Katie and Kristi who have unwittingly endured their Dad's latest crazy project. I know I am blessed to be your Dad, to know you and to enjoy your love.

"Unless the Lord build the house, they labor in vain who build it." Psalm 127:1.

BRIEF NOTE TO THE STUDENTS

I have been thinking of you the entire time that I have been writing this book, trying to decide what you really "need" to know on this topic. I believe that learning muscle design and plasticity can be fun and stimulating. I have endeavored to present you with the "truth" about muscle structure and to explain its ability to adapt. I love this topic and I hope you will catch that vision. There is so much fabulous information in the literature. I have tried to limit my presentation to those topics that I truly believe are instructive and useful. Certainly I will come up short at times and even bore you. I apologize in advance for the shortcomings of this text. Please let me know how I can make it better for you. The future of this field is in your hands. Take this presentation, process it, and advance your practice to the next level. Your patients and your students deserve your best.

Contents

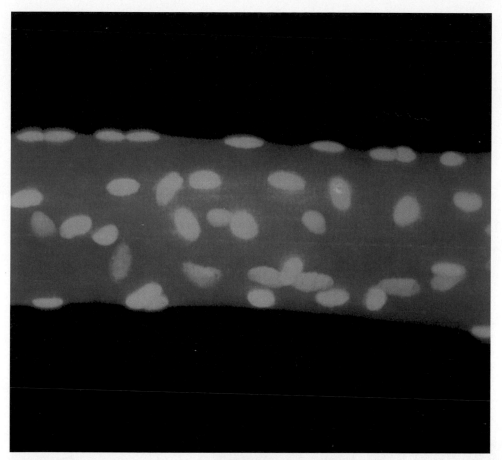

COLOR FIGURE C-1. Myonuclei identified along the length of an isolated muscle fiber. Nuclei were stained with a florescent dye that binds to DNA and then located throughout a single fiber using the method of confocal scanning laser microscopy, which is able to "reconstruct" a three-dimensional fiber based on individual optical slices. This figure forms the basis for the cover of this textbook. (Micrograph kindly provided by V. Reggie Edgerton (University of California, Los Angeles) from the publication: Allen, D. L., Monke, S. R., Talmadge, R. J., Roy, R. R., & Edgerton, V. R. (1995). Plasticity of myonuclear number in hypertrophied and atrophied mammalian muscle fibers. *Journal of Applied Physiology, 78*, 1969–1976.)

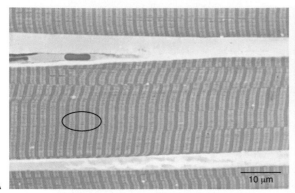

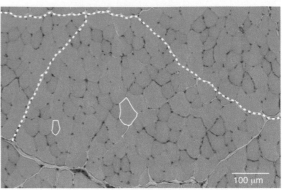

A   B

COLOR FIGURE C-2. **(A)** Longitudinal section of a tibialis anterior muscle biopsy specimen that was chemically fixed, embedded in plastic, sectioned at 1 μm thickness, stained with toluidine blue, and viewed with a light microscope. The alternating light and dark regions correspond to the sarcomere A- and I-bands. A portion of three fibers is shown in this section. The space between fibers is an artifact of the fixation process. Circled area represents the subregion shown in the electron micrograph of Figure 1-9 page 23. (Micrograph courtesy of Dr. Jan Fridén, Professor of Hand Surgery, Göteborg University, Sweden.) **(B)** Cross-section of a tibialis anterior muscle biopsy specimen that was frozen, sectioned at 8 μm thickness, and stained with hematoxylin and eosin for demonstration of normal fiber morphology. Note that, in cross-section, muscle tissue appears as a collection of densely packed polygonal muscle fibers. Each muscle fiber is surrounded by a sheath of endomysial connective tissue (shown for two individual fibers as a solid line), and groups of muscle fibers (fascicles) are surrounded by more dense perimysial connective tissue (shown for one region as dashed lines). Calibration bars correspond to a distance of 100 μm.

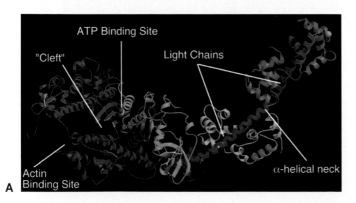

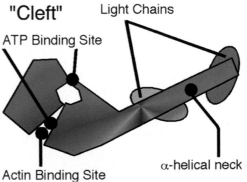

A   B

COLOR FIGURE C-3. Three-dimensional crystal structure of the S-1 portion of the myosin heavy chain molecule. **(A)** High resolution ribbon diagram of chicken S-1 myosin determined using X-ray crystallography. Labeled are the key features of the molecule, the ATP and actin binding sites, the cleft between them, and the α-helical region to which the myosin light chains binds. (Ribbon diagram kindly provided by Dr. Ivan Rayment, University of Wisconsin based on the report: Rayment, I., Rypniewski, W. R., Schmidt-Base, K., Smith, R., Tomchick, D. R., Benning, M. M., Winkelmann, D. A., Wesenberg, G., & Holden, H. M. (1993). Three-dimensional structure of myosin subfragment-1: a molecular motor. *Science, 261*, 50–58.) **(B)** Schematic drawing of the myosin S-1 portion based on the ribbon diagram presented in (A) and used to illustrate the cross-bridge cycle shown in Figure 2-10, page 70.

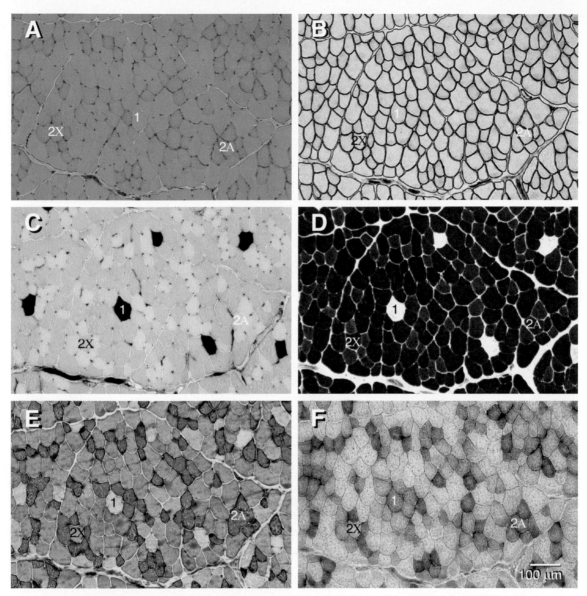

COLOR FIGURE C-4. Serial cross-sections of rabbit tibialis anterior skeletal muscles under various staining conditions. The identical fiber can be traced through each section to compare properties of fibers. **(A)** Hematoxylin and eosin, demonstrating general muscle fiber morphology. **(B)** Dystrophin immunohistochemistry showing the subsarcolemmal nature of this protein (brown deposits represent protein). **(C)** Myofibrillar ATPase under acid preincubation conditions. Under these conditions, slow fibers stain darkly as do the extracellular capillaries while fast fibers stain lightly. **(D)** Myofibrillar ATPase under alkaline preincubation conditions. Under these conditions, slow fibers stain lightly while fast fibers stain darkly. Note that in both panels C and D, fast fiber staining intensity occurs at two levels. **(E)** Immunohistochemical reaction for fast myosin heavy chain antibody. In rat skeletal muscle, this antibody (SC71, see Table 2-5, page 84) stains type 2A fibers darkly and type 2X fibers more lightly and is negative for types 2B and 1 fibers. **(F)** Succinate dehydrogenase (SDH) used to demonstrate muscle fiber oxidative capacity. Note that the slow fibers (sample fiber labeled with a ''1'') as well as the type 2A fast fibers (sample fiber labeled with a ''2A'') have higher oxidative capacity compared to the type 2X fibers (sample fiber labeled with a ''2X'').

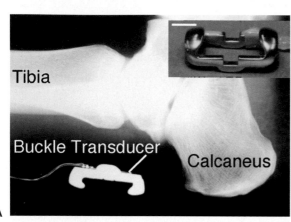

A

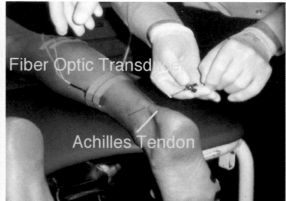

B

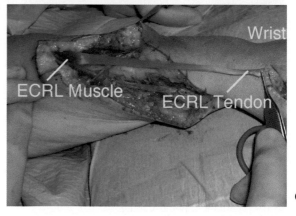

C

COLOR FIGURE C-5. Experimental methods for direct measurement of human muscle force as discussed on pages 131 to 132. **(A)** Tendon "buckle" placed on a human Achilles tendon for direct measurement of triceps surae muscle force during locomotion. (Photograph kindly provided by Professor Dr. Robert Gregor, Georgia Tech University.) **(B)** Fiber optic probe inserted into a human Achilles tendon for direct measurement of triceps surae force. (Photograph kindly provided by Professor Dr. Paavo Komi, University of Jyväskyla, Jyväskyla, Finland.) **(C)** Isolation and direct measurement of human extensor carpi radialis longus (ECRL) muscle force during hand surgery. (Photograph kindly provided by Professor Dr. Jan Fridén, Göteborg University, Göteborg, Sweden.)

CHAPTER 1

Skeletal Muscle Anatomy

Chapter Overview

Anatomy, the study of structure, forms the basis for understanding muscle function. Throughout this text, various aspects of muscle structure will be referred to continuously to understand its function. The muscle cell and muscle as a tissue represent a tremendously sophisticated arrangement of proteins. This chapter will discuss the nature of this arrangement and how it arises It will focus on muscle development and structure which will ultimately form the foundation for much of the information that will be presented later. This initial glimpse into the complex organization of skeletal muscle presents a sample of the degree to which muscle is *designed* to accomplish its task of generating force and movement. This chapter will show how the cell develops and will explore the components of the mature mammalian muscle cell. By the end of this chapter, completed muscles that perform a range of functions through a variety of novel structures will have been created.

Educational Objectives

● To understand the basic components of a muscle cell
● To understand the filament lattice structure of a muscle cell and how that results in the striation pattern
● To understand the significance of whole muscle cellular organization (architecture)
● To be familiar with the basic developmental process
● To understand structural differences between muscle fiber types

Introduction

Skeletal muscle represents the classic biological example of a structure-function relationship. At both the macroscopic and microscopic levels, skeletal muscle is exquisitely tailored for force generation and movement. Because of this structure-function relationship, studies of muscle function are intimately tied to studies of muscle structure, i.e., as muscle structures are discovered, the next goal is to determine their function. This chapter begins by discussing the skeletal muscle cell, and then describes skeletal muscle development, which will lead to a discussion of muscle cellular structure. The structural discussion begins at the microscopic level and builds to the macroscopic level, which shows the way in which the various structures contribute to muscle function both at the cellular and whole tissue levels. Muscle research is exciting and alive and full of unanswered questions. Enjoy the adventure into the study of one of the most well-understood of all biological structures.

1 Muscle Development

It is difficult to appreciate the beautifully orchestrated developmental process without first understanding the organization of mature muscle and muscle cells. The developmental sequence may make more sense after understanding muscle cellular structure presented later in the chapter. There is an intricate and specific arrangement of the neuromuscular system: Motor nerves arise from a variety of spinal cord levels, combine into a common fascicle along with nerves from other levels, and proceed peripherally to innervate specific muscles— even specific fiber types within specific muscles. How do muscles and nerves achieve this intricate arrangement? What are some of the factors that guide the process? Are nerves told exactly where to meet their muscle, or do they search into the periphery and then recognize specific muscle fibers? Do muscles attract nerves by sending specific signals? Nerve-muscle recognition is a rapidly changing and growing field; therefore, definitive answers to these questions must await further discovery. However, several exciting discoveries made over the last 3 decades provided meaningful insights into the developmental process (Kelly, 1983).

Overview of Muscle Development

For purposes of discussion, the process of muscle development will be divided into four phases (Fig. 1-1). Many of these phases occur simultaneously, coordinated in time. The four processes are (a) axonal outgrowth (the process by which axons traverse into the periphery to contact muscles), (b) myogenesis (muscle cell formation), (c) synaptogenesis (formation of neuromuscular junctions between the motor nerve and muscle fiber), and (d) synapse elimination (the process that eliminates *extra* neuromuscular connections). Studies of each step in the developmental process have used various experimental models. These include in vitro cell culture preparations (to study muscle cell differentiation) and denervation and re-innervation of mature muscle (to study nerve-muscle interaction). Taken together, these studies provide a framework on which to build our understanding of development. The following discusses each of these processes in more detail.

Axonal Outgrowth—Nerve Meets Muscle

Connections between muscles and nerves are specific. Motor nerves that exit the ventral root of the spinal cord are long processes extending from motoneuron cell bodies located along the lateral motor column of the ventral horn (Fig. 1-2). There is a rough (but not perfect) correspondence between the location of the various motoneuron pools along the spinal cord and the muscles that they innervate (Table 1-1). This correspondence is important in diagnosing the location of trauma or disease based on clinical observation of the specific patient functions that are affected. The clinician can work backwards from a determination of the altered function, to knowing which muscles affect that function, to diagnosing the level of the lesion that affects those muscles. For example, in Table 1-1 note that if elbow flexion is impaired, this can be traced to weakness or paresis of the brachialis muscles, and the nerve root exiting at the C6 level is implicated. Using this type of logic, clinical diagnoses are made regarding the level and severity of spinal cord injuries. However, it should also be noted that lesions that occur at a particular level might have different clinical presentations. Therefore, it is not extremely descriptive to state that a patient has a "C-6 lesion" without a basic description of the patient's specific sensory and motor status.

The most detailed information regarding motor axon outgrowth has been obtained from studies of the chick hindlimb. Because of the accessibility and abundance of chick embryo material, developmental biology depends on this system for the understanding of embryology. Although insights may be provided, there are certainly questions regarding the applicability of this information to mammalian systems.

Upon inspection of the complex and numerous muscle-nerve connections, one might ask, "How do all of the axons find one another and then find the appropriate muscle? After finding the muscle, how do they find the correct muscle fiber?" Before reviewing what is known, think about the potential answers to

(text continues on page 8)

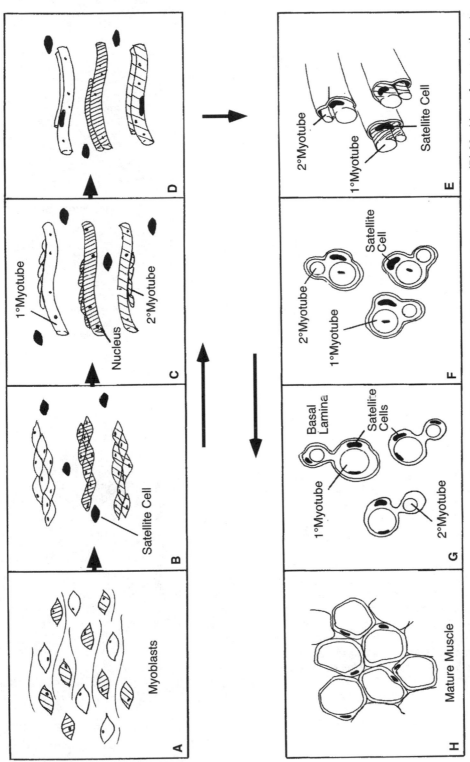

FIGURE 1-1. Schematic diagram of skeletal muscle development. **(A)** Primitive cells differentiate into myoblasts. **(B)** Myoblasts fuse together to form primary myotubes. **(C–F)** Later, secondary myotubes arise beneath the basal lamina of the primary myotubes. Fusion of myoblasts radially and longitudinally results in formation of the muscle fiber beneath basal lamina (shown in cross-section in E through H). In addition, some unfused myoblasts remain as satellite cells, which are maintained in the mature cell. **(G)** As the muscle matures, primary and secondary myotubes separate, each with myonuclei and satellite cells, to become a mature fiber. **(H)** Finally, as the muscle fibers grow, they become arranged as tightly packed polygonal cells, characteristic of adult muscle.

3

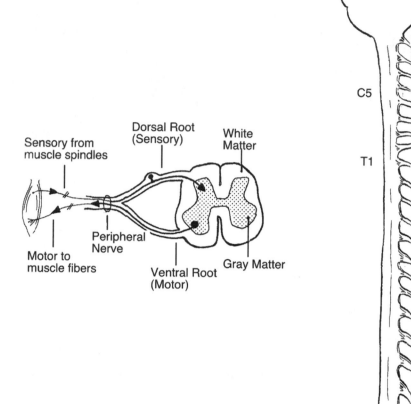

FIGURE 1-2. Left, Schematic arrangement of the spinal cord. Motoneurons have their cell bodies in the gray matter of the spinal cord and exit through the ventral root, via the peripheral nerve, to innervate skeletal muscles. Sensory nerves from muscle spindles and Golgi tendon organs have their cell bodies in the dorsal root. Sensory fibers from the muscle traverse the peripheral nerve to synapse in the spinal cord. **Right,** Cranial-caudal organization of the spinal nerve roots. Spinal nerve roots descend from the brain via specific tracts and exit the spinal cord at various locations to innervate muscle in a topographical manner (See Table 1-1). Note that nerve root level roughly corresponds with anatomic level. This is useful information clinically in that a particular muscle weakness can be associated with nerve root dysfunction at a particular spinal segment level.

| TABLE 1-1 | Anatomy of the Human Skeletal Muscles |

Muscle	Origin	Insertion	Innervation	Nerve Root	No. Joints Crossed
Extensor hallucis longus	Medial anterior fibular surface	Dorsal surface of distal phalanx	Deep peroneal	L4, L5, S1	> 3
Extensor digitorum longus	Anterior fibular surface	Dorsal surface of toes 2-5	Deep peroneal	L4, L5, S1	>3
Flexor hallucis longus	Posterior fibular surface	Planter surface of distal phalanx	Tibial	L5, S1, S2	>3
Flexor digitorum longus	Posterior fibular surface	Plantar surface of distal phalanx of toes	Tibial	L5, S1, S2	>3
Tibialis anterior	Lateral tibial surface	Medial and plantar side of medial cuneiform	Deep peroneal	L4, L5, S1	2
Tibialis posterior	Posterior surface of tibia, fibula, and interosseus membrane	Medial navicular surface	Tibial	L4, L5, S1	2
Peroneus tertius	Lower fibular anterior surface	Dorsal surface of base of 5th metatarsal	Deep peroneal	L4, L5, S1	2
Peroneus brevis	Lateral fibular surface	Dorsal surface of base of 5th metatarsal	Superficial peroneal	L4, L5, S1	2
Soleus	Posterior proximal surface of fibula and medial border of tibia	Posterior surface of calcaneus	Tibial	L5, S1, S2	1
Gastrocnemius	Posterior/superior surfaces of lateral and medial femoral condyles	Posterior surface of calcaneus	Tibial	S1, S2	3
Plantaris	Lateral supracondylar line of femur	Posterior surface of calcaneus	Tibial	L4, L5, S1	3
Popliteus	Lateral femoral epicondyle	Soleal line on posterior surface of tibia	Tibial	L4, L5, S1	1
Vastus lateralis	Lateral lip of linea aspera	Lateral patellar border	Femoral	L2, L3, L4	1
Vastus medialis	Distal half of intertrochanter line and medial lip of linea aspera	Medial patellar border	Femoral	L2, L3, L4	1
Vastus intermedius	Anterior femoral surface	Superior patellar border	Femoral	L2, L3, L4	1
Rectus femoris	Anterior inferior iliac spine	Superior patellar border	Femoral	L2, L3, L4	2
Tensor fasciae lateae	Lateral surface of anterior inferior iliac spine	Lateral tibial condyle	Superior gluteal	L4, L5, S1	2
Gracilis	Body of pubis	Medial tibial condyle	Obturator	L3, L4	2
Sartorius	Anterior superior iliac spine	Medial surface of tibia	Femoral	L2, L3, L4	2
Semimembranosus	Ischial tuberosity	Medial tibial condyle	Sciatic	L4, L5, S1, S2	2
Semitendinosus	Ischial tuberosity	Medial tibial surface	Sciatic	L4, L5, S1, S2	2

(continued)

| TABLE 1-1 | Anatomy of the Human Skeletal Muscles *(Continued)* |

Muscle	Origin	Insertion	Innervation	Nerve Root	No. Joints Crossed
Biceps femoris	*Long Head*- ischial tuberosity *Short Head*- lateral lip of linea aspera	Fibular head and lateral tibial condyle	Sciatic	L5, S1, S2, S3	2
Piriformis	Pelvic surface of sacrum	Superior border of greater trochanter	Sacral plexus	L5, S1, S2	1
Obturator internus	Pelvic surface of ischium	Medial surface of greater trochanter	Sacral plexus	L5, S1, S2	1
Obturator externus	Rami of pubis and ischium	Greater trochanter	Obturator	L3, L4	1
Gemellus superior	External surface of ischial spine	Medial surface of greater trochanter	Sacral plexus	L5, S1, S2	1
Gemellus inferior	Proximal ischial tuberosity	Medial surface of greater trochanter	Sacral plexus	L4, L5, S1	1
Quadratus femoris	Lateral border of ischial tuberosity	Intertrochanteric crest	Sacral plexus	L4, L5, S1	1
Gluteus maximus	Posterior gluteal line and dorsal sacral surface	Gluteal tuberosity of femur and iliotibial tract	Inferior gluteal	L5, S1, S2	2
Gluteus medius	Between posterior and inferior gluteal lines of ilium	Lateral surface of greater trochanter	Superior gluteal	L4, L5, S1	2
Gluteus minimus	Between anterior and inferior gluteal lines of ilium	Anterior surface of greater trochanter	Superior gluteal	L4, L5, S1	2
Psoas major	Transverse processes of vertebral bodies	Lesser femoral trochanter	Lumbar plexus	L1, L2, L3, L4	3
Iliacus	Illiac fossa of ilium	Lesser femoral trochanter	Femoral	L2, L3, L4	1
Adductor longus	Inferior ramus of pubis	Linea aspera of femur	Obturator	L3, L4	1
Adductor brevis	Inferior ramus of pubis	Linea aspera of femur	Obturator	L3, L4	1
Adductor magnus	Ischial tuberosity and inferior ramus of pubis	Entire linea aspera and adductor tubercle of femur	Obturator and sciatic	L2, L3, L4	1
Pectineus	Superior ramus of pubis	Pectineal line of femur	Femoral	L2, L3, L4	1
Deltoid	Clavicle and scapula	Deltoid tuberosity of humerus	Axillary	C5, C6	1
Pectoralis major	*Clavicular*- medial half of clavicle *Sternal*- anterior surface of sternum and cartilages of ribs 2-6.	Crest of greater tubercle and lateral lip of intertubercular groove of humerus	Pectoral	C5–T1	2
Coracobrachialis	Tip of coracoid process	Medial surface of humerus	Musculocutaneous	C5, C6, C7	1

TABLE 1-1	Anatomy of the Human Skeletal Muscles

Muscle	Origin	Insertion	Innervation	Nerve Root	No. Joints Crossed
Latissimus dorsi	Lower thoracic and lumbar vertebrae	Intertubercular groove of humerus	Thoracodorsal	C6, C7, C8	2
Teres major	Inferior angle of scapula	Medial lip of inter-tubercular groove of humerus	Lower subscapular	C5, C6	1
Supraspinatus	Supraspinous fossa	Greater tubercle of humerus	Suprascapular	C5	1
Teres minor	Lateral scapular border	Greater tubercle of humerus	Axillary	C5	1
Infraspinatus	Infraspinous fossa	Greater tubercle of humerus	Suprascapular	C5, C6	1
Subscapularis	Subscapular fossa	Lesser tubercle of humerus	Subscapular	C1–C6	1
Biceps brachii	*Short Head*- tip of cora-coid process *Long Head*- supra-glenoid tubercle	Radial tuberosity	Musculocutaneous	C5, C6	3
Triceps brachii	*Lateral Head*- lateral margin of humerus *Long Head*- Infraglenoid tubercle of scapula *Medial Head*- posterior surface of humerus	Common tendon: supe-rior aspect of olecranon process	Radial	C5, C6	1
Brachialis	Anterior surface of humerus	Tuberosity of ulna	Musculocutaneous and radial	C5–C8	1
Brachioradialis	Lateral epicondyle of humerus	Lateral aspect of styloid process of radius	Radial	C5, C6	2
Anconeus	Lateral epicondyle of humerus	Lateral margin of olec-ranon process of ulna	Radial	C5, C6	1
Supinator	Lateral epicondyle of humerus and supina-tor crest of ulna	Lateral surface of radius	Deep Radial	C6, C7, C8	1
Pronator teres	Medial epicondyle of humerus	Lateral surface of radius	Median	C6, C7	1
Pronator quadratus	Medial surface of ulna	Anterior surface of radius	Median	C8–T1	1
Flexor carpi radialis	Medial epicondyle of humerus	2nd and 3rd metacarpal	Median	C6, C7	1
Flexor carpi ulnaris	Medial epicondyle of humerus	Pisiform, hamate, and 5th metacarpal	Ulnar	C8–T1	1
Palmaris longus	Medial epicondyle of humerus	Palmar aponeurosis	Median	C6, C7	1
Extensor carpi radialis longus	Supracondylar humeral ridge	2nd metacarpal	Radial	C6, C7	1

(continued)

TABLE 1-1 **Anatomy of the Human Skeletal Muscles** *(Continued)*

Muscle	Origin	Insertion	Innervation	Nerve Root	No. Joints Crossed
Extensor carpi radialis brevis	Lateral epicondyle of humerus	3rd metacarpal	Radial	C6, C7	1
Extensor carpi ulnaris	*Humeral Head-* lateral epicondyle of humerus *Ulnar Head-* posterior surface of ulna	5th metacarpal	Deep Radial	C6, C7, C8	1
Extensor digitorum communis	Lateral epicondyle of humerus	*Central-* posterior aspect of middle phalanx 2 *Collaterals-* posterior aspect of distal phalanx	Radial	C7	>3
Extensor indicis proprius	Lower dorsal surface of ulna	Unites with index finger tendon of ext. dig. Comm. on middle phalanx 2	Deep Radial	C6, C7, C8	>3
Extensor digiti minimi	Lateral epicondyle of humerus	Posterior aspect of middle phalanx 5	Deep Radial	C6, C7, C8	>3
Flexor digitorum superficialis	*Humeral Head-* medial epicondyle *Radial Head-* anterior shaft of ulna and radius	Sides of middle phalanx 2-5	Median	C7–T1	>3
Flexor digitorum profundus	Anterior surface of ulna	Distal phalanges 2-5	Palmar, median, and ulnar	C8–T1	>3
Abductor pollicis longus	Metacarpal and carpal bones	Proximal phalanx of thumb	Ulnar	C8–T1	2
Extensor pollicis brevis	Posterior surface of radius	Posterior surface of proximal phalanx of thumb	Deep Radial	C6, C7	3
Extensor pollicis longus	Posterior and lateral surfaces of ulna	Base of distal phalanx of thumb	Deep Radial	C6, C7, C8	>3
Flexor pollicis longus	Anterior radial surface	Base of distal phalanx of thumb	Median	C8–T1	>3

these questions. Perhaps nerves do not know where they are supposed to go and instead go everywhere. Or perhaps the nerves that do find the appropriate destination (i.e., the appropriate target muscle) survive, and all other nerves degenerate, or the process of neuronal cell death (which is known to occur in the CNS) creates a specific innervation pattern out of one that starts randomly. On the other hand, maybe nerves are programmed with a particular *destination* and simply meet the target muscle fibers at that location.

Landmesser and her colleagues (Landmesser, 1980) demonstrated that, early in development, nerves that project into muscle masses are composed almost entirely of the appropriate spinal nerves. This neural outgrowth occurs before the primitive muscle masses even contain any muscle fibers so these nerves know where they are supposed to end up and are not

Box 1-1. How do I Describe a Spinal Cord Injury?

Because of the consistent relationship between the level at which nerve roots exit the spinal cord and the particular muscle innervated, it is possible to create classification schemes for patients with spinal cord injuries. The most commonly used scheme is based on the consensus arising from an international meeting in which these factors were discussed. To describe the injury, the level of injury and the accompanying sensory ability of the patient is presented.

attracted there by muscle fibers because, at the time of their arrival, no mature muscle fibers are present. Thus, specificity begins when nerves first grow out from the ventral horn. The nerve performs this remarkable navigation virtually without error because all nerves find the correct muscles.

An interesting experiment by Landmesser and colleagues emphasized the interaction between muscle and nerve (Lance & Landmesser, 1978). They surgically switched the topographic location of two muscle masses before nerve outgrowth to see if outgrowing axons would innervate whichever muscle mass was found at the end location, or, instead, would search for the correct muscle mass. In fact, the outgrowing axons detoured and innervated the correct muscles. Therefore, even though the nerves knew the basic location for outgrowth, there was some type of cueing that existed between nerves and muscles. The nature of the cueing between nerves and muscles is an active area of research. Imagine the variety of experiments that could be performed to identify molecules needed to establish neuromuscular connections. Identification of such factors is not only important to define the basic science of neuromuscular development, but may also result in future clinical application to injured patients who require reinnervation of muscle by nerves that have been interrupted due to injury, disease, or inappropriate development

(Lundborg, 1988). By understanding the molecular signals between nerves and muscles, scientists may develop therapeutic treatments to aid in recovery of function by patients with spinal cord injuries.

Myogenesis—Birth of the Muscle Fiber

Skeletal muscles are derived from the somites of the embryo (somites are the masses of primordial muscle tissue that occur at regular intervals along the embryo's length). As myogenesis proceeds within the somites, primitive cells become *determined* to be muscle tissue. The process of determination is regulated in skeletal muscle by two proteins that turn on the developmental program, enabling these stem cells to become myoblasts. These proteins were named myoD (which stands for "myogenic determination") and myf5 (myogenic factor 5) and were discovered using an extremely clever application of molecular methods in a variety of cell types (Edmonson & Olson, 1989; Scales, Olson, & Perry, 1990). In fact, these investigators were able to show that, if myoD expression was forced in nonmuscle cells such as fibroblasts, they would become myoblasts. Myoblasts are the primitive, single-celled mononucleated muscle fiber precursor cells (Fig. 1-1A; you will see the prefix "myo" in many locations throughout this book. *Myo* is the Latin prefix for "muscle"; "blast" refers to a precursor cell. Thus, "osteoblasts" become bone cells, "fibroblasts" become tendon cells, etc.) One of the first steps in myogenesis is the aggregation of myoblasts into clusters (Fig. 1-1B). Further development of myoblasts (known as differentiation and maturation) is accompanied by the expression of two other myogenic regulatory factors known as mrf4 and myogenin. In fact all of the myogenic regulatory factors have a similar structure and precisely controlled timing of expression that enables them to cause stem cells to ultimately become whole muscles. The most significant structural feature they share is a specific region within the protein that directly binds DNA. It is this DNA binding process that turns on the muscle development program during development. This is a fascinating area of current research because it has the potential to provide therapeutic development of artificial or diseased muscle to improve patient function. Clusters of myoblasts begin to fuse to form small, multinucleated cells known as myotubes, which are about 100–300 µm in length (0.1–0.3 mm). Further length increase (which is necessary because mature fibers may extend several centimeters in length) occurs by fusion of more myoblasts onto the myotube ends. The earliest myotubes formed are known as primary myotubes. With further development, primary myotubes, and some associated, less differentiated cells, separate from the other primary myotubes into clusters that are surrounded by a sheath known as the basement membrane or basal lamina (Fig. 1-1C). At this time, more myoblasts begin to aggregate beneath the primary myotube's basal lamina, using the primary myotube as a structural scaffold. These subsequent myoblasts also fuse into myotubes, known as secondary myotubes. Now, the cell cluster is composed most noticeably of the primary myotube, its associated secondary myotube, and unfused myoblasts known as satellite cells. With further development, the primary myotube begins to look more like a mature muscle fiber, with the nuclei being forced from the fiber center to the periphery because of the progressive *filling* of the fiber with contractile proteins (Fig. 1-1D, E). If a muscle fiber is stained at this point for the contractile protein myosin, the most abundant muscle protein, the fiber appears as a doughnut shape because the contractile proteins first fill the periphery, leaving the central cell core devoid of contractile proteins and, therefore, unstained. Secondary myotubes also begin to mature into fibers at this stage so that the satellite cell, and the primary and secondary myotubes are contained within a single basement membrane (Fig. 1-1F). At this time, the motor nerve is ready to form a connection with the muscle—a neuromuscular junction.

Synaptogenesis—Birth of the Neuromuscular Junction

The neuromuscular junction (or motor endplate) is a true synapse in the sense that a chemical neurotransmitter (acetylcholine, abbreviated ACh) is used to convey information from the nerve (presynaptically) to the muscle (postsynaptically) across a synaptic cleft. Thus, the neuromuscular junction (NMJ) is a specific example of a cholinergic synapse (a synapse where the neurotransmitter is ACh). Later in the discussion of muscle contraction (Chapter 2, page 47) you will see that ACh is intimately involved in the contractile process. Early in development, ACh receptors diffusely cover the entire muscle fiber (Fig. 1-3). These receptors are specific proteins that integrate themselves into the muscle membrane (sarcolemma). As the nerve contacts the muscle fiber, ACh receptors begin to cluster around the site of nerve contact and become *trapped* by the nerve (Fig. 1-3). The mechanism of this trapping process is not known, but two interesting observations have been made that may provide insights into the trapping mechanism. Poo (1982) demonstrated that ACh receptors migrate in a specific way when exposed to external electrical fields. He suggested that nerve excitation itself, which generates small electrical fields at the endplate (the so-called endplate potential) may *attract* and trap ACh receptors in a positive feedback fashion: As ACh receptors are trapped, larger endplate potentials are generated, trapping more receptors, causing larger endplate potentials, etc. Another interesting observation was that, following nerve-muscle contact, the nuclei beneath the ACh receptor (recall that muscle cells are multinucleated and, therefore, have literally hundreds of nuclei along their length) began to direct the synthesis of ACh receptor mRNA and the ACh receptor. The overall effect of nerve contact with the fiber, therefore, is to decrease the number of extrajunctional ACh receptors and to increase the number of junctional ACh receptors (Fig. 1-3). Once these receptors are localized, the nuclei in the region of

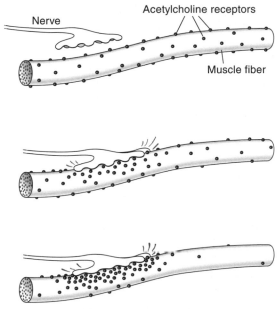

FIGURE 1-3. Distribution of ACh receptors on the muscle cell during development. Prior to innervation ACh receptors are distributed across the muscle fiber surface (*top*). As the nerve contacts the muscle fiber and electric activity ensues (denoted by lines around the neuromuscular junction), receptors aggregate in the region of the neuromuscular junction (*middle*). As maturation progresses, extrajunctional receptors decrease significantly while junctional receptors increase in number and density (*bottom*).

the NMJ take on a specialized role, expressing the genes responsible for normal NMJ function.

In the adult neuromuscular system, denervation results in a reversal of this process—an increase in extrajunctional ACh receptors. This is one reason that the mature muscle denervation-reinnervation model has been used to study some aspects of development. The processes that control normal nerve-muscle interaction are believed to also control reinnervation of muscle. It is also intriguing that the increase in extrajunctional ACh receptors that occurs following denervation can be prevented by direct muscle fiber electrical stimulation. Does this mean that electrical stimulation of denervated muscles may prevent or inhibit re-

innervation? This possibility is considered later in Chapter 5 (pages 272–275).

After the NMJ forms, the muscle fiber loses its receptivity to the formation of an NMJ at other sites. Thus, as long as a muscle is normally innervated, it is not receptive to innervation by other axons. The activity of the muscle fiber seems to be a crucial factor in this lack of receptivity because if a normally innervated muscle is chemically paralyzed, an ectopic synapse (a synapse at a location other than the NMJ) is easily formed (Bennett, 1983). This intimate association between nerve and muscle is readily demonstrated when the nerve to a muscle is cut or its ability to communicate with the muscle is interrupted chemically. In such cases, the denervated muscle responds differently to incoming electrical signals and goes to extraordinary measures to achieve reinnervation and restoration of communication. These events are considered in detail in Chapter 4.

After the initial NMJ formation, several other motoneurons may form synapses at the same location. The actual number of motoneurons per synapse ranges from two to six, depending on the muscle, and begins to decline just after birth. It declines so that, at maturity, all mammalian fibers have only a single motoneuron per fiber. This decrease is specific and is

> **Box 1-2 How Can Electrodiagnosis Reveal Denervation?**
>
> Small needles placed into a denervated muscle result in extremely large electrical potentials, known as *giant potentials*. This is due to two factors: (1) overexpression of Acetyl Choline receptors across the surface of denervated muscle fibers that increase action potential magnitude and (2) clustering of muscle fibers that occurs upon reinnervation forming *fiber type groups* where many fibers from a motor unit are in one physical location as opposed to the *spread out* mosaic distribution of normal motor units (See Color Plate C4).

accomplished by the process of synapse elimination (Jansen & Fladby, 1990).

Synapse Elimination—The Finishing Touches

The reason muscle fibers are initially hyperinnervated is not clear. Early thinking suggested that hyperinnervation followed by synapse elimination served as a mechanism to correct for hardwiring errors that occurred during haphazard axonal outgrowth. In other words, the outgrowth process would be viewed as relatively "random" but synapse elimination would correct such random outgrowth. However, as discussed earlier, axonal outgrowth is a well-defined process in which few mistakes are made. (It was known that synapse elimination occurred elsewhere in the CNS to correct for "wiring errors," so that, at the time, this was a plausible hypothesis.) Thus, the precise teleological explanation for synapse elimination is still unclear. What are the factors that determine which motoneuron will win "the battle of the synapse"? Clearly, competition between the hyperinnervating motoneurons exists, because when competing motoneurons to a particular muscle are surgically removed, the motoneurons remaining innervate a larger number of fibers than usual. However, these surviving motoneurons do not simply innervate all available fibers. There is thus some other factor (perhaps the metabolic capacity of the cell body) that limits the final innervation ratio (number of muscle fibers per axon) (Sanes & Lichtman, 1999).

In addition to the internal *programmed* changes that are scheduled to occur during development, it is clear that environmental cues also play a role. One important environmental cue is the tension experienced by the fusing and developing muscle. Dr. Vandenburgh (Vandenburgh et al. 1991) developed an ingenious method for mechanically stretching cultured muscle cells in vitro to observe the effects of stretch timing and magnitude on the developmental process. He found that cells subjected to stretch increased their rates of protein synthesis, causing an increase in cell size, and

> **Therapist's Comments**
>
> Understanding muscle development is important for the therapist who is trying to treat neuromuscular disorders such as cerebral palsy, stroke, head injury, and other traumatic Injuries. This is because, as Dr. Lieber will point out in Chapter 6, regeneration after disease or injury is basically a re-enactment of the developmental process. Similarly, recovery after denervation injury is basically a re-enactment of the original innervation of the muscle. Clearly, to develop rational treatments for these maladies, interventions must be designed that affect specific physiological processes. One example of such an intervention is the use of botulinum toxin for treatment of spasticity in diplegic cerebral palsy.

changed their orientation to become parallel to the stretch axis (Chapter 6). Although it was not clear exactly how this mechanical event was transduced by the cell, it was clear that the mechanical events strongly influenced the cellular machinery and its developmental fate. This sets up another positive feedback system in that movement enhances differentiation, which increases movement, which then increases differentiation, etc. In fact, the mechanical control of development and differentiation has become important for many cell types and is currently an exciting area of research (Banes, 1993).

Development of Specific Muscle Fiber Types

Most mammalian muscles contain a mixture of fiber types and motor units (See Chapter 2). Generally, whole muscles contain a heterogeneous mixture of fast-contracting and slow-contracting fibers, and fibers with high endurance and low endurance. This diversity allows muscles to perform a range of tasks from standing for long periods of time, to explosive power production in sprinting, to fine motor control of the fingers while taking notes in class. Thus, the processes of myogenesis, axonal outgrowth, and synapse elimination usually produce a muscle of mixed fiber type. At what stage is a fiber type determined? What is the influence, if any, of the nerve in determining fiber type? In a classic experiment, Buller and colleagues (Buller, Eccles, & Eccles, 1960a) clearly demonstrated the influence of motor nerves on mature muscle fiber types by surgically reattaching a motor nerve from a fast-contracting muscle to a slow-contracting muscle and vice versa. This experiment is described as a *cross-innervation* experiment and is commonly used to improve our understanding of nerve-muscle interaction. They found that, after cross-reinnervation, the fast-contracting muscle became slow and the slow-contracting muscle became fast (Buller, Eccles, & Eccles, 1960b). This experiment has been influential in the field of muscle physiology and formed the basis for the idea that nerves strongly influence the fate of muscle fibers. Using molecular biology techniques, Miller and Stockdale (Miller and Stockdale, 1986a,b, 1987) demonstrated that, even at the myoblast stage, myoblasts can exist as different types. Using histochemical and immunohistochemical fiber typing techniques in avian muscle, they demonstrated that even primary and secondary myotubes existed as *fast* and *slow* types. By isolating a single type of myoblast, allowing it to proliferate, and then causing it to form myotubes, they confirmed this idea because the resulting myotubes were all of a single type. Innervation was not required in this avian preparation for the different embryonic myoblast populations to arise, proliferate, and form distinct myotube populations, although further differentiation required innervation. This suggested that during development, the arriving nerve encounters a population of muscle fibers that are already heterogeneous.

Because in mature mammals, all fibers within a motor unit are of a particular type (Chapter 2, page 94), axons must either initially innervate the correct fibers, innervate the wrong muscle fiber type and then change the fiber type, or innervate randomly and use synapse elimination to correct the faulty connections. Again, experiments in this area demonstrate that the initial innervation is fairly specific.

Thompson and colleagues (Thompson, Sutton, & Riley, 1984) experimentally tested this question. Fiber type composition of developing rat soleus motor units was investigated at two different postnatal ages—8 and 16 days. At 8 days postnatally, every fiber of the rat soleus is innervated by at least two motoneurons. Over the next 8 days, synapse elimination occurs and results in the ultimate single innervation of each fiber. If the initial fiber innervation had occurred randomly, Thompson et al. predicted that muscle fibers belonging to a single motor unit aged 8 days would be composed of approximately 50% fast and 50% slow fibers, since an equal number of fast and slow fibers were present at this time. Then, after synapse elimination, he predicted that motor units would become predominantly fast or slow as the *wrong* connections were deleted. However, this was not the case. Thompson et al. found that the fiber type composition of motor units at both ages was largely of one type. In fact, although the innervation ratio fell from around 250 to 100 during the period of synapse elimination, the preponderance of a particular fiber type in a given motor unit did not change. This implied selective initial innervation of muscle fibers by specific axons. The precise mechanism for such a process is not yet clear, and many details of neuromuscular specificity await the results of future studies.

2 Skeletal Muscle Cell Microstructure

Skeletal muscle fibers are cells that, in many ways, are like any other body cell. However,

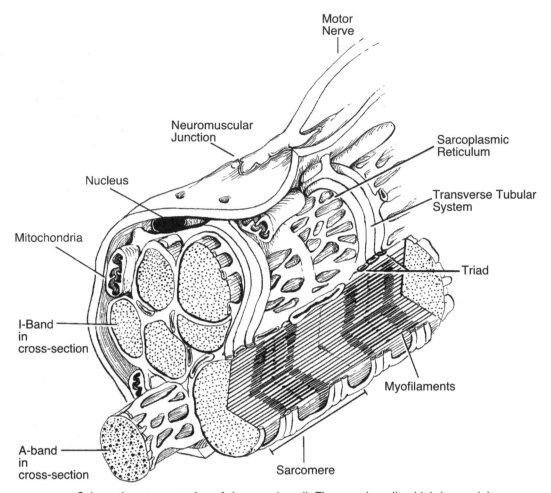

FIGURE 1-4. Schematic representation of the muscle cell. The muscle cell, which is specialized for the production of force and movement, contains an array of filamentous proteins as well as other subcellular organelles such as mitochondria, nuclei, satellite cells, sarcoplasmic reticulum, and transverse tubular system. Note the formation of "triads," which represent the T-tubules flanked by the terminal cisternae of the sarcoplasmic reticulum. Also note that when the myofilaments are sectioned longitudinally, the stereotypic striated appearance is seen. When myofilaments are sectioned transversely at the level of the A- or I-bands, the hexagonal array of the appropriate filaments is seen.

because muscle cell function is highly specialized to produce force and movement, the cellular components are also highly specialized (Fig. 1-4). Muscle cells (fibers) are cylindrical, with a diameter ranging from about 10 μm to about 100 μm—less than the diameter of a human hair. Muscle fiber diameter is profoundly important for at least two reasons: First, a muscle fiber's diameter determines its strength, and second, when altered fiber diameters are observed in mature muscle, this suggests that the level of muscle use has changed. Muscle fiber length is also highly variable, depending on the muscle's architecture (See below). Fiber length has a profound influence on fiber contraction velocity and the distance over which the fiber can shorten (*i.e.*, muscle fiber excursion).

The scaffolding that surrounds the muscle cell is known as the basal lamina. The normal physiologic role of the basal lamina is poorly understood. However, it is clear the basal lamina plays an important role in muscle fiber recovery from injury. In injuries in which the basal lamina remains intact (*i.e.,* crush injury), recovery is relatively complete. Conversely, in cases in which the basal lamina is destroyed (*i.e.,* traumatic cut), fiber regeneration first requires the laying down of a new scaffold. In fact, if a muscle fiber is destroyed and denervated, but the basal lamina remains intact, when the motor nerve reinnervates the fiber, it will do so at the original site dictated by the basal lamina, even though no muscle fiber is present. Thus the basal lamina, which demarcated functional myotubes during development, retains a good deal of identity later in cellular life (See discussion in Chapter 6). It is likely that the basal lamina expresses a variety of proteins that create a "molecular fingerprint" that remains even if the muscle fiber itself is destroyed.

A mesh-like sheath of collagenous tissue, called the endomysium, surrounds the muscle fiber. The endomysium might play some role in the passive mechanical properties of the fiber, but presently this has not been clearly determined. Beautiful scanning electron micrographs of the muscle endomysium have been presented by Trotter (1990) that portray a complex structure with intimate interaction between the endomysium and the muscle fiber (Fig. 1-5). In fact this type of picture has raised a number of questions regarding the nature of muscle fiber-muscle fiber interaction. Recent studies suggest that muscle fibers are intimately associated with this connective tissue matrix and that muscle fibers themselves do not simply extend from one tendon to the other (Loeb, Pratt, Chanaud, & Richmond, 1987; Ounjian et al., 1991). In fact, it appears that there are some muscle fibers that actually begin and end within the muscle belly itself. Thus, the connective tissue matrix may play a central role in muscle fiber-to-tendon tension transmission and not merely a supportive role.

This important function will be discussed in greater detail in Chapters 2 and 3. Bundles of fibers, each surrounded by endomysial tissue, are organized into muscle fascicles, each surrounded by a more stout perimysium (literally, *around muscle*). Finally, bundles of fascicles are organized into muscles, surrounded by epimysium connective tissue (literally, *on top of muscle*).

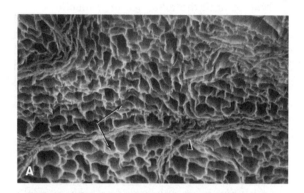

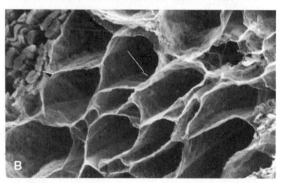

FIGURE 1-5. Scanning electron micrograph of the endomysial connective tissue within skeletal muscle. This image was generated by scanning electron microscopy of a muscle whose fibers were removed by acid digestion. **(A)** Lower magnification view of connective tissue. Arrowhead points to perimysial connective tissue. Arrows point to individual endomysial tubes. **(B)** Higher magnification view. Arrowhead points to undigested muscle fibers while arrow points to a single endomysial plane. (Original micrograph kindly provided by John Trotter (University of New Mexico) and reprinted with permission from: Trotter, J. A., & Purslow, P. P. (1992). Functional morphology of the endomysium in series fibered muscles. *Journal of Morphology, 212,* 109–122.)

Therapist's Comments

As Dr. Lieber points out, the role of the endomysium and perimysium in the passive mechanical properties of the muscle are not completely known. Many physical therapists assume that the connective tissue in the muscle accounts for the passive tension during elongation of the muscle. Although the perimysium may help to limit the extent of the muscle elongation or extensibility, the passive tension in the muscle is determined primarily by the protein titin, which is discussed extensively in Chapter 2, pages 55–60.

Cellular Organelles—Discreet Components with Specific Jobs

NUCLEI—THE BRAIN OF THE CELL

As with any other eukaryotic cell, muscle cells contain collections of organelles that are responsible for meeting the day-to-day needs of the cell. However, unlike other eukaryotic cells, muscle cells are multinucleated. There are literally hundreds of these nuclei located at intervals along the cell length (See Color Plate Section, Fig. C-1). The scheduling of synthesis and thus the type of cellular material that is distributed throughout the cell is controlled by the cell's nucleus. As a result of the many nuclei present within the cell, there is probably some form of internuclear communication to ensure that cellular properties are compatible along the cell length. Interestingly, as a muscle cell adapts to a new condition (for example, to chronic electrical stimulation), changes that occur along the cell length occur at slightly different rates. Each nucleus must, therefore, retain some degree of autonomy. For example, it was already noted that, during development, nuclei in the region of the NMJ specified the synthesis of ACh receptor mRNA whereas adjacent nuclei did not. Now you have a picture of a community of subcellular structures in communication with one another to meet the needs

of the cell. Apparently, the number of nuclei within a cell is not a constant value. A current concept is that each nucleus is "responsible" for a particular volume of cytoplasm, known as a *nuclear domain*. As the cell grows in length or diameter, new myonuclei are recruited from the satellite cells at the fiber's periphery. Conversely, if the cell experiences serious atrophy due, for example, to immobilization, space flight, or tenotomy (all of these *decreased use* models are discussed in detail in Chapter 4) the number of nuclei within the cell decreases by a process of "programmed cell death," a mechanism elucidated in modern molecular experiments (Jacobson, Weil, & Raff, 1997; Steller, 1995). Satellite cell recruitment and loss will be discussed in further detail in subsequent chapters.

SYNTHETIC MACHINERY

Associated with the cell nucleus is the endoplasmic reticulum (ER), which, as with any other cell, is responsible for the transportation of cellular material outside the cell. Because the muscle cell primarily manufactures components for local use (as opposed to the adrenal glands, for example, which synthesize hormones for general body use), this system is not well developed. Ribosomes are associated with the poorly developed ER, on which the numerous muscle proteins are synthesized. Protein synthesis that is coordinated by the nucleus is performed on ribosomes and is tremendously important to the cell. The amount and type of muscle proteins present confer on the cell its strength, speed, and endurance properties. Therefore, the regulation of protein synthesis is of paramount importance to the cell in surviving the many different environments in which it finds itself, whether it is one of increased use (exercise, electrical stimulation, stretch) or decreased use (denervation, spaceflight, spinal cord injury, immobilization, tenotomy). Specific studies that highlight the impressive upward and downward regulation of the synthetic machinery will be detailed in Chapters 4 and 5, respectively and are important because simple interventions such as exercise or passive stretch can increase muscle rates of protein synthesis and thus alter muscle function.

MITOCHONDRIA—SOURCES OF AEROBIC ENERGY

Muscle mitochondria are responsible for generation of the main cellular energy molecule, adenosine triphosphate (ATP). Mitochondria contain all the enzymes that are responsible for oxidation of the high-energy precursor (*i.e.,* nicotinamide adenine dinucleotide [NADH]) into molecular oxygen and water. During this process, much chemical energy is trapped as ATP that is used throughout the cell for muscle contraction, ion transport, protein synthesis, cellular repair, etc. (In Chapter 2 metabolism will be described in more detail and its importance to muscle function discussed.) The location and distribution of mitochondria depend on the particular muscle fiber type (see below). There is also evidence that muscle mitochondria are not actually discrete organelles but rather interconnected by a reticular network (Kayar, Hoppeler, Mermod, & Weibel, 1988; Kirkwood, Munn, & Brooks, 1986). This network might provide a means by which mitochondria in one portion of the cell communicate intracellularly with others. Because mitochondria generate ATP aerobically, their presence in the cell permits it to function continuously in the presence of oxygen. Therefore, it is not surprising that mitochondrial density is extremely plastic in the cell, responding rapidly and adequately to exercise training. It is also not surprising that mitochondrial density is important in determining the muscle fiber's endurance properties. The actual amount of mitochondria in the highly oxidative fibers may exceed 20% of the total cell volume (Eisenberg, 1983).

Cytoplasmic Components

The cytoplasm of the muscle cell is rich in soluble proteins, filamentous cytoskeletal components, and other substances. Some of the more important of these substances are the muscle fiber energy sources: glycogen and lipids. The machinery that is used to generate ATP anaerobically from glucose is also present in the cytoplasm. Glycogen is a polymer of linked glucose molecules used by muscle cells as the immediate source of glucose, which can be metabolized with or without oxygen. Large glycogen granules are located in two main locations within the cell: near the terminal cisternae of the sarcoplasmic reticulum (SR) (See below) and in between the myofibrils. Soluble enzymes within the cytoplasm perform glycolysis. Because oxygen is required to metabolize lipids (See metabolism in Chapter 2), lipid droplets are most prevalent in cells with high mitochondrial densities. Finally, numerous free-floating ribosomes synthesize proteins at locations throughout the cell.

Filamentous Components—The Defining Characteristics of a Muscle Cell
MYOFIBRILS

The discussion of the filamentous systems in the cell will be discussed from the largest scale to the smallest scale. At each stage, note that there is a precise arrangement of proteins that form the particular structure of interest. Perhaps the most distinctive feature of the muscle cell is the ordered array of contractile filaments that are arranged throughout the cell (Fig. 1-6; Table 1-2). There is a well-defined hierarchy of filament organization that proceeds from a large scale (on the order of microns, 10^{-6} m, abbreviated μm) to a small scale (on the order of angstroms, 10^{-10} m, abbreviated Å). The largest functional unit of contractile filaments is the myofibril (literally, *muscle thread*). Myofibrils are simply a string of sarcomeres arranged in series. Myofibrillar diameter is about 1μm, which means that thousands of myofibrils can be packed into a single muscle fiber. One way in which a muscle fiber grows is to increase the number of myofibrils that it contains. Myofibrils are arranged in parallel (side-by-side) to make up the muscle fiber. However, their arrangement might not resemble a bundle of spaghetti; there is some evidence that myofibrils within the fiber are arranged similar to

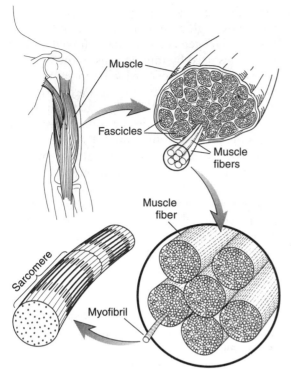

FIGURE 1-6. Structural hierarchy of skeletal muscle. Whole skeletal muscles are composed of numerous fascicles of muscle fibers. Muscle fibers are composed of myofibrils arranged in parallel. Myofibrils are composed of sarcomeres arranged in series. Sarcomeres are composed of interdigitating actin and myosin filaments.

the weave in a rope (Peachey & Eisenberg, 1978). (The functional consequence of this arrangement is that various myofibrils may not act independently of one another during normal contraction).

Myofibrils are interconnected with one another by a set of specialized proteins known as "intermediate filaments." In mature skeletal muscle, the major intermediate filament is named desmin and provides a cytoskeletal support system that permits efficient mechanical coupling of the force generated by one myofibril to the adjacent myofibril (Lazarides, 1980). You will see when the mechanisms of muscle injury (Chapter 6) is discussed, this intermediate filament network can dynamically remodel in response to intense exercise and may be pro-

foundly important to a muscle's ability to grow in response to mechanical stress.

SARCOMERES—FUNCTIONAL UNIT OF CONTRACTION

Myofibrils can also be subdivided into their subunits known as sarcomeres (Fig. 1-6), the functional unit of muscle contraction. A myofibril is therefore a number of sarcomeres (literally, *muscle segment*) arranged in series (end-to-end). The total number of sarcomeres within a fiber depends on the muscle fiber length and diameter and is the most important determinant of muscle fiber function. Because of the series arrangement of sarcomeres within a myofibril, the total distance of myofibrillar shortening is equal to the sum of the shortening distances of the individual sarcomeres. This is why a whole muscle may shorten several centimeters even though each sarcomere can only shorten about 1μm. It should also be stated that the number of sarcomeres in a mature muscle can change given the appropriate stimulus (Chapter 4, pages 179–189). This means that muscle fibers have a great capacity for adaptation, which is the subject of the last half of this book.

Sarcomeres are composed of contractile filaments termed *myofilaments*. Two major sets of contractile filaments exist in the sarcomere: One set is relatively thick, and the other set is relatively thin (Fig. 1-7). These thick and thin filaments represent large polymers of the proteins named myosin and actin, respectively. The myosin-containing filaments (thick filaments) and the actin-containing filaments (thin filaments) interdigitate to form a hexagonal lat-

TABLE 1-2	Hierarchy of Skeletal Muscle Organization

Structure	Size
Whole skeletal muscles	cm
Muscle fascicles	mm
Muscle fibers	μm × 100
Myofibrils	μm
Myofilaments	nm

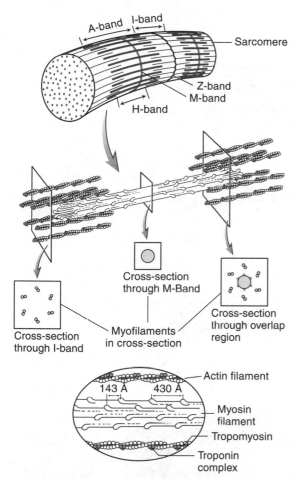

FIGURE 1-7. Hexagonal array of interdigitating myosin and actin filaments, which comprise the sarcomere. The myosin filament is composed of myosin molecules, and the actin filament is composed of actin monomers. Arranged at intervals along the actin filament are the regulatory proteins troponin and tropomyosin. See text for details.

tice (Fig. 1-7). It is the active interdigitation of these microscopic filaments that produces muscle shortening (Chapter 2, page 52). It is also this interdigitated pattern that gives the muscle its striated or striped appearance and is observable using the light microscope (See Color Plate Section, Fig. C-2). In fact, another term for skeletal muscle is "striated muscle" because of this repetitive dark and light banding pattern.

Various regions of the sarcomere are named based on their appearance so that reference can

be made to them (Figs. 1-7 and Color Plate C-2). For example, the sarcomere region containing the myosin filaments is known as the A-band (A stands for *anisotropic*, which is an optical term describing what this band does to incoming light). The region containing the actin filament is known as the I-band (I stands for "isotropic"). The region of the A-band in which there is no actin-myosin overlap is called the H-zone (H stands for *helle*, which is German for "light"). The dark narrow line that bisects the I-band is the Z-band (Z stands for *zwitter*, which is German for "between"). Finally, the relatively dense zone in the center of the A-band is known as the M-band. Most investigators who quantify sarcomere dimensions use the distance from one Z-band to the next as the definition of the sarcomere length, which is an important variable relative to force generation (Chapter 2, pages 52–55).

MYOSIN—HOME OF THE CROSS-BRIDGE

The myosin-containing filament is a polymer of myosin molecules known as the myosin heavy chain. This relatively large protein (about 220 kDaltons) is one of the most widely studied proteins in all of biology because it is found in cells other than muscle cells (Pollard, Doberstein, & Zot, 1991; Squire, 1981). Myosin proteins are arranged in a so-called antiparallel fashion to make up the myosin filament (Fig. 1-8). The myosin molecule is highly asymmetrical. At one end, is a globular "motor" domain, which powers muscle contraction, and at the other end is a long rodlike "tail" that permits multiple molecules to assemble into the thick filament described above. As individual myosin molecules polymerize to form the thick filament, one molecule rotates about 60° relative to the molecules on either side (this arrangement varies slightly among vertebrate muscles) and is displaced longitudinally by about 1.4 nm. Due to the antiparallel (tail-to-tail) arrangement of these molecules, as the filament is formed, it takes on a characteristic feathered appearance, with projections coming out at either end of the filament, but with the middle portion of the filament void of these projec-

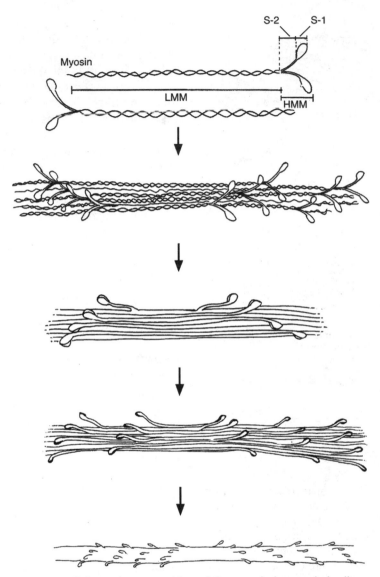

FIGURE 1-8. Schematic composition of the myosin heavy chain dimer. A single myosin molecule can be digested enzymatically into its fragments. Subfragments one and two (S-1 and S-2) are composed of the globular head and neck regions of the cross-bridge, respectively. Together, S-1 and S-2 comprise the heavy meromyosin (HMM), while the remainder of the molecules comprise the light meromyosin (LMM). Myosin monomers spontaneously polymerize into myosin filaments that are placed within the sarcomere as in Fig. 1-7.

tions. Because of the systematic packing of the myosin molecules into a filament, every 430 Å, the myosin molecules make a complete revolution (Figs. 1-7 and 1-8), which means that myosin heads are spaced approximately 143 Å along the length of the myosin filament. This antiparallel arrangement of myosin gives the sarcomere symmetry down the middle so that each half-sarcomere is functionally identical and has a mirror image on the opposite side of the sarcomere.

Myosin was one of the first proteins to be isolated from muscle. Although muscle tissue was the first shown to contain "motors," it is now clear that all cells contain some form of a "motor molecule" used to move cellular components or transport materials across the cell membrane. Thus, the lessons learned from studies of the myosin molecule have been applied to all cell types and have taken on added significance.

Experimentally, it is known that when myosin is placed in solution with a mild protease (an enzyme that digests proteins, e.g., chymopapain, the same enzyme that makes up meat tenderizer), the myosin molecule "falls apart" into two discrete components (Fig. 1-8): the so-called light meromyosin (LMM) and heavy meromyosin (HMM), terms reflecting the fact that LMM has a molecular weight of only 90 kDaltons whereas HMM weighs about 140 kDaltons. Further incubation of HMM in protease results in the production of two subfragments: subfragment 1 (S-1; molecular weight 90 kDaltons) and subfragment 2 (S-2; molecular weight 50 kDaltons). The reason that this sequential digestion of the myosin molecule furthered our understanding of muscle contraction was that each "piece" of the molecule could be tested individually to determine how myosin itself causes muscle contraction to occur. For example, it was determined that the protein's tail is the LMM whereas the portion of the molecule projecting from the backbone is the HMM. S-2 was shown to be the portion of HMM that projects out from the LMM backbone, whereas S-1 is the globular "head" that is

the actual motor molecule that powers muscle contraction. It is the combination of S-1 and S-2 that forms the well-known "cross-bridge," so central to the theory of force generation in muscle (See below). Also associated with the myosin heavy chain are two light chains (not shown in Fig. 1-8). The precise function of these proteins is not known. It is believed that they may provide structural support for the S-1 head and there is evidence that light chains can change the speed of contraction of the myosin heavy chain molecule (Bottinelli, Betto, Schiaffino, & Reggiani, 1994; Staron & Pette, 1987). It is known that various forms of the same light chain, so-called isoforms, exist in different muscle fibers. In Chapter 4 the analysis of the myosin isoform distribution provides insights into the nature of muscle adaptation (Chapter 4, pages 175–178). Isoforms of most of the sarcomere proteins exist. Myosin isoforms, however, have been the most widely studied.

MYOSIN ISOFORMS—THE BASIS OF "FIBER TYPES":

Several forms of myosin heavy chain and myosin light chain proteins may exist within the same muscle. It is interesting to speculate on the reason for the existence of these isoforms. Although it is true that the various myosin heavy chain isoforms have different functional properties, the magnitude of the differences in not necessary for survival (Bottinelli, Betto, Schiaffino, & Reggiani, 1994). Thus, detailed molecular analysis of different isoforms within the same species show that two very small regions of the myosin heavy chain are the "most different" regions between isoforms (Lutz, Razzaghi, & Lieber, 2000; Weiss, Schiaffino, & Leinwand, 1999). Detailed biophysical experiments on myosin heavy chain molecules that have been altered in these regions using modern molecular techniques support the idea that these small regions are functionally significant (Uyeda, Ruppel, & Spudich, 1994). The discussion of this most important protein will continue as the function of muscle is discussed in Chapter 2 and the plasticity of muscle in Chapters 4 and 5. At this point, studies of the structure and function of the myosin heavy chain play a central role in our understanding of muscle contractile mechanisms.

ACTIN—REGULATION OF CONTRACTION

The structure of the actin-containing filament is equally as elegant as that of myosin. Although the myosin-containing filament generates tension during muscle contraction, the actin-containing filament regulates tension generation. (Not all muscle systems are regulated by the actin-containing filament. In several invertebrate systems, force regulation and generation are both performed on the myosin-containing filament (Ebashi, Maruyama, & Endo, 1980). These so-called thick-filament-regulated systems are common. However, mammals use only thin-filament-based regulation). The actin filament is composed of a long α-helical arrangement of actin monomers. In contrast to the myosin-containing filament, there is no directional symmetry to this helix (i.e., the filament does not have a distinct middle section as does the myosin filament) although the filament does have a "+" and a "−" end that are based on the direction of polymerization.

Actin is an ubiquitous protein found in virtually all cells as part of the cell's cytoskeleton. (Interestingly, the discovery of actin filaments in cells other than muscle was first confirmed by "decorating" the actin-containing microfilaments with HMM. This was done by adding HMM to cytoskeletal cellular components and observing the feathered appearance of the HMM heads that were located at regular intervals along the actin filaments). Actin monomers are relatively small compared to myosin (only about 40 kDaltons) and are roughly spherical in shape. As a result of their helical arrangement, a long groove is created along the filament's length (Fig. 1-7). The regulatory protein, tropomyosin, fits nicely into this groove along the filament length. At intervals along the filament (approximately every seven actin monomers), the protein troponin is located. Troponin is the protein that is responsible for

turning on contraction. Troponin (abbreviated Tn) is composed of three subunits: Tn-I, Tn-C, and Tn-T. The functions of these subunits will become clearer following discussion of the cross-bridge cycle (Chapter 2, pages 66–71). At this point, note that Tn-T binds troponin to tropomyosin (hence "T"), Tn-C binds calcium during contraction (hence "C"), and Tn-I exerts an inhibitory influence on tropomyosin when calcium is not present (hence the "I").

In summary, contractile proteins within the muscle cell are arranged according to an elegant hierarchy. From the myosin molecule to the myofibril, structural hierarchy and organization are the rule, not the exception. A clear understanding of their physical relationship to one another makes understanding their function (presented in Chapter 2) much easier.

Membrane Components—A Way to Excite Muscle

In addition to the well-defined arrangement of force-generating components present in muscle cells, there exists an intricate system for activating these force generators. Recall that the skeletal muscle fiber is a highly differentiated cell that is specialized for producing force and movement. The membrane system present is actually a specially designed version of the membrane systems within normal cells. Although longitudinal micrographs of muscle provide a dramatic representation of the contractile filaments, the membrane system that activates them is less obvious. The two main components of this system are the transverse tubular system (abbreviated as the "T-system") and the sarcoplasmic reticulum (abbreviated as the "SR").

TRANSVERSE TUBULAR SYSTEM AND SARCOPLASMIC RETICULUM

The T-system begins as invaginations of the surface membrane and is therefore physically contiguous with the sarcolemma. If one observes a surface "scan" of a muscle fiber at very high magnification, periodic invaginations of the surface membrane will appear as "holes" that extend deep into the muscle fiber. These invaginations extend transversely across the long axis of the muscle fiber (hence their name). The function of the T-system is to convey the activation signal received from the motoneuron to the myofibrils, which are not in direct contact with the motoneuron (Chapter 2, page 48). The T-system thus acts as an electrical conduit for the nervous signal that ends up reaching deep into the fiber. This provides a means for myofibrillar activation that is much faster than would occur if activation relied on simple diffusion of molecules from the cell surface. It is thought that the T-system is an electrically excitable membrane much like the sarcolemma and the membranes surrounding neurons. To gain an accurate view of the T-system extent and orientation, sections of muscles are obtained at a variety of angles and, either reconstructed using computer technology or mathematically interpreted to yield information regarding their extent and orientation (Peachey & Franzini-Armstrong, 1983).

The SR is a much more complex membrane system than the T-system, which is directly involved in the storage of calcium that switches on muscle activation and the removal of calcium from the myofilaments to cause muscle relaxation. Embedded in the SR membrane are specific calcium channels and calcium pumps that accomplish the functions of calcium release and uptake, respectively. The SR envelops each myofibril to permit intimate contact between the activation and force-generation systems (Fig. 1-4). The SR is also in contact with the T-system and therefore acts as the "middleman" in skeletal muscle activation and relaxation. Physical structures that link the T-system to the SR were identified some time ago and were named the "junctional feet" of the SR, based on their close association between the T- and SR-systems (Peachey & Eisenberg, 1978; Peachey & Franzini-Armstrong, 1983). Since that time, the junctional feet have been shown to be composed of two discrete protein components. The first component, the ryanodine receptor (RyR) is a voltage sensing protein embedded into the SR that senses the action potential traveling across the T-system. The second component, the dihydropyridine receptor (DHP) is the calcium release channel through which the myofilament activating calcium passes (Franzini-Armstrong, 1999).

Although the sheer quantity of T-system and SR is not well appreciated on most muscle micrographs, because they are dominated by contractile filaments, the relative position of the T-system and SR relative to sarcomeres gives rise to a characteristic pattern that is observable in a high magnification longitudinal section (a section parallel to the long axis) of a muscle cell (Fig. 1-9) (this is usually seen by chemically fixing the tissue, embedding it in plastic, and thin

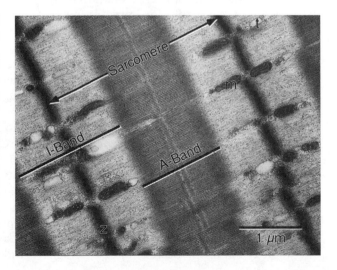

FIGURE 1-9. Longitudinal electron micrograph of a human vastus lateralis muscle which was fixed in glutaraldehyde, embedded in plastic, sectioned at about a 60 nm thickness, and stained with heavy metal. This severe processing is necessary to view the tissue with an electron microscope. Note the much greater magnification of the A- and I-bands in this electron micrograph compared to the longitudinal light micrograph shown in Color Plate Section, Figure C-2A. The region in this micrograph corresponds roughly to the circled region of the Color Plate Section, Figure C-2A. Calibration bar corresponds to a distance of 1 μm. (m-mitochondrion, z-Z-band, and t-Transverse tubular system.) Micrograph courtesy of Dr. Jan Fridén, Göteborg University, Sweden.

sectioning, staining, and viewing it under the electron microscope such as in Figure 1-9). The stereotypic arrangement, apparent to the trained eye, is that of a single T-tubule surrounded by two SR tubules at each Z-disk (Fig. 1-4). This arrangement of the three observable membrane components is so common that it has been named the "triad." As described above, the triad is the true interface between the extracellular and intracellular worlds about the muscle fiber. Extending longitudinally from either side of the triad are membrane systems that appear as flattened sacs. These represent longitudinal extensions of the SR that surround the myofibril. Remember, although these flattened sacs appear as a relatively minor area fraction in the longitudinal view, this is only because they have a complex three-dimensional arrangement that is not adequately represented by one slice in two-dimensions. The various portions of the T-system and SR are so distinct that they can be physically isolated and experimentally manipulated using modern fractionation techniques now commonly used in cell biology.

Studies of Muscle Filament and Sarcomere Structure

The uncanny degree of order of the contractile proteins that was described above permits detailed investigations of muscle that, in many ways, serve as the model for investigation of other biological systems. For example, modern electron microscopy, light microscopy, ion transport, membrane isolation, and metabolic investigational methods were developed specifically to understand muscle. Some of these tools developed to study muscle structure will now be presented, along with the evidence they provide for the structural descriptions given above.

Light Microscopy

Numerous microscopic methods have been used to examine skeletal muscle structure. In fact, many of the modern-day electron and light microscopic techniques implemented throughout biology were pioneered by Dr. Hugh

Huxley and Sir Andrew Huxley, respectively (no relation) to elucidate the mechanism of muscle contraction. Obviously, these methods have provided unique insights into the structure of many biologic tissues; however, since this book is about muscle, muscle structural studies will continue to be the major focus.

Early light microscopes did not provide much insight into the structure of the living muscle fiber. This was because, unstained, the muscle fiber appeared as a translucent cylinder without discrete subcellular order. However, in the early 1950s, Andrew Huxley developed an interference microscope that enhanced the contrast of different muscle fiber regions. Recall that the different "bands" within the sarcomere were so named (A- and I-bands) based on the way they affected incident light. Huxley's microscope exploited this difference and, under the interference microscope, instead of appearing translucent, the muscle fiber adapted a striped or striated appearance (Color Plate Section, Fig. C-2A). This striation pattern, which is so well-known today, was hypothesized to result from the interdigitation of the sarcomere thick and thin filaments. In their now classic report, Huxley and Niedergerke (1954) demonstrated that, as muscle length changed, the striation pattern also changed. Thus in their interference microscope they knew that they had a tool that enabled investigation of contractile mechanisms on isolated, living muscle fibers.

Huxley and Niedergerke performed a series of experiments in which a muscle was caused to contract and was observed using the interference microscope. They observed that, during muscle shortening, the width of the A-band remained constant while the I-band length changed. Based on what is known about the A- and I-bands, how can this observation be explained? Huxley and Niedergerke hypothesized that this observation might result from interdigitation of filaments that themselves maintained a constant length. They claimed that A-band stayed a constant length because it represents the myosin filaments, which remain at a constant length. The I-band decreased in width because it represents the non-overlap region of the actin filament. I have not detailed the experiments, but the highly technical nature of the microscopy, along with the clever interpretation of their data (especially considering the thinking at that time) are truly awe-inspiring. At that time in history, most muscle contraction theories were thermodynamic or chemical in nature, reflecting the intellectual climate. This turns out to be a continuing theme in science—to make a big advance, one must think "outside the box."

Electron Microscopy

During the same period as Andrew Huxley and colleagues were studying single muscle fibers with the interference microscope, Dr. Hugh Huxley and his coworker, Dr. Jean Hanson, were developing preparative methods for the then-new electron microscope (EM; Fig. 1-9). The advantage of the EM over the light microscope was that it had a greater magnification power (over 50,000X compared with the light microscope's 500X capability). Unfortunately, the material to be viewed under the EM could not be living—all of the water had to be extracted because the specimen was viewed in a vacuum chamber. Thus, Huxley and Hanson (1954) developed methods for dehydrating, embedding, and sectioning skeletal muscles at various lengths. When sectioned longitudinally, the banding pattern described above was observed. In addition, as muscle length was changed, the banding pattern observed in longitudinal and cross-sections changed as would be expected by two sets of interdigitating filaments. Although this result seems obvious to us in retrospect, it should be emphasized that most scientists at the time thought that this banding pattern was simply an artifact of the rather harsh dehydration and embedding procedures. However, Huxley and Hanson succeeded in demonstrating that this almost crystalline array of contractile proteins was truly representative of living muscle. They also succeeded in sectioning the muscle fiber transversely to the long muscle fiber axis and demonstrated hexagonal arrays of myofilaments (Fig. 1-7). The interesting point was that if they

sectioned through the H-band, only a myosin filament lattice was observed (See sections shown in Fig. 1-7). If they sectioned through the I-band, only a thin filament lattice was observed. However, if they sectioned through the overlap region of the A-band, an interdigitating hexagonal array of actin and myosin filaments was observed. Again, based on your understanding of sarcomere structure, you should be able to explain this result. In fact, you should also be able to explain how these results would change with varying sarcomere length.

Huxley and Hanson's findings were complementary to Huxley and Niedergerke's and were equally as surprising. Both groups of investigators independently proposed (and, showing an impressive degree of profession collegiality and mutual respect, published the results side-by-side in the prestigious scientific journal *Nature*) that muscle contraction occurred by the relative sliding of the thick and thin filaments past one another. This became known as the "sliding filament hypothesis" and has since been elevated to the "sliding filament theory" as much data have been acquired that provide support. Note that all scientists are not in complete agreement with the sliding filament theory. For an example, refer to Pollack, 1983.

X-ray Diffraction

A third tool for structural investigation of muscle that was highly influential in developing theories of muscle contraction was the method of X-ray diffraction. The principle of X-ray diffraction is similar to that observed in the ripple pond experiment from basic physics. If an X-ray beam is projected onto a living muscle, the X-rays are scattered by the tissue. If some of the scattering elements are arranged in a regular array (as the myofilaments are), an interference pattern results that represents constructive and destructive interference of the scattered X-rays. This diffraction pattern appears as a series of lines (the so-called layer lines) that can be quantified in terms of their position and intensity. For an excellent discussion of X-ray diffraction in muscle, refer to Squire, 1981. The spacing between these layer lines can then be directly related to microscopic spacing contained in the sarcomere itself.

As with all diffraction methods, the size of the structures "seen" by the X-rays is close to the wavelength of the X-rays themselves. Since most X-rays fall in the Å range, X-ray diffraction resolves spacing between objects with molecular dimensions. Consider what some of these dimensions might represent in muscle. Structures with relatively large spacing, on the order of microns have been discussed up until this point. For example, the A-band is about 1.6 μm in length and sarcomeres are 2–3 μm in length. Myofibrils are about 1 μm in diameter. None of these dimensions would be resolved using X-ray diffraction.

In a series of experimental studies, Hugh Huxley and colleagues transilluminated whole muscles and obtained layer lines that represented strong periodicities along and across the muscle fiber axis. For example, across the muscle fiber axis, they measured the spacing between the actin and myosin filaments as sarcomere length was increased from resting length to very long lengths. Interestingly, as sarcomere length was increased, filament spacing decreased in a way that kept total sarcomere volume constant. Along the fiber axis, they demonstrated that the spacing between the various myosin heads was shown to be 143 Å and 430 Å distances and was consistent with the myosin filament structure described above. The 143 Å spacing represented the displacement of one myosin molecule relative to the next one in the filament and the 430 Å spacing represented the displacement of the myosin molecule after a complete turn around the filament had been made (Fig. 1-7). Even the spacing between the monomers of the actin molecule as well as the troponin subunits was obtained. Needless to say, these studies had a tremendous influence on theories of muscle contraction (Haselgrove, 1983). Sophisticated analysis of the intensities of these layer lines during passive muscle length change and active muscle contraction was consistent with a theory of muscle contraction whereby force generation occurred by the relative sliding of filaments past one another

and provided direct support for the idea of a portion of the myosin molecule extending out toward the actin filament during force generation. More recent studies have confirmed these earlier studies on a much faster time scale and with much better spatial resolution (Huxley, 1990; Huxley, Simmons, Faruqi, Kress, & Koch, 1981) than the original studies by Huxley and colleagues.

Thus, although X-ray diffraction may not be a familiar technique, in muscle structural studies it has provided some of the most direct, quantitative data available on normal muscle structure and muscle structural changes during contraction and has had a tremendous influence in developing the molecular theory of contraction that is discussed in Chapter 2.

Satellite Cells: Reserves for Injury and Repair

An important but rarely observed component of skeletal muscle tissue is the satellite cell. These small cells are located beneath the fiber basal lamina (See page 3) and are approximately the same size as a muscle cell nucleus. Although the satellite cell plays no known role in normal cell function, it plays the central role in recovery of muscle fibers from injury. Satellite cells are "stem cells" that have the ability to differentiate into myoblasts and to form new muscle fibers. Clearly such ability is central to the formation of new muscle fibers after injury. This regeneration process will be discussed in some detail in Chapter 6 as muscle injury and recovery are considered. In addition, molecular manipulation of satellite cells may form the basis for gene therapy of muscular and other genetic disorders in the future.

3 Whole Skeletal Muscle Structure

Even though skeletal muscles and bodies have a variety of shapes and sizes, there are several recurring universal themes. Skeletal muscles attach to bones via connective tissue structures known as tendons, which have a variety of shapes and sizes. Often, the origin of a muscle is associated with a well-defined tendon such as in the case of the biceps brachialis muscle. Sometimes, the tendinous origin is fairly broad and thin and may be poorly defined such as the common origin of the digital flexors on the medial epicondyle. At times, the amount of tendon is so small that the muscle fibers appear to arise from bone. However, microscopic analysis of the muscle fiber end shows connective tissue such as tendon interposed between fibers and bones. At the gross anatomic level, each muscle has an origin (the proximal muscle end) and insertion (the distal muscle end, Table 1-1). Often the muscle origin is broader than the insertion, in which the fibers converge onto a stout tendon (*e.g.*, flexor digitorum profundus). Knowing a muscle's origin and insertion anatomy provides the first evidence for a muscle's function. However, in spite of knowing a muscle's origin and insertion, it is not possible to simply describe a motion resulting from muscle contraction based only on this information. This is because muscles often cross more than one joint and may therefore exert an influence at multiple locations (inspection of Table 1-1 shows that most muscles cross multiple joints). For example, the rectus femoris crosses both the knee and hip joints. If the knee was fixed and the hip was free to move, rectus femoris contraction would cause hip flexion. Conversely, if the hip was fixed and the knee free to move, rectus femoris contraction would cause knee extension. Should the rectus femoris then be described as a hip flexor or a knee extensor or both? It is not possible to answer this question unambiguously without specifying a movement. For example, in standing from a squat, the rectus femoris is activated and generates tension, and clearly acts during knee and hip extension. Therefore, anatomically the rectus is a hip flexor and knee extensor, but this does not specify the conditions under which a muscle may be used. Therefore, resist the temptation to classify muscles simply in terms of

---

Box 1-3. How Are Multi-joint Muscles Designed?

Many if not most muscles cross multiple joints. For example, the rectus femoris can cause both knee extension and hip flexion. Digital extensors are also wrist extensors. The design of these multi-joint muscles appears to be customized for the task required. For example, digital extensors have relatively long fibers to enable simultaneous wrist and finger extension. However, this design is not necessary for the rectus muscle because hip flexion is accompanied by knee extension during normal movement (See Chapter 3, pages 153–156). Thus, muscle design is reflected in the normal functional use pattern of that muscle.

---

anatomy. Instead, state that the rectus femoris always acts to generate a hip flexion moment and a knee extension moment but reserve creating general categories in the absence of specifying a motion (Zajac & Gordon, 1989). This point will be discussed further in analyzing biarticular muscle function in Chapter 3.

Muscle Architecture—Organization of Muscle Fibers

Skeletal muscle is not only highly organized at the microscopic level; the arrangement of muscle fibers at the macroscopic level also demonstrates a striking degree of organization. In making comparisons among various muscles, certain factors such as fiber type distribution are important, but there is no question that an important factor in determining a whole muscle's contractile properties is the muscle's architecture.

Skeletal muscle architecture can be defined as "the arrangement of muscle fibers relative to the axis of force generation." Although muscle fibers have a relatively consistent fiber diameter among muscles of different sizes, the arrangement of these fibers can be quite different. It would be completely impossible then, to estimate the force a muscle would generate if you measured fiber diameter from a muscle biopsy because there would be no estimate of the num-

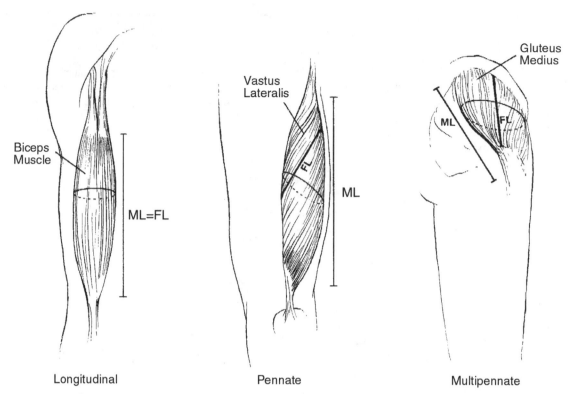

FIGURE 1-10. Generalized picture of muscle architectural types. Skeletal muscle fibers may be oriented parallel to the muscle's force-generating axis (left, known as "longitudinal" architecture), at a fixed angle relative to the force-generating axis (middle, known as "pennate" architecture), or at multiple angles relative to the force-generating axis (right, known as "multipennate" architecture). Each of these drawings represents an idealized view of muscle architecture and probably does not adequately describe any single muscle. (ML, muscle length. FL, fiber length.)

ber of muscle fibers generating the force. Similarly, even if there was an estimate of the total muscle volume, the myriad ways to arrange fibers within that volume would preclude producing a valid force estimate. In fact, the various types of muscle fiber arrangement within whole muscles are as numerous as the muscles themselves, but for convenience there are three general types of fiber architecture.

Muscles with fibers that extend parallel to the muscle force-generating axis are termed parallel or longitudinally arranged muscles (Fig. 1-10, left). Although the fibers extend parallel to the force-generating axis, they never extend the entire muscle length (Tables 1-3 and 1-4). Muscles with fibers that are oriented at a single angle relative to the force-generating axis are termed unipennate muscles (Fig. 1-10, middle). The angle between the fiber and the force-generating axis generally varies from 0° to 30°. It is obvious when preparing muscle dissections that most muscles fall into the final and most general category, multipennate muscles—muscles composed of fibers that are oriented at several angles relative to the axis of force generation (Fig. 1-10, right). As will be discussed in the next chapter, an understanding of muscle architecture is critical to understanding the functional properties of different muscles.

(text continues on page 31)

TABLE 1-3	Architectural Properties of the Human Arm and Forearm[a,b]					
Muscle	Muscle Mass (g)	Muscle Length (mm)	Fiber Length (mm)	Pennation Angle (°)	Cross-Sectional Area (cm^2)	FL/ML Ratio
BR (n=8)	16.6±2.8	175±8.3	121±8.3	2.4±.6	1.33±.22	.69±.062
PT (n=8)	15.9±1.7	130±4.7	36.4±1.3	9.6±.8	4.13±.52	.28±.012
PQ (n=8)	5.21±1.0	39.3±2.3	23.3±2.0	9.9±.3	2.07±.33	.58±.021
EDC I (n=8)	3.05±.45	114±3.4	56.9±3.6	3.1±.5	.52±.08	.49±.024
EDC M (n=5)	6.13±1.2	112±4.7	58.8±3.5	3.2±1.0	1.02±.20	.50±.014
EDC R (n=7)	4.70±.75	125±10.7	51.2±1.8	3.2±.54	.86±.13	.42±.023
EDC S (n=6)	2.23±.32	121±8.0	52.9±5.2	2.4±.7	.40±.06	.43±.029
EDQ (n=7)	3.81±.70	152⊥9.2	55.3±3.7	2.6±.6	.64±.10	.36±.012
EIP (n=6)	2.86±.61	105±6.6	48.4±2.3	6.3±.8	.56±.11	.46±.023
EPL (n=7)	4.54±.68	138±7.2	43.6±2.6	5.6±1.3	.98±.13	.31±.020
PL (n=6)	3.78±.82	134±11.5	52.3±3.1	3.5±1.2	.69±.17	.40±.032
FDS I(P) (n=6)	6.0±1.1	92.5±8.4	31.6±3.0	5.1±0.2	1.81±.83	.34±.022
FDS I(D) (n=9)	6.6±0.8	119±6.1	37.9±3.0	6.7±0.3	1.63±.22	.32±.013
FDS I(C) (n=6)	12.4±2.1	207±10.7	67.6±2.8	5.7±0.2	1.71±.28	.33±.025
FDS M (n=9)	16.3±2.2	183±11.5	60.8±3.9	6.9±0.7	2.53±.34	.34±.014
FDS R (n=9)	10.2±1.1	155±7.7	60.1±2.7	4.3±0.6	1.61±.18	.39±.023
FDS S (n=9)	1.8±0.3	103±6.3	42.4±2.2	4.9±0.7	0.40±.05	.42±.014
FDP I (n=9)	11.7±1.2	149±3.8	61.4±2.4	7.2±0.7	1.77±.16	.41±.018
FDP M (n=9)	16.3±1.7	200±8.2	68.4±2.7	5.7±0.3	2.23±.22	.34±.011
FDP R (n=9)	11.9±1.4	194±7.0	64.6±2.6	6.8±0.5	1.72±.18	.33±.009
FDP S (n=9)	13.7±1.5	150±4.7	60.7±3.9	7.8±0.9	2.20±.30	.40±.015
FPL (n=9)	10.0±1.1	168±10.0	45.1±2.1	6.9±0.2	2.08±.22	.24±.010

[a]Data from: Lieber, R.L., Fazeli, B.M., & Botte, M.J. (1990). Architecture of selected wrist flexor and extensor muscles. *Journal of Hand Surgery, 15A*, 244–250, and Lieber, R.L., Jacobson, M.D., Fazeli, B.M., Abrams, R.A., & Botte, M.J. (1992). Architecture of selected muscles of the arm and forearm: anatomy and implications for tendon transfer. *Journal of Hand Surgery, 17A*, 787–798.

[b]BIC: biceps brachialis; BR: brachioradialis; EDC I, EDC M, EDC R, and EDC S: extensor digitorum communis to the index, middle, ring and small fingers, respectively; ECRB: extensor carpi radialis brevis; ECRL: extensor carpi radialis longus; ECU: extensor carpi ulnaris; EDQ: extensor digiti quinti; EIP: extensor indicis proprious; EPL: extensor pollicis longus; FCR: flexor carpi radialis; FCU: flexor carpi ulnaris, FDP I, FDP M, FDP R, and FDP S: flexor digitorum profundus muscles; FDS I, FDS M, FDS R, and FDS S: flexor digitorum superficialis muscles; FDS I (P) and FDS I (D): proximal and distal bellies of the FDS I; FDS I (C): the combined properties of the two bellies as if they were a single muscle; FPL: flexor pollicis longus; PQ: pronator quadratus; PS: palmaris longus; PT: pronator teres; TRI: triceps brachii.

TABLE 1-4	Architectural Properties of Human Lower Limb[a,b]					
Muscle	Muscle Mass (g)	Muscle Length (mm)	Fiber Length (mm)	Pennation Angle (°)	Cross-Sectional Area (cm²)	FL/ML Ratio
RF (n=3)	84.3±14	316±5.7	66.0±1.5	5.0±0.0	12.7±1.9	.209±.002
VL (n–3)	220±56	324±14	65.7±0.88	5.0±0.0	30.6±6.5	.203±.007
VM (n=3)	175±41	335±15	70.3±3.3	5.0±0.0	21.1±4.3	.210±.005
VI (n=3)	160±59	329±15	68.3±4.8	3.3±1.7	22.3±8.7	.208±.007
SM (n=3)	108±13	262±1.5	62.7±4.7	15±2.9	16.9±1.5	.239±.017
BF$_l$ (n=3)	128±28	342±14	85.3±5.0	0.0±0.0	12.8±2.8	.251±.022
BF$_s$ (n=3)		271±11	139±3.5	23±0.9		.517±.032
ST (n=2)	76.9±7.7	317±4	158±2.0	5.0±0.0	5.4±1.0	.498±0.0
SOL (n=2)	215 (n=1)	310±1.5	19.5±0.5	25±5.0	58.0 (n=1)	.063±.002
MG (n=3)	150±14	248±9.9	35.3±2.0	16.7±4.4	32.4±3.1	.143±.010
LG (n=3)		217±11	50.7±5.6	8.3±1.7		.233±.016
PLT (n=3)	5.30±1.9	85.0±15	39.3±6.7	3.3±1.7	1.2±0.4	.467±.031
FHL (n=3)	21.5±3.3	222±5.0	34.0±1.5	10.0±2.9	5.3±0.6	.154±.010
FDL (n=3)	16.3±2.8	260±15	27.0±0.58	6.7±1.7	5.1±0.7	.104±.004
PL (n=3)	41.5±8.5	286±17	38.7±3.2	10.0±0.0	12.3±2.9	.136±.010
PB (n=3)	17.3±2.5	230±13	39.3±3.5	5.0±0.0	5.7±1.0	.170±.006
TP (n=3)	53.5±7.3	254±26	24.0±4.0	11.7±1.7	20.8±3	.095±.015
TA (n=3)	65.7±10	298±12	77.3±7.8	5.0±0.0	9.9±1.5	.258±.015
EDL (n=3)	35.2±3.6	355±13	80.3±8.4	8.3±1.7	5.6±0.6	.226±.024
EHL (n=3)	12.9±1.6	273±2.4	87.0±8.0	6.0±1.0	1.8±0.2	.319±.030
SAR (n=3)	61.7±14	503±27	455±19	0.0±0.0	1.7±0.3	.906±.017
GR (n=3)	35.3±7.4	335±20	277±12	3.3±1.7	1.8±0.3	.828±.017
AM (n=3)	229±32	305±12	115±7.9	0.0±0.0	18.2±2.3	.378±.013
AL (n=3)	63.5±16	229±12	108±2.0	6.0±1.0	6.8±1.9	.475±.023
AB (n=3)	43.8±8.4	156±12	103±6.4	0.0±0.0	4.7±1.0	.663±.036
PEC (n=3)	26.4±6.0	123±4.5	104±1.2	0.0±0.0	2.9±0.6	.851±.040
POP (n=2)	20.1±2.4	108±7.0	29.0±7.0	0.0±0.0	7.9±1.4	.265±.048

[a]Data from: Wickiewicz, T.L., Roy, R.R., Powell, P.L., & Edgerton, V.R. (1983). Muscle architecture of the human lower limb. *Clinical Orthopaedics and Related Research, 179,* 275–283.

[b]AB, adductor brevis; AL, adductor longus; AM, adductor Magnus; BF$_l$, biceps femoris, long head; BF$_s$, biceps femoris, short head; EDL, extensor digitorum longus; EHL, extensor hallucis longus; FDL, flexor digitorum longus; GR, gracilis; FHL, flexor hallucis longus; LG, lateral gastrocnemius; MG, medial gastrocnemius; PEC, pectineus; PB, peroneus brevis; PL, peroneus longus; PLT, plantaris; POP, popliteus; RF, rectus femoris; SAR, sartorius; SM, semimembranosus; SOL, soleus; ST, semitendinosus; TA, tibialis anterior; TP, tibialis posterior; VI, vastus intermedius; VL, vastus lateralis; VM, vastus medialis.

Experimental Determination of Skeletal Muscle Architecture

Early studies of muscle architecture were pioneered by the anatomist Dr. Carl Gans. Gans and his colleagues (Gans & Bock, 1965) developed precise methods for muscle architecture determination based on microdissection of whole muscles. These muscles were chemically fixed to maintain their integrity during dissection. Ideally, the muscle was fixed while attached to the skeleton to roughly preserve its physiologic length. After fixation, muscles were dissected from the skeleton, their mass determined, and their pennation angle (i.e., the fiber angle relative to the force-generating axis) and muscle length were measured.

Currently, pennation angle is usually measured by determining the average pennation angle of fibers on the superficial muscle surface. Although more sophisticated methods could be devised, it is doubtful they would provide a great deal more information for reasons presented below. In measuring muscle length, it is important to note that muscle length is defined as the distance from the origin of the most proximal muscle fibers to the insertion of the most distal fibers. As mentioned above, this distance is not the same as the whole muscle length. Muscle fiber length can only be determined by microdissection of individual fibers from the fixed tissues. In general, unless investigators are explicit, when they refer to muscle fiber length, they are actually referring to muscle fiber bundle length. It is extremely difficult to isolate intact fibers, which run from origin to insertion, especially in mammalian tissue (Loeb, Pratt, Chanaud, & Richmond et al., 1987; Ounjian et al., 1991; Sacks & Roy, 1982).

The final experimental step in performing architectural analysis is to determine the sarcomere length within the isolated bundles. This is necessary to compensate for differences in muscle lengths that occur during fixation. In other words, if it was concluded that a muscle was "long," it must be certain that it is truly "long" and that it was not simply fixed in a stretched position. Similarly, muscles measured to be "short" must be further investigated to ensure that they were not simply fixed at a short sarcomere length. To permit such conclusions, architectural measurements should always be expressed after being normalized or "adjusted" to a constant sarcomere length.

Having measured muscle mass, fiber length, sarcomere length, muscle length, and pennation angle, a number of parameters are then calculated that summarize the muscle architecture. These parameters have a direct relation to the whole muscle's contractile properties.

PHYSIOLOGIC CROSS-SECTIONAL AREA

After measurement of the typical architectural parameters, the so-called physiologic cross-sectional area (PCSA) can be calculated. What is the significance of such a calculation? In short, the PCSA is directly proportional to the maximum tetanic tension that can be generated by the muscle. This value is almost never the cross-sectional area of the muscle in any of the traditional anatomic planes, as would be obtained, for example, using a noninvasive imaging method such as magnetic resonance imaging (MRI) or computerized tomography (CT) or ultrasound. Theoretically, PCSA represents the sum of the cross-sectional areas of all of the muscle fibers within the muscle. It is calculated using Equation 1-1, which was pioneered by Gans and verified experimentally by Roy, Edgerton, and colleagues. This equation is important to understand normal muscle and to make valid estimates of PCSA in human studies in which the attempt is to evaluate patient performance in a physiological context. In Equation 1-1, ρ represents muscle density (1.056 g/cm^3 for mammalian muscle) and θ represents surface pennation angle.

$$PCSA\ (cm^2) = \frac{Muscle\ Mass\ (g) \cdot cosine\ \theta}{\rho\ (g/cm^3) \cdot Fiber\ Length\ (cm)} \quad (Eq.\ 1\text{-}1)$$

If you partition the equation into its components, the rationale for this expression becomes clearer. First, note that muscle mass divided by density equals muscle volume (Equation 1-2). If the muscle was roughly cylindrical in shape, dividing volume by length (fiber length) would represent the cylinder cross-sectional area (Equation 1-3). Since, in our example, fiber length does not equal cylinder length, the area is not an actual area; rather, it is a theoretical area that would be occupied by a cylinder with a length equal to that of the fibers. Since the fibers may be oriented at some angle relative to the axis of force generation, the cosine term must be included (Equation 1-4). For those of you with a background in physics, the basis for this term is obvious. Because this is a concept that will be useful at a later stage, consider the situation shown in Figure 1-11.

$$\text{Volume (cm}^3) = \frac{\text{Muscle Mass (g)}}{\rho \text{ (g/cm}^3)} \qquad \text{(Eq. 1-2)}$$

$$\text{CSA (cm}^2) = \frac{\text{Volume (cm}^3)}{\text{Fiber Length (cm)}} \qquad \text{(Eq. 1-3)}$$

Suppose a muscle fiber pulls with × units of force at an angle θ relative to the muscle axis of force generation. Clearly, some of the force of the fiber will not be transmitted along the axis but will be lost. Thus, only a component of muscle fiber force will actually be transmitted along the muscle axis. Noting the right triangle in Figure 1-11A, it can be seen that the component of muscle force transmitted will be x · cosθ, since cosθ = x/F, which will *always* be less than x since cosθ is always less than 1. In other words, pennation itself as described here results in a loss of muscle force relative to a muscle with the same mass and fiber length but with zero pennation angle. Why would the system be designed in such a way that force was lost? Consider the alternative: If the pennation angle was zero, the absolute size of the muscle would prohibit placing it in many bodily locations due to the large number of fibers that would have a PCSA equal to an anatomic CSA in, for example, the transverse plane (Fig. 1-11B). Thus, it appears that pennation is a space-saving strategy even though it costs a bit in force generation. Pennation angle (θ) does not appear to have a large detrimental influence on PCSA in spite of this argument. This is be-

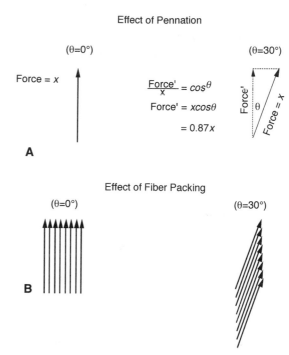

FIGURE 1-11. Schematic illustration of the effect of muscle fiber pennation. **(A)** A single fiber oriented parallel to the axis of force generation transmits all of its force in the same direction as the tendon while a muscle fiber oriented at a 30° angle relative to the force-generating axis transmits only a portion of its force (cosine 30° = 0.87, or 87%) along the muscle force-generating axis. **(B)** Generalizing the single fiber in **(A)** to the whole muscle shows how pennation may increase the packing of many fibers into a smaller space compared to fibers packed without pennation.

cause, the cosine of 0° is 1 and the cosine of 30°(which would be a very large pennation angle and is rarely encountered) is 0.87 which represents only a 13% force loss for a huge increase in fiber packing ability.

$$\text{PCSA (cm}^2) = \text{CSA (cm}^2) \cdot \cos\theta \qquad \text{(Eq. 1-4)}$$

The usefulness of this equation was recently highlighted by Roy, Edgerton, and colleagues (Powell, Roy, Kanim, Bello, & Edgerton, 1984) in an experimental comparison between the *estimated* maximum muscle tetanic tension (based on PCSA calculations) and *measured* maximum tetanic tension (measured using traditional physiologic testing techniques). These investigators found that the estimations and predictions agreed within experimental error. The only exception to that conclusion was that the soleus muscle (a monoarticular plantarflexor of the deep calf) did not seem to agree. Interestingly, this was the only muscle tested that contained a large proportion of slow muscle fibers (See Chapter 2). These data may suggest that slow fibers generate less tension per unit area compared with fast fibers, but the evidence is not conclusive in this regard.

A potential problem with Equation 1-1 is that it assumes muscle fiber pennation angle is constant during muscle contraction. Detailed experimental measurement of muscle fiber pennation angle in the unipennate rat gastrocnemius muscle have revealed that this is not the case. Huijing and colleagues (Zuurbier & Huijing, 1992) placed small wire markers across the rat gastrocnemius posterior surface and filmed the marker movement during muscle contraction. Using this approach, they measured fiber pennation angle and showed that it varied considerably as muscle length was altered throughout the normal physiological range of motion. Although resting pennation angle was approximately 30°, during isotonic contraction, it increased to almost 60° and the angle between the muscle aponeurosis and the muscle axis rotated from about 10° to 15°. The fact that muscle fibers appear to be free to rotate during contraction has a number of implications. First, PCSA calculations as obtained from Equation 1-1 may be inexact in their ability to predict force. Second, fiber rotation has a significant impact on the estimation of muscle fiber contraction velocity based on the measurement of whole muscle velocity. During shortening of the rat gastrocnemius, if one calculates fiber contraction velocity holding pennation angle constant, it will simply scale with whole muscle velocity. However, if fiber rotation is included, fiber velocity is actually much lower than whole muscle velocity, which, functionally, results in prediction of greater

force generation by the muscle fibers. This may be one reason that muscle force estimates from isokinetic testing are so poor. More will be said about isokinetic testing in Chapter 3 (pages 147–153).

Does significant fiber rotation occur in human muscles? An affirmative answer to this question was provided in a most dramatic example by Fukunaga and colleagues (Fukunaga, Ichinose, Ito, Kawakami, & Fukashiro, 1997; Kawakami, Ichinose, & Fukunaga, 1998) who have measured fascicle plane orientation during voluntary contraction of the human quadriceps, dorsiflexor and plantarflexor muscles. Their measurements revealed that, during low level voluntary contraction, vastus lateralis pennation angle increased from 14° with the knee extended to 21° with the knee flexed and during this voluntary contraction, fascicle length decreased tremendously from 126 mm to 67 mm. Similarly, the medial gastrocnemius increased from about 20° to 45° with a similar significant degree of shortening (Fig. 1-12). These data provide a real-time picture indicating that muscle fiber shortening and rotation are simultaneous and normal events that occur during muscle contraction.

Fiber rotation during muscle contraction permits tensile force transmission to occur even when muscle fibers are oriented at an angle relative to the muscle's force-generating axis. The fact that pennation angles are small at muscle resting lengths (0–30°) probably ac-

---

Box 1-4. Can Muscle Fibers Rotate During Muscle Contraction?

For many muscles, the answer is clearly, *yes*. Direct, real-time measurements of muscle fiber bundle angle have been made during *isometric* as well as *isokinetic* contractions. In both cases (and probably during normal movement) fiber angle can change by as much as 45° depending on the particular muscle and the specific movement studied.

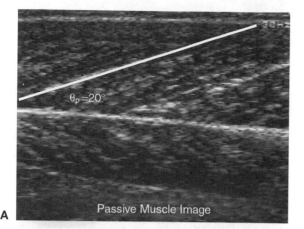

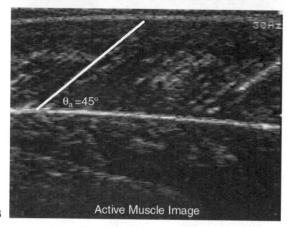

FIGURE 1-12. Ultrasound image of human medial gastrocnemius measured in the saggital plane (hip joint to right, knee joint to left). **(A)** Muscle image at rest demonstrating passive fiber angle (θ_p) of 20° relative to the aponeurosis that borders the deep medial gastrocnemius. **(B)** Muscle image with the muscle activated with the ankle joint fixed, demonstrating fiber rotation and an active fiber angle (θ_a) of 45° relative to the aponeurosis. (Ultrasound images courtesy of Drs. Tetsuo Fukanaga and Yasuo Kawakami (Tokyo University). Unpublished images from study published as: Kawakami, Y., Ichinose, Y., & Fukunaga, T. (1998). Architectural and functional features of human triceps surae muscles during contraction. *Journal of Applied Physiology, 85,* 398–404.)

counted for the agreement between experiment and theory previously reported (Powell, Roy, Kanim, Bello, & Edgerton, 1984). Thus, in predicting maximum muscle force producing capacity, correction for fiber angulation may not

be necessary and may even be conceptually incorrect.

It is important to emphasize the point that PCSA (and therefore maximum muscle tension) is *not* simply proportional to muscle mass (as is clear from the equation). In other words, given information on muscle mass or on muscle mass change (for instance, due to immobilization or spinal cord injury), *no* statement can be made with respect to muscle force. This is another way of saying that although mass is proportional to the amount of contractile material in the muscle, the *arrangement* of that material is of critical importance. It should also be stated that in some pathologic conditions, mass may change because of noncontractile proteins (*e.g.*, increased connective tissue or inflammatory cells). In such cases, even calculated PCSA will not accurately predict tetanic tension.

MUSCLE FIBER LENGTH

Unfortunately, even though it is often stated that muscle fiber length is proportional to fiber excursion (or velocity), there has not been a comprehensive study in mammalian muscle, analogous to the study described above for PCSA that confirms this relationship quantitatively. However, there is a good deal of experimental evidence available in the literature to suggest that this relationship is valid. First, in mechanical studies of isolated frog single muscle fibers, in which fiber length and thus, the number of sarcomeres in series, is easily measured, maximum contraction velocity is directly proportional to fiber length as is the width of the isometric length-tension relationship. This is the reason that muscle contraction velocities are often normalized and expressed in "fiber lengths/sec" or "sarcomere lengths/sec." Second, in a mechanical and anatomical study of the cat semitendinosus muscle, which represents a unique model in that it is composed of distinct proximal and distal heads separated by a tendinous inscription and which has distinct innervation to each head, the maximum contraction velocity of the two heads stimulated simultaneously was the same as the sum of the maximum contraction velocity of the two heads stimulated individually (Bodine et al., 1982).

The relationship between fiber length and whole muscle properties is also complicated by the observation that some long feline muscles have been shown to be composed of relatively short muscle fibers arranged in series. The cat sartorius, tenuissimus and semitendinosus muscles, that may extend 10–15 cm in length were microdissected and shown to be composed of relatively short fibers 2–3 cm in length that were arranged in series (Loeb, Pratt, Chanaud, & Richmond, 1987). By staining these specimens with acetylcholinesterase, the authors also showed that the endplates occurred in about the same serial arrangement. These data were combined with electromyographic data that demonstrated that the "in series" fibers were innervated by branches of axons also arranged in series so that all serial fibers would be expected to activate simultaneously. This led to the suggestion that short fibers arranged in series are simultaneously activated to effectively act like single long muscle fibers. The reason this was viewed as a good design is that it is known electrical conduction along muscle fibers is relatively slow (2–10 m/s). The long length of these cat muscles (10–15 cm) could set up the scenario whereby a portion of the fiber was activated and, by the time the action potential reached the end of the fiber, the central region would already be relaxing. Mechanically, this is clearly unfavorable. This is not to say that longer fibers do not exist within cat muscles. In a histological study of the cat tibialis anterior, Edgerton and colleagues (Ounjian et al., 1991) traced single muscle fibers within single motor units along the muscle belly cross-section and clearly demonstrated that the fibers did not run the entire muscle length, nor even the entire fascicle length (Fig. 1-13). Fibers within motor units ranged from ~8 mm to ~50 mm. Furthermore, they elucidated the general pattern that slow (S) units tended to have more uniform fiber lengths compared with fast (F) units. (This concept will be revisited in Chapter 2; save the informa-

tion that architecture and motor unit type may be related). Additionally, some units began and ended within a fascicle whereas others extended all or part of the length of a fascicle (Fig. 1-13). Thus, at the high-resolution level, single fiber arrangement within muscle may be very complex. The functional significance of such arrangements is discussed in Chapter 2.

Architecture of Human Skeletal Muscles

Experimental measurement of human muscle architecture has significant importance not only in understanding normal muscle function but also in understanding muscle adaptation (Chapters 4–6). Understanding the architecture of muscle may be the single most important fact to learn from this book.

Several architectural investigations have been performed in human upper and lower limbs. Tables of the relevant architectural features are presented in Tables 1-2 and 1-3. These tables look intimidating at first but will serve primarily as a reference. Take some time to look at the normal range of parameters seen. For example, notice that pennation angles normally range from about 0° to 30°. Thus, as mentioned above, pennation probably has a relatively small influence on muscle PCSA calculations (and function). Note also that the ratio of muscle fiber length to muscle length (FL/ML ratio) typically ranges from about 0.2 to about 0.6. In other words, even the most longitudinally oriented muscles have fibers that extend only approximately 60% of the muscle length. Finally, note that there is a poor correlation between muscle mass and muscle PCSA. Again, mass gives little information that is relevant to function.

Muscles of the Lower Limb
Although each muscle is unique in terms of its architecture, taken as functional groups (e.g., hamstrings, quadriceps, dorsiflexors, plantarflexors), several generalizations can be made (Fig. 1-14). In terms of architecture, the typical

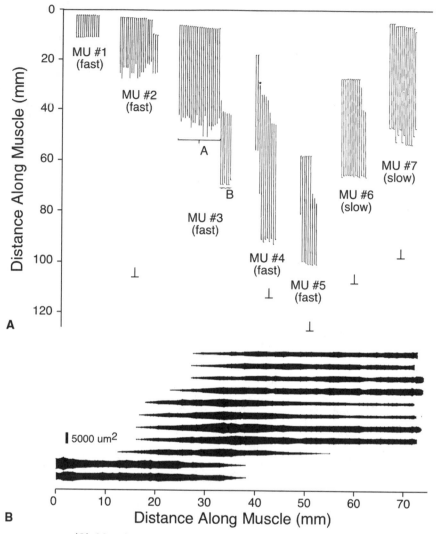

FIGURE 1-13. (A) Muscle fiber length determined by glycogen depletion within seven different single motor units of the cat tibialis anterior muscle. Motor units 1–5 were typed physiologically as fast and motor units 6 and 7 were physiologically typed as slow. The most proximal end of the muscle is defined as 0 mm while the most distal portion of the muscle is denoted by the "⊥" symbol. Fibers that taper at their end are shown as normal thin lines whereas fibers that end in blunted fashion are indicated by a right angle at the end of the line. Note that some muscle fibers actually begin and end within the muscle fascicle itself. **(B)** Higher magnification view of the cross-sectional area of fibers within motor unit #4 shown in **(A)**. Note that, typically, fibers taper at their end within the fascicle. (Figure modified from Ounjian, M., Roy, R. R., Eldred, E., Garfinkel, A., Payne, J. R., Armstrong, A., Toga, A. W., & Edgerton, V. R. (1991). Physiological and developmental implications of motor unit anatomy. *Journal of Neurobiology, 22,* 547–559.)

properties of the various groups can be articulated (compare properties shown in Table 1-3) (Wickiewicz, Roy, Powell, & Edgerton, 1983). Quadriceps femoris are characterized by their relatively high pennation angles, large PCSAs, and short fibers. In terms of design, these muscles appear suited for the generation of large forces (because force is proportional to PCSA). The hamstrings, on the other hand, by virtue of their relatively long fibers and intermediate PCSAs, appear to be designed for large excursions (because excursions are proportional to fiber length). A similar generalization can be made for the plantarflexors and dorsiflexors—plantarflexors appear to be designed for high force production whereas dorsiflexors appear to be designed for moderate forces, but high excursions. A general (and a bit dangerous) conclusion might be that the antigravity extensors are more designed for force production, whereas the flexors are more designed for high excursions. This generalization

will break down upon close scrutiny but might provide a useful memory tool. Be careful when considering muscles alone when trying to deduce function because normally muscles act via a moment arm to produce joint torque. Moment arms and clinical manifestations of strength will be discussed in Chapter 3.

Probably the two most important muscle architectural parameters are muscle PCSA (which is proportion to maximum muscle force) and muscle fiber length (which is proportional to maximum muscle excursion). These two parameters are shown in graphical form for each muscle (Figs. 1-15 and 1-16) and can be used to make general comparisons between muscles in terms of design. For example, note that the sartorius, semitendinosus, and gracilis muscles have extremely high fiber lengths and low PCSAs, which permit high excursions at low forces (Fig. 1-15). At the other end of the spectrum is the soleus muscle, with its high PCSA and short fiber length, suitable

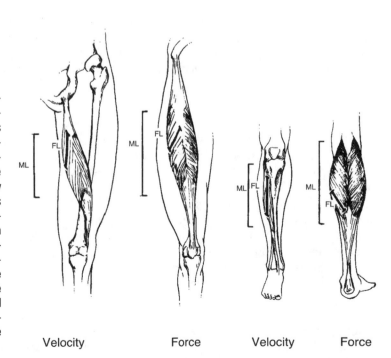

Hamstring   Quadriceps   Dorsiflexor   Plantarflexor

FIGURE 1-14. Schematic illustration of muscle architectural properties in the large muscle groups of the human lower limb. Functionally, quadriceps and plantarflexors are designed for force production based on their low fiber length/muscle length ratios and large physiological cross-sectional areas. Conversely, in general, hamstrings and dorsiflexors are designed for high excursions and velocity by nature of their high fiber length/muscle length ratios and relatively small physiological cross-sectional areas. Abbreviations: ML, muscle length; FL, fiber length.

Velocity   Force   Velocity   Force

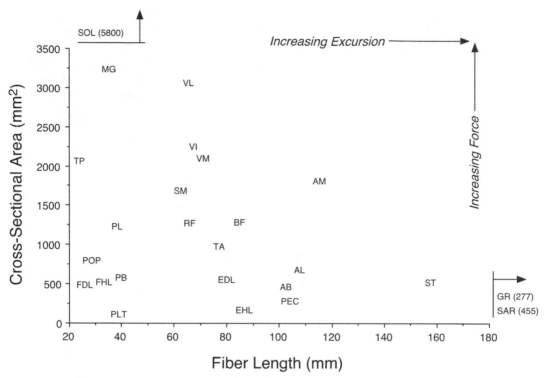

FIGURE 1-15. Scatter graph of fiber length and physiological cross-sectional areas of muscles in the human lower limb. Fiber length is proportional to muscle excursion while physiological cross-sectional area is proportional to maximum muscle force. Thus, this graph can be used to compare the relative forces and excursions of leg muscles. See Table 1-3 for abbreviations. Muscles placed at extremes of graph (SOL, GR, and SAR) would be plotted off this scale at the position shown. (Data from: Wickiewicz, T. L., Roy, R. R., Powell, P. L., & Edgerton, V. R. (1983). Muscle architecture of the human lower limb. *Clinical Orthopaedics and Related Research, 179,* 275–283.)

for generating high forces with small excursions. Based on our understanding of the normal use of each of these muscles in the gait cycle (Chapter 3, page 153), these designs are reasonable.

A particularly striking comparison between architecturally derived muscle properties and anatomically derived properties was provided by Edgerton and colleagues (Wickiewicz, Roy, Powell, & Edgerton, 1983; Fukunaga et al., 1992) for the human triceps surae muscle group. These investigators used the sophisticated method of MRI to image the entire volume of the triceps surae in 2 cm slices along its entire length. Then, using the architectural estimates of fiber length that their laboratory had

previously published, they calculated the PCSA of the soleus, medial gastrocnemius and lateral gastrocnemius muscles. They further compared these PCSA estimates to the anatomical measurements of cross-sectional area (ACSA) obtained from slices in the coronal plane, *i.e.,* those directly provided from the MRI image. Compare these two "measures" of area. The PCSA value is based on the entire muscle volume and includes the estimate of fiber length to arrive at the value for area across the entire muscle. The ACSA is only valid for one slice, and, in fact, varies from slice-to-slice depending on how much of the muscle happens to be located at that slice level. Also, the ACSA value has no information regarding fiber length. Not

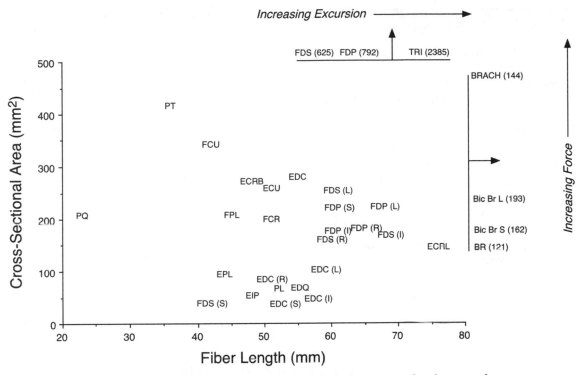

FIGURE 1-16. Scatter graph of the fiber length and physiological cross-sectional areas of muscles in the human arm. Fiber length is proportional to muscle excursion while physiological cross-sectional area is proportional to maximum muscle force. Thus, this graph can be used to compare the relative forces and excursions of arm and forearm muscles. See Table 1-2 for abbreviations. Muscles placed at extremes of graph (FDS, FDP, TRI, BRACH, BR, and Bic Br) would be plotted off this scale at the position shown. (Data from: Lieber, R. L., Fazeli, B. M., & Botte, M. J. (1990). Architecture of selected wrist flexor and extensor muscles. *Journal of Hand Surgery, 15A,* 244–250, and Lieber, R. L., Jacobson, M. D., Fazeli, B. M., Abrams, R. A., & Botte, M. J. (1992). Architecture of selected muscles of the arm and forearm: anatomy and implications for tendon transfer. *Journal of Hand Surgery, 17A,* 787–798.)

surprisingly, these authors demonstrated a poor correlation between ACSA and PCSA and urged investigators not to try to imply muscle function based on simple anatomical images of muscle.

Muscles of the Upper Limb

In light of the specialization observed in the lower limb and the interest in upper extremity surgical procedures, it is important to understand the architectural features of muscles in the human arm and forearm. Although no such clear-cut generalizations regarding functional group design could be made for upper extrem-

ity muscles as were made above for the lower limb, it is possible to demonstrate a high degree of architectural specialization present in many upper limb muscles (Jacobson et al., 1992; Lieber, Fazeli, & Botte, 1990; Lieber, Jacobson, Fazeli, Abrams, & Botte, 1992). The details of these results are presented in Table 1-2. Again, note the high degree of specialization *built into* each of these muscles by virtue of their design. For example, the superficial and deep digital flexors to each digit are similar to one another but different from the digital extensors (Fig. 1-16). As with the lower extremity, this type of scatter plot can be used to compare functional

Therapist's Comments

This section on muscle architecture is important because students often struggle with application at this point. They read the texts and can understand that muscle architecture is important for understanding isolated muscle function. The question is, "how can they use this information for patient care?" However, I believe that knowing what a muscle in designed for, *i.e.*, excursion (in the same way that a muscle is a knee flexor) assists the clinician in evaluating the movement dysfunction of the patient. Ultimately, knowing muscle architecture assists in the evaluation of the patient, and potentially in designing the most appropriate exercise.

properties between muscles of the forearm. Clearly, such differences could be considered in surgical and rehabilitative procedures involving the upper limb or in designing artificial muscles that might restore lost function. One might expect that when a muscle is surgically transferred to perform the function of another muscle whose function has been lost, matching of architectural properties may prove beneficial. This is a popular area of study that will be discussed in Chapter 3.

Significance of Muscle Architecture

After this relatively lengthy discussion of architecture, one might ask, "So what? What do I know now that I didn't know before?" The answer to that question is two-fold. First, the fact that muscles composed of identical building blocks (sarcomeres) can have such dramatically different force-generating properties highlights the clever design of the human body. The body uses identical components and arranges them in different ways to construct different "motors," that produce movement across a range of forces and speeds. Second, by virtue of architectural specialization, it is clear that the

neuromuscular system does not simply modify muscular force and excursion by changing the nervous input to the muscles. Muscles are designed for a specific function—large excursion, for example. The nervous system provides the signal for the muscle to "do its thing" but does not necessarily specify the details of that action. It is as if the nervous system acts as the central control while the muscle interprets the control signal into an external action by virtue of its intrinsic design. This elegant design is but one of many that will be encountered in the examination of the neuromusculoskeletal system. This theme will be revisited in Chapter 3 by providing some specific examples. However, first, the physiological properties of muscle (Chapter 2) and the mechanics of the skeletal system (Chapter 3) must be discussed.

Architectural Implications for Electromyogram (EMG) Measurements

The relatively high pennation angles reported for some muscles has implications for muscle biopsy analysis and electromyogram (EMG) measurement. Because muscle fibers may be relatively short, a biopsy obtained along the length of the muscle may not be representative of all the fibers along the muscle.

Experimental quantification of repeated biopsies from four rhesus monkeys were studied by Roy and colleagues (1991) in three different

Box 1-5. Are EMG Measurements Affected by Architecture?

Yes. EMG electrodes may not provide an adequate sample along the entire length of a muscle if it is highly pennated. In addition, the natural gradation in muscle fiber type from deep to superficial might provide nonrepresentative activation patterns. Finally, some muscles demonstrate compartmentalization that may require multiple electrodes in the same muscle to obtain adequate sampling. Clinicians must be careful in extrapolating from EMG to whole muscle function.

locations along the length of the soleus, medial gastrocnemius, and tibialis anterior muscles. The authors demonstrated a much greater fiber type percentage variability between animal subjects than between biopsies within a subject. However, they did demonstrate that, in spite of sampling different fibers along muscles with very different architectures (fiber length-to-muscle length ratios ranging from 0.23–0.35) it was possible to obtain representative percentages within these different muscle regions. Fiber type variability was 5–10% within a muscle but as much as 30% between the same muscles of different animal subjects.

With regard to EMG measurements, a similar sampling problem may arise as a result of muscle fiber stagger. Electrodes placed in one region of the muscle may not provide an electrical signal that is representative of motor units from different regions of the same muscle (Loeb & Gans, 1986). This is due to two factors, first and most obvious, is the fact that muscle fibers do not extend the length of the muscle and second, there is a natural gradation in fiber type percentage and thus motor unit types from superficial to deep within a muscle. Since motor units are activated in a stereotypical fashion from slow to fast, this may affect duration and amplitude of EMG signals measured at different depths. It should be noted, however, the extent to which this inability to sample uniformly affects either clinical judgment or our understanding of muscle activation has not been clearly determined. A second level of complexity that may affect the extent to which an EMG signal is representative of muscle function arises from the fact that some muscles, such as the cat lateral gastrocnemius, demonstrate what is known as "compartmentalization." English and his colleagues (1984) have shown discrete compartments within the cat lateral gastrocnemius that may have unique functions during normal movement. Under these conditions, separate portions of muscles with unique fiber type distributions are innervated by distinctly different motor nerve branches. As a result, their activa-tion pattern and general level of use can differ, in spite of the fact that they are in the same muscle.

■ Chapter Summary

Skeletal muscles arise by a unique developmental process that includes axonal outgrowth, myogenesis, neuromuscular junction formation, and synapse elimination. The fully differentiated muscle cell is uniquely suited to perform force generation and movement. A stereotypical view of the muscle fiber can be presented in which force-generating, force-regulating, and force-activating roles are assigned to various structures. The structural muscle hierarchy proceeds from the whole muscle all the way to the myofilaments and even to individual molecules. Skeletal muscle fibers can be differentiated into various types, which provide further ability for the muscular system to customize structure to function. Finally, the arrangement of muscle fibers within whole muscles is known as muscle architecture and is an important factor in determining whole muscle properties.

REFERENCES

Banes, A.J. (1993). Mechanical strain and the mammalian cell. In J A, Frangos, ed. *Physical Forces and the Mammalian Cell* (pp. 81–123). San Diego: Academic Press, San Diego.

Bennett, M.R. (1983). Development of neuromuscular synapses. *Physiological Review, 63,* 915–1048.

Bodine, S.C., Roy, R.R., Meadows, D.A., Zernicke, R.F., Sacks, R.D., Fournier, M., Edgerton, V.R. (1982). Architectural, histochemical, and contractile characteristics of a unique biarticular muscle: the cat semitendinosus. *Journal of Neurophysiology, 48,* 192–201.

Bottinelli, R., Betto, R., Schiaffino, S., Reggiani, C. (1994). Unloaded shortening velocity and myosin heavy chain and alkali light chain isoform composition in rat skeletal muscle fibres. *Journal of Physiology (London), 478,* 341–349.

Buller, A.J., Eccles, J.C., Eccles, R.M. (1960a). Differentiation of fast and slow muscles in the cat hindlimb. *Journal of Physiology (London)*, *150*, 399–416.

Buller, A.J., Eccles, J.C., Eccles, R.M. (1960b). Interactions between motorneurons and muscles in respect to the characteristic speeds of their responses. *Journal of Physiology (London)*, *150*, 417–439.

Ebashi, S., Maruyama, K., Endo, M. (1980). Muscle contraction: Its regulatory mechanisms (pp. 104–122). New York: Springer Verlag.

Edmonson, D.G., Olson, E.N. (1989). A gene with homology to the myc similarity region of myoD is expressed during myogenesis and is sufficient to activate the muscle differentiation program. *Genes Development*, *3*, 628–640.

Eisenberg, B.R. (1983). Quantitative ultrastructure of mammalian skeletal muscle. In L. D. Peachey, Adrian, R.H. and Geiger, S.R., (Ed.). *Skeletal Muscle. Vol. 10.* (pp. 73-112). Baltimore, MD: American Physiological Society.

English, A.W. (1984). An electromyographic analysis of compartments in cat lateral gastrocnemius muscle during unrestrained locomotion. *Journal of Neurophysiology*, *52*, 114–125.

Franzini-Armstrong, C. (1999). The sarcoplasmic reticulum and the control of muscle contraction. *FASEB Journal*, S266–S270.

Fukunaga, T., Roy, R.R., Shellock, F.G., Hodgson, J.A., Day, M.K., Lee, P.L., Kwong, F.H., Edgerton, V.R. (1992). Physiological cross-sectional area of human leg muscle based on magnetic resonance imaging. *Journal of Orthopedic Research*, *10*, 928–934.

Fukunaga, T., Ichinose, Y., Ito, M., Kawakami, Y., Fukashiro, S. (1997). Determination of fascicle length and pennation in a contracting human muscle in vivo. *Journal of Applied Physiology*, *82*, 354–358.

Gans, C., Bock, W.J. (1965). The functional significance of muscle architecture: a theoretical analysis. *Advances in Anatomy, Embryology and Cell Biology*, *38*, 115–142.

Haselgrove, J.C. (1983). Structure of vertebrate striated muscle as determined by x-ray-diffraction studies. In *Handbook of Physiology* (pp. 143–171). Bethesda, MD: American Physiological Society.

Huxley, A.F., Niedergerke, R. (1954). Structural changes in muscle during contraction. Interference microscopy of living muscle fibers. *Nature*, *173*, 971–973.

Huxley, H.E. (1990). Sliding filaments and molecular motile systems. *Journal of Biological Chemistry*, *265*, 8347–8350.

Huxley, H.E., Hanson, J. (1954). Changes in the cross-striations of muscle during contraction and stretch, and their structural interpretation. *Nature*, *173*, 973–976.

Huxley, H.E., Simmons, R.M., Faruqi, A.R., Kress, M., Koch, M. (1981). Millisecond time-resolved changes in x-ray reflections from contracting muscle during rapid mechanical transients, recorded using synchrotron radiation. *Proceedings of the National Academy of Sciences of the United States of America*, *78*, 2297–2301.

Jacobson, M.D., Raab, R., Fazeli, B.M., Abrams, R.A., Botte, M.J., Lieber, R.L. (1992). Architectural design of the human intrinsic hand muscles. *Journal of Hand Surgery*, *17A*, 804–809.

Jacobson, M.D., Weil, M., Raff, M.C. (1997). Programmed cell death in animal development. *Cell*, *88*, 347–354.

Jansen, J.K.S., Fladby, T. (1990). The perinatal reorganization of the innervation of skeletal muscle in mammals. *Progress in Neurobiology*, *34*, 39–90.

Kawakami, Y., Ichinose, Y., Fukunaga, T. (1998). Architectural and functional features of human triceps surae muscles during contraction. *Journal of Applied Physiology*, *85*, 398–404.

Kayar, S.R., Hoppeler, H., Mermod, L., Weibel, E.R. (1988). Mitochondrial size and shape in equine skeletal muscle: a three-dimensional reconstruction study. *Anatomical Record*, *222*, 333–339.

Kelly, A.M. (1983). Emergence of specialization in skeletal muscle. In L. D. Peachey, (Ed.) *Handbook of Physiology* (pp. 417–486). Baltimore, MD: American Physiological Society.

Kirkwood, S.P., Munn, E.A., Brooks, G.A. (1986). Mitochondrial reticulum in limb skeletal muscle. *American Journal of Physiology*, *86*, C395–C402.

Lance, J.C., Landmesser, L. (1978). Effect of spinal cord deletions and reversals on motoneuron projection patterns in the embryonic chick hindlimb. *Society for Neuroscience Abstracts*, *4*, 118.

Landmesser, L.T. (1980). The generation of neuromuscular specificity. *Annual Review of Neuroscience*, *3*, 279–302.

Lazarides, E. (1980). Intermediate filaments as mechanical integrators of cellular space. *Nature*, *283*, 249–256.

Lieber, R.L., Fazeli, B.M., Botte, M.J. (1990). Architecture of selected wrist flexor and extensor muscles. *Journal of Hand Surgery, 15A*, 244–250.

Lieber, R.L., Jacobson, M.D., Fazeli, B.M., Abrams, R.A., Botte, M.J. (1992). Architecture of selected muscles of the arm and forearm: anatomy and implications for tendon transfer. *Journal of Hand Surgery, 17A*, 787–798.

Loeb, G.E., Gans, C. (1986). Electromyography for experimentalists. Chicago: University of Chicago Press.

Loeb, G.E., Pratt, C.A., Chanaud, C.M., Richmond, F.J.R. (1987). Distribution and innervation of short, interdigitated muscle fibers in parallel-fibered muscles of the cat hindlimb. *Journal of Morphology, 191*, 1–15.

Lundborg, G. (1988). Nerve injury and repair. New York: Churchill Livingstone, New York.

Lutz, G.J., Razzaghi, S., Lieber, R.L. (2000). Cloning and characterization of the S1 domain of four myosin isoforms from functionally divergent fiber types in adult *Rana pipiens* skeletal muscle. *Gene, 250*, 97–107.

Miller, J.B., Stockdale, F.E. (1986a). Developmental origins of skeletal muscle fibers; clonal analysis of myogenic cell lineages based on expression of fast and slow myosin heavy chains. *Proceedings of the National Academy of Science of the United States of America, 83*, 3860–3864.

Miller, J.B., Stockdale, F.E. (1986b). Developmental regulation of the multiple myogenic cell lineages of the avian embryo. *Journal of Cell Biology, 103*, 2197–2208.

Miller, J.B., Stockdale, F.E. (1987). What muscle cells know that nerves don't tell them. *Trends in Neurosciences, 10*, 10–14.

Ounjian, M., Roy, R.R., Eldred, E., Garfinkel, A., Payne, J.R., Armstrong, A., Toga, A.W., Edgerton, V.R. (1991). Physiological and developmental implications of motor unit anatomy. *Journal of Neurobiology, 22*, 547–559.

Peachey, L.D., Eisenberg, B.R. (1978). Helicoids in the T system and striations of frog skeletal muscle fibers seen by high voltage electron microscopy. *Biophysical Journal, 22*, 145–154.

Peachey, L.D., Franzini-Armstrong, C. (1983). Structure and function of membrane systems of skeletal muscle cells. In *Handbook of Physiology* (pp. 23–73). Baltimore, MD: American Physiological Society.

Pollack, G.H. (1983). The cross-bridge theory. *Physiological Review, 63*, 1049–1113.

Pollard, T.D., Doberstein, S.K., Zot, H.G. (1991). Myosin-I. *Annual Review of Physiology, 53*, 653–681.

Poo, M.M. (1982). Rapid lateral diffusion of functional ACh receptors in embryonic muscle cell membrane. *Nature, 295*, 333–334.

Powell, P.L., Roy, R.R., Kanim, P., Bello, M., Edgerton, V.R. (1984). Predictability of skeletal muscle tension from architectural determinations in guinea pig hindlimbs. *Journal of Applied Physiology, 57*, 1715–1721.

Roy, R.R., Bodine-Fowler, S.C., Kim, J., Haque, N, de Leon, D., Rudolph, W., Edgerton, V.R. (1991). Architectural and fiber type distribution properties of selected rhesus leg muscles: feasibility of multiple independent biopsies. *Acta Anatomica (Basel), 140*, 350–356.

Sacks, R.D., Roy, R.R. (1982). Architecture of the hindlimb muscles of cats: functional significance. *Journal of Morphology, 173*, 185–195.

Sanes, J.R., Lichtman, J.W. (1999). Development of the vertebrate neuromuscular junction. *Annual Review of Neuroscience, 22*, 389–442.

Scales, J.B., Olson, E.N., Perry, M. (1990). Two distinct Xenopus genes with homology to MyoD1 are expressed before somite formation in early embryogenesis. *Molecular and Cellular Biology, 10*, 1516–1524.

Squire, J. (1981). The structural basis of muscular contraction. New York: Plenum Press.

Staron, R.S., Pette, D. (1987). The multiplicity of combinations of myosin light chains and heavy chains in histochemically typed single fibres. Rabbit soleus muscle. *Biochemical Journal, 243*, 687–693.

Staron, R.S., Pette, D. (1987). The multiplicity of combinations of myosin light chains and heavy chains in histochemically typed single fibres. Rabbit tibialis anterior muscle. *Biochemical Journal, 1243*, 695–699.

Steller, H. (1995). Mechanisms and genes of cellular suicide. *Science, 267*, 1445–1449.

Thompson, W.J., Sutton, L.A., Riley, D.A. (1984). Fibre type composition of single motor units during synapse elimination in neonatal rat soleus muscle. *Nature, 309*, 709–711.

Trotter, J.A. (1990). Interfiber tension transmission in series-fibered muscles of the cat hindlimb. *Journal of Morphology, 206*, 351–361.

Uyeda, T.Q.P., Ruppel, K.M., Spudich, J.A. (1994). Enzymatic activities correlate with chimaeric substitutions at the actin-binding face of myosin. *Nature, 368,* 567–569.

Vandenburgh, H.H., Swasdison, S., Karlisch, P. (1991). Computer-aided mechanogenesis of skeletal muscle organs from single cells in vitro. *FASEB Journal, 5,* 2860–2867.

Weiss, A., Schiaffino, S., Leinwand, L.A. Comparative sequence analysis of the complete human sarcomeric myosin heavy chain family: implications for functional diversity. *Journal of Molecular Biology, 290,* 61–75.

Wickiewicz, T.L., Roy, R.R., Powell, P.L., Edgerton, V.R. (1983). Muscle architecture of the human lower limb. *Clinical Orthopaedics and Related Research, 179,* 275–283.

Zajac, F.E., Gordon, M.E. (1989). Determining muscle's force and action in multi-articular movement. In John Hollozy (Ed.) *Exercise and Sport Sciences Review* (pp. 187–230). Baltimore, MD: Williams & Wilkins.

Zuurbier, C.J., Huijing, P.A. (1992). Influence of muscle geometry on shortening speed of fibre, aponeurosis and muscle. *Journal of Biomechanics, 25,* 1017–1026.

CHAPTER 2

Skeletal Muscle Physiology

Chapter Overview

This chapter describes the relationship between the muscle structure, which was discussed in Chapter 1, and muscle function. This information is generally classified under "physiology," and, to organize this relatively broad area of study, the chapter is divided into three parts. The first part discusses the activation and contraction sequence of muscle, along with some functional and clinically relevant consequences of this scheme. Second, two important mechanical properties of muscle—the length-tension (isometric) and force-velocity (isotonic) properties—are highlighted. The basis for all muscle contraction is presented as well as the details of the cross-bridge cycle. The manner in which whole muscle architecture affects isometric and isotonic mechanical properties is included. Finally, the important topics of muscle fiber types and motor units are presented, which enables discussion of recruitment, locomotion, and fatigue.

Educational Objectives

● To understand the structures involved in excitation-contraction coupling along with their physical relationships.
● To understanding the underlying events giving rise to the force-frequency relationship in skeletal muscle.
● To understand the structural basis for the length-tension relationship.

● To be able to describe the way in which muscle force depends on velocity.
● To understand motor unit structure/function relationships.
● To be able to describe structural and functional differences among fiber types.
● To be able to describe possible causes of muscle fatigue.
● To understand the physiological basis of the electromyogram and limitations of interpretations of it.

Introduction

In this chapter, anatomy meets physiology; the functional importance of the physical arrangement of the muscle components presented in the last chapter will now become apparent. An understanding of muscle physiology is predicated upon a good understanding of muscle macroanatomy and microanatomy. Thus, it was important to lay the anatomical groundwork in Chapter 1. Note that anatomic studies are rarely performed in isolation of physiologic studies and vice versa. In fact, anatomists routinely refer to physiologic data to infer the significance of their findings, whereas physiologists routinely refer to anatomic studies when proposing structural bases for their observations. Thus, the distinction between muscle anatomy and physiology is often one of orientation with both disciplines studying similar phenomena. Significant cross-referencing between muscle anatomic and physiologic studies will be required as we continue our discussion of skeletal muscle structure and function.

1 Muscle Fiber Activation

Excitation-Contraction Coupling

The discussion of skeletal muscle physiology begins with the process of muscle activation itself. It is well known that peripheral nerves innervate skeletal muscles and that neural activation precedes muscle contraction. The precise process by which this neural activation signal culminates in muscle contraction is known as

excitation-contraction coupling, or EC coupling (Fig. 2-1). EC coupling is a sequence of microscopic events, each of which is necessary for contraction to occur. If any single step of EC coupling is impaired, muscle contraction does not occur normally. This impairment might be interpreted as muscle paralysis or fatigue. However, such a general classification is not useful unless the underlying cause is known (Ebashi, Maruyama, & Endo, 1980).

The Action Potential

The first step in the EC coupling chain is the generation of the peripheral nerve action potential. An action potential results from activation of the peripheral nerve axon that innervates the muscle. Of course the "normal" way to

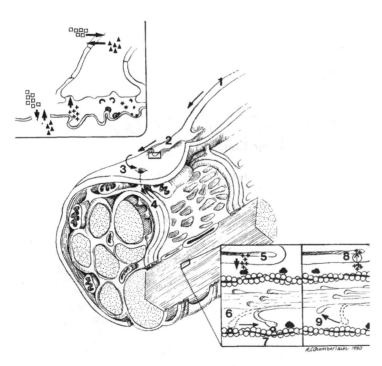

FIGURE 2-1. Sequence of events involved in excitation-contraction coupling of a nervous impulse to muscle contraction. 1. Action potential conducted by nerve to muscle (inset, squares represent Na^+ ions entering nerve, and triangles represent K^+ ions leaving the nerve to conduct the action potential). 2. Nervous impulse transmitted across neuromuscular junction to muscle fiber (inset, crosses represent Ca^{++} ions entering nerve end, half-moons represent the neurotransmitter ACh, and asterisks represent the enzyme acetylcholinesterase degrading ACh). 3. Action potential conducted along fiber surface (inset, squares represent Na^+ ions entering fiber, and triangles represent K^+ ions leaving the fiber to conduct the action potential). 4. Action potential conducted deep into fiber via the T-system. 5. Ca^{++} released from SR to bind troponin and thus activate the actin filament. 6 and 7. Cross-bridge produces force and filament sliding. 8. Ca^{++} is pumped back into SR when electrical impulses cease. 9. Cross-bridges relax due to lack of Ca^{++} filament activation.

Box 2-1. Artificial Activation of Muscles is Good Therapy!

Electrical activation of peripheral nerves using external devices is often used to substitute function when the patient cannot activate the muscle themselves. This may be due to nerve injury, spinal cord injury, or because of the "inhibition" that seems to occur after many types of surgery. Such use of external devices, known as "functional electrical stimulation" or "neuromuscular electrical stimulation" can be exploited by therapists to improve muscle function after injury or disuse.

---

activate an axon is by generation of a signal from the CNS to initiate movement. However, the axon may be depolarized in a number of additional ways, including trauma to the peripheral nerve or application of an external electrical stimulating device. In fact, the use of an electrical stimulating device is used clinically to substitute lost function in cases of paralysis, muscle weakness that occurs after surgery, or the lost ability of the motor system to activate a muscle after surgery (see Chapter 4 for more details on clinical use of muscle stimulation). Regardless of the manner of initiation, the resulting action potentials that propagate down the peripheral nerve are identical. The action potential arrives at the neuromuscular junction, the interface between muscle and nerve. As we saw in Chapter 1, the neuromuscular junction is itself a complex structure composed of the presynaptic motor neuron and the postsynaptic muscle membrane. The indentation on the muscle fiber surface in which the motor nerve rests, is known as the synaptic cleft.

Acetylcholine Release—The Neurotransmitter

The end of the peripheral nerve contains packets of the neurotransmitter acetylcholine (ACh), which causes muscle fiber excitation. ACh is synthesized by the cell body of the motor nerve and is transported down the axon where it is stored at nerve endings for later use.

Following nerve activation, the resulting depolarization causes a quantum or unit of ACh to be released into the synaptic cleft (Fig. 2-1). ACh then diffuses across the synaptic cleft and binds to the ACh receptor, which is integrated into the muscle membrane (refer to the discussion of synaptogenesis in Chapter 1). ACh binding results in depolarization of the muscle fiber sarcolemma and an action potential that propagates from the neuromuscular junction outwardly in all directions. Communication between the nerve and muscle therefore occurs via a standard synapse in which the neurotransmitter is acetylcholine and, therefore, this type of synapse is referred to as cholinergic. (There are other neurotransmitters used within the body and they are named as a class based on the type of neurotransmitter used.)

The storage and release of ACh to cause muscle activation is accomplished by the interaction of numerous active enzymes. The function of these enzymes has been studied in isolation and a therapy for "overactive" or "spastic" muscles was developed based on discoveries made. One method for blocking neuromuscular transmission is to inject Botulinum toxin into the muscle, near the motor point. This

---

Box 2-2. Bacterial Poison Used for Therapy?

α-bungarotoxin, commonly referred to as "botox," is used clinically to provide a temporary block of neuromuscular function. This compound is produced by bacteria and causes the disease known as Botulism. It acts by entering the presynaptic nerve terminal and blocking the normal release of acetylcholine into the synaptic cleft thus blocking muscle contraction. One of the most common uses of α-bungarotoxin in physical therapy is to decrease the symptoms of "spasticity" that accompany such disorders as cerebral palsy. However, its use is not without controversy because many believe that this compound induces changes in muscle that resemble denervation.

Therapist's Comments

It may be helpful to point out to students that the disease, myasthenia gravis represents an overexpression of acetylcholine receptors as a consequence of general anesthetic and the rise in body temperature. The clinical presentation of this patient is muscle fasciculation, weakness and, on occasion, uncontrolled fever. Myasthenia gravis represents one example in which we are fortunate enough to have knowledge of the precise neuromuscular malfunction and now must work on effective treatments to help these patients.

---

toxin enters the presynaptic nerve terminal and blocks ACh release by interrupting the activity of one of the enzymes involved in the release process. Such chemical "blocks" typically act for 3–6 months before they are no longer needed or before another dose is required. Is this good for the muscle? This question will be answered in greater detail in Chapter 4. Briefly, the answer is that this is one of the best current therapies available, but certainly the muscle is upset with interrupted neuromuscular transmission.

Transverse Tubular-System and Sarcoplasmic Reticulum Involvement in Excitation-Contraction Coupling

At various intervals along the fiber surface, the action potential encounters invaginations of the sarcolemma that extend into the fiber—the transverse tubular system, T-system, Fig. 2-1 (Peachey & Franzini-Armstrong, 1983). The action potential is conducted deep into the fiber by the T-system. The interface between the "outside world" of the muscle fiber and the "inside world" of the contractile apparatus occurs at the next step where the T-system signals the sarcoplasmic reticulum (SR) to release calcium. This is accomplished by the specialized voltage receptors and calcium release channels that ap-

pear as the "SR feet," that anchor the terminal region of the SR to the T-system (Eisenberg, 1983). An important observation that allows you to test your understanding of the three-dimensional nature of the muscle fiber is that the lumen of the T-system contains extracellular fluid because it is ultimately continuous with the extracellular space whereas the lumen of the SR contains intracellular fluid. Thus, extracellular fluid is contained deep within the muscle fiber. This fact has been exploited by muscle anatomists and physiologists to better understand fiber structure and function.

Calcium Release Results in Muscle Contraction

After the T-system signals the SR that the fiber has been activated, the SR releases calcium ions in the region of the myofilaments (Fig. 2-1). This release process is fast—much faster than the resulting contraction/relaxation cycle. The calcium ions bind to troponin, the actin filament regulatory protein, which in turn releases the inhibition on the actin filament, permitting interaction between the myosin and actin filaments, which results in cross-bridge cycling (see details below) and, therefore, in force generation and movement.

Calcium Uptake Results in Muscle Relaxation

As long as neural impulses arrive at the neuromuscular junction and calcium concentrations remain high in the region of the myofilaments, force generation continues. However, when the impulses cease, calcium levels drop and force decreases as calcium is pumped back into the SR by the calcium-activated adenosine triphosphatase (ATPase) enzyme. The calcium-activated ATPase enzyme is an integral protein that is embedded within the bilayer of SR membrane. The mechanism of action of this enzyme has been thoroughly studied and is one of the best understood of the ion transport enzymes (Entman & Van Winkle, 1986). The calcium pumping process is energy dependent and requires ATP. When calcium levels in the region of the myofilaments drop below a critical level, thin filament inhibition again resumes, and actin-myosin interaction is prevented. Muscle fiber relaxation parallels the drop in calcium levels. Muscles with high SR/calcium pumping ability can thus relax faster compared with muscles with less SR/calcium pumping ability. This ultrastructural difference among muscles allows some muscles to function at extremely high contraction/relaxation rates (Rome & Klimov, 2000).

The chain of events required for muscle contraction to occur after nerve depolarization has been outlined. Picture the structure and its location as you review this sequence:

1. Generation of the peripheral nerve action potential
2. Release of ACh from the presynaptic nerve terminal
3. Binding of ACh to the muscle fiber ACh receptor on the postsynaptic membrane
4. Depolarization of the sarcolemma after ACh receptor binding
5. Conduction of the action potential into the fiber by the T-system
6. Signaling of the SR by the T-system to release calcium
7. Binding of calcium to the regulatory protein troponin, permitting actin-myosin interaction
8. Force generation resulting from actin-myosin interaction
9. Pumping of calcium back into the SR when neural activation ceases
10. Decreased SR calcium concentration resulting in inhibition of actomyosin interaction and muscle relaxation

Temporal Summation

A well-known muscle contractile property follows directly from an understanding of the EC coupling sequence presented above. First, it should be obvious that the time required for activation, contraction, and relaxation to occur is finite. That is, excitation (with accompanying calcium release) is relatively rapid (~5 msec)

whereas contraction and relaxation are relatively slow (~100 msec). The mechanical consequence of the activation process (i.e., the muscle twitch) lags far behind the activation process itself.

To discuss the functional effects of multiple muscle impulses, suppose the entire EC coupling process requires 100 msec. If, after the first impulse, a second impulse is delivered before 100 msec has elapsed, the muscle will be signaled to contract before it has fully relaxed. In other words, the second impulse will be superimposed upon part of the cycle that was initiated by the first impulse, resulting in some degree of summation of the two impulses. Because the two events have summated because of their relative temporal relationship, this process is referred to as temporal summation. The specific functional effect of temporal summation depends on the number of impulses and proximity to each other. The overall idea is that multiple impulses result in higher forces than single impulses alone. This is partly because of the different mechanical conditions encountered by the first and subsequent pulses. The effect of the first stimulus is to cause the contracting sarcomeres to "stretch out" the passive structures that lie in series with them (e.g., tendons or passive sarcomeres). When the second impulse arrives, it is not required to stretch out any of these structures and all of the cross-bridge interaction can be transmitted through the "pre-tightened" series elastic structures, resulting in a greater force being generated at the ends of the muscle fiber. Thus, two impulses that are delivered to a muscle fiber and separated by approximately 50 msec result in more force than the same two pulses delivered to the muscle but separated by more time. If a "train" of such pulses (e.g., 50 pulses in a row) is delivered to the muscle, separated in time by different amounts, this results in what is known as a tetanic contraction, and the force generated is quite different (Fig. 2-2). Higher forces result when stimuli are delivered at higher frequencies because there is less time for relaxation (frequency = 1/interpulse interval; low intervals correspond to high frequencies).

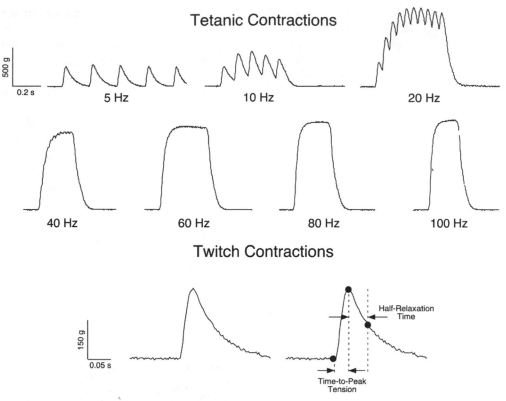

FIGURE 2-2. Upper Panel: Contractile records from a rabbit tibialis anterior muscle demonstrating fusion of mechanical twitches as stimulation frequency increases from 5 Hz to 100 Hz (temporal summation). Lower Panel: Twitch contraction record from a rabbit tibialis anterior muscle, which includes definitions of parameters often measured from twitch contractions, namely, half-relaxation time and time-to-peak twitch tension. Note different tension calibration bars for tetani and twitches. (Unpublished experimental data acquired by Jennifer Davis, University of California, San Diego).

In Figure 2-2, notice that at relatively low frequencies (*e.g.,* 10 Hz), the contractile record almost completely relaxes between successive pulses. This is referred to as an unfused tetanic contraction, because it is still possible to distinguish individual contractile events within the force record. However, note that as stimulation frequency increases, the tetanic record becomes more fused, until at high frequencies (*e.g.,* 100 Hz), the contractile record becomes a fused contraction. A fused tetanic contraction appears as such because calcium is released onto the myofilaments much faster than the rate at which the myofilaments can relax.

Rate Coding: The Physiological Significance of Temporal Summation

The strategy for varying force by altering activation frequency is known as frequency or rate coding. Because muscle force varies as a function of activation frequency, this is one method the CNS can use to alter muscle force. If high forces are required at the periphery, the CNS can deliver high-frequency pulses. Conversely, if only low forces are required, the CNS can deliver low-frequency pulses. Of course, this type of effect is difficult to demonstrate directly. In a technical procedure involving single motor unit recording, ventral root recording, and muscle tension recording in situ during locomotion (as well as some fancy post-experimental data processing), Hoffer and colleagues (Hoffer, O'Donovan, Pratt, & Loeb, 1981, 1987) demonstrated what they interpreted to be rate coding, during normal locomotion. (This series of experiment required measurement of muscle action potentials as well as neural action potentials during free locomotion.) In spite of the fact that rate coding can control muscle force, it is easy to see that this would not be a great strategy to control muscle force in general for at least two reasons: The first reason is that the range over which force can be changed due to rate coding is only four-fold. For most muscles, the ratio of peak tetanic force to twitch force is only 3–4 (compare peak twitch to peak tetanic force in Figure 2-2). However, it is easy to show that, fingertip grip force can vary by 1,000-fold. This large range is necessary to accomplish the variety of tasks required in activities of daily living. Temporal summation alone cannot provide such a range. The second reason that rate coding is not a great control strategy is that, at low stimulation frequencies, where force is lower and, presumably, control would be most important, the tension record fluctuates tremendously (see 10 Hz trace in Figure 2-2). Therefore, with rate coding alone, steadiness decreases as force decreases, which is exactly opposite of what is desired.

Later in this chapter it will become apparent that the control of muscle force by the CNS is much more sophisticated than simple rate coding. The area of study that includes the control of muscles by the nervous system is known as neuromotor control (Binder & Mendell, 1990). For now, suffice it to say that muscle and nerve properties are matched in a sophisticated fashion through the motor unit structure within muscle to provide a tremendous degree of control under a variety of conditions. Rate coding is only one of the methods by which this match is accomplished.

2 Skeletal Muscle Mechanics

Length-tension Relationship: Isometric Muscle Contraction

Since the late 1800s, it has been known that the force developed by a muscle during isometric contraction (*i.e.*, when the muscle is not allowed to shorten) varies with its starting length (See review in Podolsky and Shoenberg, 1983). The isometric length-tension curve is generated by maximally stimulating a skeletal muscle at a variety of discrete lengths and measuring the tension generated at each length (Fig. 2-3).

FIGURE 2-3. Individual isometric contractions permit experimental determination of the length tension curve. Each trace represents a schematic isometric tetanic contraction at a particular length. AT-active tension; PT-passive tension shown as the distance between the dotted line and beginning of curve (only significant at lengths above L_o where L_o is optimal length). Each AT and PT value from each contraction is plotted as a single data point to create the length-tension relationship in Figure 2-4.

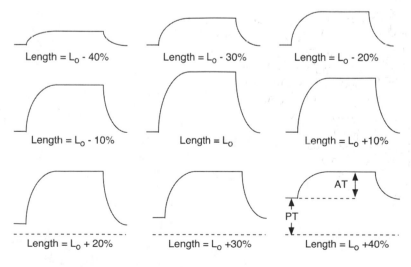

Length = L_o - 40% Length = L_o - 30% Length = L_o - 20%

Length = L_o - 10% Length = L_o Length = L_o +10%

Length = L_o + 20% Length = L_o +30% Length = L_o +40%

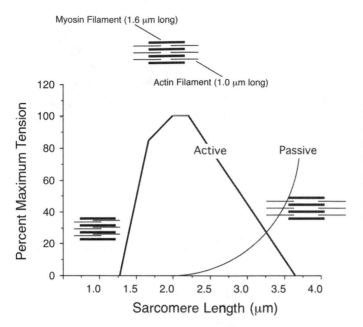

FIGURE 2-4. The sarcomere length-tension curve for frog skeletal muscle obtained using sequential isometric contractions in single muscle fibers. Insets show schematic arrangement of myofilaments in different regions of the length-tension curve. Curved line represents passive muscle tension.

When maximum tetanic tension at each length is plotted against length, a relationship such as that shown in Figure 2-4 is obtained. Although a general description of this relationship was established early in the history of biologic science, the precise structural basis for the length-tension relationship in skeletal muscle was not elucidated until the sophisticated mechanical experiments of the early 1960s were performed. It was these experiments that defined the precise relationship between myofilament overlap and tension generation, which is referred to today as the length-tension relationship. In its most basic form, the length-tension relationship reflects the fact that tension generation in skeletal muscle is a direct function of the magnitude of overlap between the actin and myosin filaments.

Sarcomere Length-Tension Relationship

In the late 1950s and early 1960s, Drs. Andrew Huxley, Albert Gordon, and Fred Julian, working in England (1966) and Dr. Paul Edman, working in Sweden (1966), defined what might be one of the most explicit structure-function relationships in all of biology. It was obvious to these investigators that, to determine the de-

tailed structural basis for the length-tension relationship, isolated, intact single skeletal muscle fibers would be required. This is because whole muscles, with their variety of fiber sizes and types "smeared out" the precise properties of individual fibers. To elucidate detailed mechanisms, single fibers (i.e., single cells) were studied. The only species from which isolated intact fibers could be obtained was the frog and, at that time, a great deal was known about its structure. Picture the experimental setup: The following experiments were performed on tissue (single muscle cells) approximately 3 mm long and 75 μm in diameter! Studies in mammalian systems have lagged behind when it comes to understanding structure-function relationships of intact muscle and they have served largely to confirm what was discovered in frog muscle. At several times throughout this text, references to studies of frog muscle will be made even though it is understood that your main interest is in human muscle. This is done to permit a detailed discussion of mechanisms, but an attempt to generalize to human muscle will follow as soon as possible after the mechanistic point is made.

Sir Andrew Huxley (who by this time had

already received a Nobel Prize in collaboration with Sir Alan Hodgkin for determining the mechanism of the nerve action potential) invented a mechanical version of his voltage clamp apparatus that had previously been used in the nerve studies. This apparatus was designed to keep a small segment of the fiber at a constant length (and therefore keep a region of the fiber at a constant sarcomere length). This enabled him to make a unique correlation between muscle tension and sarcomere length. However, it was much easier said than done because it turned out that "isometric" force generation in a single muscle fiber was anything but isometric. Sarcomeres in the end region of the fiber tended to stretch sarcomeres in the central region, so the apparatus Huxley developed was designed to stabilize such mechanical instabilities (Gordon, Huxley, & Julian, 1966).

The results of these classic experiments (Gordon, Huxley, & Julian, 1966) are summarized in Figure 2-4. In this figure, muscle relative tetanic tension (as a percentage of maximum) is plotted as a function of sarcomere length (in μm). This was one case in which anatomy met physiology in dramatic fashion because knowledge of the precise anatomic lengths of the myosin and actin filaments was crucial for understanding the basis of this relationship. This relationship has tremendous implications for understanding normal movement and even for imposing therapeutic treatment.

Descending Limb of the Length-Tension Curve

As the muscle fiber was highly stretched by the investigators to a sarcomere length of 3.65 μm, the muscle developed no active force. Why did the muscle develop zero force at this length? The answer was because the myosin filament is 1.65 μm long and the actin filament is 2.0 μm long, at a sarcomere length of 3.65 μm there is no overlap (interdigitation) between the actin and myosin filaments. Therefore, although the EC coupling process might permit actin-myosin interaction by removing the inhibition of the actin filament, because no myosin cross-

bridges are in the vicinity of the actin active sites, no force generation can occur.

As the muscle was allowed to shorten, overlap between actin and myosin was possible, and the amount of force generated by the muscle increased as sarcomere length decreased. Increasing force with decreasing sarcomere length occurred until the muscle reached a sarcomere length of 2.2 μm. Why did tension slowly increase? Over the range of sarcomere lengths from 2.2–3.65 μm, as sarcomere length decreased, the number of cross-bridges between actin and myosin increased, resulting in increased force. This region of the length-tension curve is known as the descending limb. This result extended to the whole muscle indicates that, if a muscle is normally operating across the descending limb of the length-tension curve, as it gets shorter, it will get stronger (see Chapter 3, page 141, for a specific example of such an operating range).

Plateau Region of the Length-Tension Curve

As sarcomere length changed from 2.0 μm to 2.2 μm, muscle force remained constant. Again, it was possible to directly relate this result to knowledge of thick filament structure. Recall from Chapter 1 that the myosin filament is a polymeric arrangement of myosin molecules arranged in an antiparallel fashion. Because many myosin "backbones" (the light meromyosin portion of the myosin molecules) come together in the center of the myosin filament, there exists a bare region of the myosin molecule that is devoid of cross-bridges. In fact, the length of the bare region is 0.2 μm. Although sarcomere length shortening over the range 2.2–2.0 μm results in greater filament overlap, it does not result in increased force generation because no additional cross-bridge connections are made. The region of the length-tension curve over which length change results in no change in force is known as the plateau region. The maximum tetanic tension generated by the muscle in this region is abbreviated P_o. The length at which P_o is attained is known as a muscle's optimal length and is abbreviated L_o. There are some very interesting specific biological examples in which muscles appear to be "designed" to operate on the plateau of the length-tension curve. The best understood of these examples is fish swimming, in which fish muscle on either side of the body appear to "vibrate" back and forth in opposition to power swimming (Lieber, Raab, Kashin, & Edgerton, 1992; Rome, Swank, & Corda, 1993).

Ascending Limb of the Length-Tension Curve

At a sarcomere length of 2.0 μm, notice that the actin filaments from one side of the sarcomere juxtapose the actin filaments from the opposite side of the sarcomere (Fig. 2-4). It might be predicted that shortening past this point would be impossible. However, as sarcomere length decreases below 2.0 μm, actin filaments from one side of the sarcomere overlap with the actin filaments on the opposite side of the sarcomere. That is, at these lengths, actin filaments exist in a "double overlap" state as they overlap both with the opposite actin filament as well as with the myosin filament. Under these double-overlap conditions, the actin filament from one side of the sarcomere interferes with cross-bridge formation on the other side of the sarcomere, and this causes decreased muscle force output. This occurs from 2.0–1.87 μm in frog muscle and this region is known as the shallow ascending limb of the length-tension curve. The word "shallow" distinguishes it from the next portion of the length-tension curve, which is known as the steep ascending limb, because at such short lengths (<1.7 μm), the myosin filament begins to interfere with shortening as it abuts the sarcomere Z-disk, reducing force precipitously.

An interesting observation relative to muscle force generation at short lengths was made in the late 1960s by Taylor and Rüdel (1970). They observed that when an intact muscle fiber was stimulated at very short sarcomere lengths (*i.e.*, sarcomere lengths on the ascending limb), electrical failure of the EC coupling apparatus occurred. This raised the question as to whether the decreased force at short sarcomere lengths was because of myofilament properties or if it was simply an electrical failure phenomenon. To address this question, these investigators ensured maximal single fiber activation by bathing the fiber in caffeine (which enhances calcium release from the SR) and obtained the same relationship that Gordon, Huxley, and Julian had obtained. This experiment was repeated in an elegant fashion by Moss, who argued that, even with caffeine bathing, there might be insufficient calcium around the myofilaments to maximally activate them. To circumvent this problem, Moss (1979) repeated the experiment on small pieces of single muscle fibers that were activated chemically using a calcium buffering system. Again, the same relationship was obtained. Therefore, although shortening deactivation as described by Rüdel and Taylor could occur, it did not seem to detract from the elegance and truth of the sarcomere length-tension relationship itself. Shortening deactivation may be a mechanism that exists in muscle to prevent activation at excessively short lengths, which can produce damage (Ramsey & Street, 1940).

To summarize, the length-tension relationship states that active muscle force varies as a function of sarcomere length (myofilament overlap). This is a physiologic property of the force-generating system and should not simply be viewed as an anatomic artifact. Recent experimental studies suggest that this length-tension relationship can be advantageous to the musculoskeletal torque-generating system, as will be described in Chapter 3. Before leaving discussion of the active length-tension relationship, be aware of this: never try to describe a shortening muscle using the length-tension relationship. In other words, looking at Figure 2-4, one might be tempted to predict that as a muscle shortens from a long length, force increases. However, one must remember that the length-tension relationship is strictly valid only for isometric contractions. Thus, the curve represents the artificial connection of individual data points from isometric experiments. To de-

Therapist's Comments

It is important to warn the therapist that knowledge of the muscle-length tension curve cannot simply be applied to a patients' muscle-joint system. Although this idea will be covered in detail in Chapter 3 it should be emphasized that the joint movement and placement of the muscle will have a major effect on a muscle's "joint angle-tension" relationship and a therapist must gather all of the appropriate muscle, joint, and tendon information before making decisions regarding the basis for a patient's dysfunction.

scribe motion will require an understanding of the force-velocity relationship, which is presented below.

Origin of the Passive Portion Length-Tension Curve—Titin

The solid line in Figure 2-4 represents the tension generated if a muscle is stretched to various lengths without stimulation. Note that near the optimal length, passive tension is almost zero. However, as the muscle is stretched to longer lengths, passive tension increases dramatically. These relatively long lengths can be attained physiologically, and therefore, passive tension can play a role in providing resistive force even in the absence of muscle activation. What is the origin of passive tension? Obviously, the structure(s) responsible for passive tension are outside of the cross-bridge itself because muscle activation is not required. Several recent studies have shed light on what has turned out to be a fascinating and huge protein with skeletal muscle—aptly named, "titin." A seminal study performed by Magid and Law, demonstrated convincingly that the origin of passive muscle tension is within the myofibrils themselves. This is extremely significant because, before this study, most had assumed that

extracellular connective tissue in striated muscle caused the majority of its passive properties. However, Magid, and Law (1985) measured passive tension in whole muscle, single fibers and single fibers with membranes removed and showed that each relationship scaled to the size of the specimen. In other words, the source for passive force bearing in muscle was within the normal myofibrillar structure, not extracellular as had previously been supposed. Parallel to these studies, Podolsky and colleagues (Horwitz, Kempner, Bisher, & Podolsky, 1986) demonstrated that the size of the protein responsible for passive force bearing in muscle was huge—in the megadalton range. Because most proteins are in the tens to hundreds of kilodaltons, this was a startling observation. It either meant that a qualitatively new type of protein had been discovered or that there was some interesting polymeric arrangement of smaller proteins that "appeared" to act as a giant protein.

The discovery of titin has tremendous clinical significance because during the traditional physical examination, it is the passive properties of skeletal muscles that are the most readily appreciated and quantified and which are used to make clinical decisions. Because passive properties are dominated by titin, it is probably the titin molecule that most strongly influences such an examination. Although it is certainly premature to make definitive statements, it's probable that the titin molecule will become as important for clinicians as the myosin molecule has become for physiologists.

Fantastic micromechanical studies have been performed that provide detailed information on titin structure and function. A creative experiment that quantified the mechanical properties of the titin complex was reported by Wang and colleagues (Wang, McCarter, Wright, & Ramirez-Mitchell, 1993). Using isolated segments of rabbit muscle fibers, they mechanically peeled back the surface membrane of the fiber leaving only the myofibrillar lattice intact. They then measured the relationship between sarcomere length and tension in the in-

---

Box 2-3. Can You Feel "Titin" on a Physical Exam?

Of course, this is a provocative and speculative idea. But it is based in fact. The giant intramuscular protein, that is aptly named "titin," is the primary source of passive tension in skeletal muscle. This means that, during normal range of motion manipulations, in the absence of bony or ligamentous abnormalities, the "feel" of a patient may be dominated by this intramuscular protein. It is possible that the increased stiffness that is sensed in spastic patients suffering from cerebral palsy, stroke, or head injury is because of alterations in and amount or type of titin that is expressed throughout the muscle itself. Perhaps joint contractures themselves, which are a tremendous clinical problem, are exacerbated by altered amount and type of titin isoforms expressed.

---

tact fiber and obtained a biphasic response where the muscle was initially relatively compliant (at a sarcomere length designated SL_o) then stiffness increased until a yield point (at a sarcomere length designated SL_y) until, at very long lengths, it became less stiff again (Fig. 2-5A). To determine the structural basis of this phenomenon, they performed a clever study in which the titin molecule was labeled in two different regions of the molecule using two different monoclonal antibodies—one that labeled the portion of titin molecule located in the I-band and a second antibody that labeled titin in the A-band (Fig. 2-5B). By measuring the distance between either the A-band and M-line or the distance between the I-Band and Z-line, the authors measured the "stretch" of the titin molecule in both the A-band and I-band regions. They found dramatic differences—titin in the I-band region was stretched easily and to a much greater extent than titin in the A-band region. This suggested to them that titin acted as a two-part molecular spring with a "stiff" component in the A-band region that was arranged in series with a more "compliant" component in the I-band region. (As an aside, in the original study, it was not clear whether the high

stiffness in the A-band was due to titin's intrinsic properties or whether it was because of its association with the myosin filament. By selectively extracting thick filaments from the titin lattice and again measuring titin properties in the region that used to contain the A-band, they found that the titin molecule had a relatively constant compliance along its entire length, but that it was the association between titin and myosin that gave it the increased stiffness in the A-band).

TITIN SEQUENCE PROVIDES INSIGHTS INTO FUNCTION:

Penetrating insights into titin structure-function relationships were recently provided based on examination of the titin amino acid pattern predicted by the DNA sequence of the cloned titin molecule (Labeit & Kolmerer, 1995). Cloning a novel protein these days is really not much of an accomplishment, however cloning titin was a tremendous project and its results were high-profile. This is for three reasons: First, the tremendous size of the molecule made assembling the sequence a tremendous bookkeeping task; second, the sequence obtained provided tremendous insights into the structural basis for function; and third, the sequence explained several aspects of muscle anatomy that were previously poorly understood.

Even though this is not a molecular biology text, the methods used for this study are so powerful and so common, that they are worth mentioning. The primary structure (i.e., sequence of amino acids) was determined in the usual way—making complimentary DNA (cDNA) copies of the messenger RNA (mRNA) encoding the synthesis of titin using reverse transcription (RT). Reverse transcription involves incubating the cell's mRNA with a special enzyme that converts mRNA to cDNA copies. Although mRNA is unstable (may be degraded in minutes) DNA is extremely stable. The cDNA that specifically corresponded to titin was amplified millions of fold using the powerful polymerase chain reaction (PCR) and then cloned for subsequent study. Because the

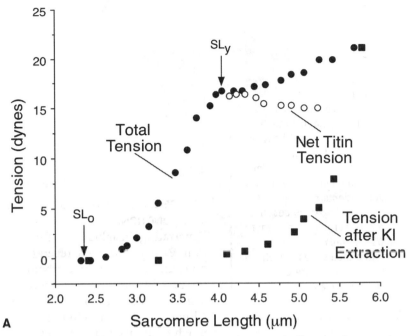

A

FIGURE 2-5. Mechanical measurement of passive muscle fiber tension as a function of sarcomere length. **(A)** Passive tension, at an initial sarcomere length designated SL_o is low but increases until the yield point at a sarcomere length designated SL_y. Filled Circles: total passive tension; Open Circles: passive tension of muscle calculated with intermediate filament contribution subtracted. Filled squares: tension measured after everything but intermediate filaments were extracted. (Data from: Wang, K., McCarter, R., Wright, J., Beverly, J., Ramirez-Mitchell, R. (1993). Viscoelasticity of the sarcomere matrix of skeletal muscles. The titin-myosin composite filament is a dual-stage molecular spring. *Biophysical Journal, 64*, 1161–1177). *(continued)*

titin molecule is so large, sequencing the entire molecule was accomplished by piecing together information from about 50 overlapping clones. The results were astounding! Titin, the largest protein known, is composed of a single chain of over 27,000 amino acids with a molecular weight of about 3 million daltons. This is greater than 10 times the molecular weight of the average protein. Translation of a single titin molecule requires about 45 minutes compared with 3 minutes for the average protein. The sequence obtained also revealed why titin serves so well as a muscular "spring." Interestingly, about 90% of the titin protein consists of 244 repeating copies of the fibronectin type III (FN3) and immunoglobulin (Ig) domains (Fig. 2-5C). These are well-known structures that

are designed to be "sticky" in other cell types. Therefore, titin is a good molecule for sticking things (such as sarcomere components) together. It was also interesting that these authors discovered a so-called "super repeat" pattern of Ig and FN3 motifs that was repeated 11 times within the A band region—this correlated exactly with the many accessory proteins known to be arranged in eleven stripes across the myosin-containing A band. Of course, these stripes have all been named and studied but here is a situation in which one discovery sheds light onto another area that was poorly understood. This increases the significance of the finding. It is thus believed that titin acts as an "organizer" of sarcomere structure. When considering the tremendous spatial regularity of

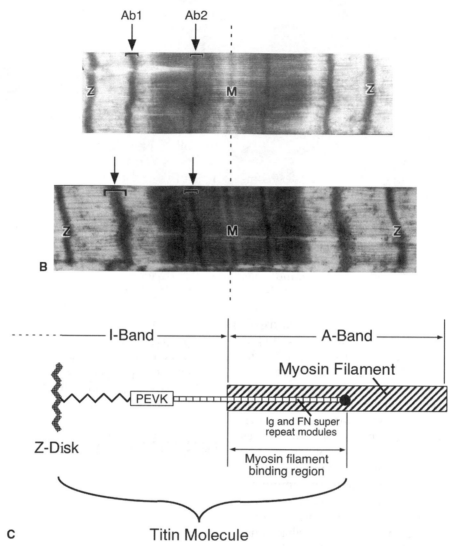

FIGURE 2-5. *(CONTINUED)* **(B)** Longitudinal electron micrograph of rabbit psoas muscle labeled with an antibody to the titin I-band region (Ab1) and A-band region (Ab2). This labeling appears as additional vertical stripes in the sarcomeres (arrows). Upper micrograph is from a shortened muscle while lower micrograph is from a lengthened muscle. (Micrograph kindly provided by Dr. Henk Granzier, Washington State University). **(C)** Schematic representation of the primary structure of titin. Ninety percent of titin consists of 244 repeating copies of the FN3 and Ig domains. A special I band region containing primarily the amino acids protein, glutamate, valine, and lysine (PEVK) appears to be the primary elastic region of the molecule (Drawing modified from Labeit, S., and Kolmerer, B. (1995). Titins: Giant proteins in charge of muscle ultrastructure and elasticity. *Science (Washington D.C.), 270,* 293–296.)

the sarcomere presented in Chapter 1, the question arises as to how that regularity arises. Probably (although definitive studies have yet to be performed) titin acts as a molecular template for sarcomere organization. Indeed, titin is one of the earliest proteins expressed during development (Horowits, 1999).

Another extremely novel region within the I-band was defined by Labeit and Kolmerer. Unlike the well understood FNIII and Ig domains, it was completely unique when compared with all known protein sequences. This region also demonstrated tremendous variation between muscle types in contrast to the FNIII and Ig domains that were consistent between muscles. The sequence of this region included a majority (70%) of the amino acids proline (whose one-letter abbreviation is P), glutamate (whose one-letter abbreviation is E), valine (whose one-letter abbreviation is V) and lysine (whose one-letter abbreviation is K) and was the region that corresponded to the compliant region. This region was thus named the "PEVK" region of titin. In support of the correlation between muscle stiffness and the size of the PEVK region, titins were compared between cardiac and skeletal muscle. It was demonstrated that PEVK region in cardiac muscle (which is known to be much stiffer than skeletal muscle) was only 163 amino acids long, whereas the PEVK region in the human soleus muscle (which is nearly 10 times more compliant compared with cardiac muscle) was more than 2000 amino acids long. This finding may provide a structural basis for the known difference in elasticity between different skeletal muscles. Whether all skeletal muscles are the same or whether systematic differences in passive elasticity between skeletal muscles can also be explained by differences in the PEVK region remains to be determined. It is also possible that altered muscle stiffness that is observed secondary to chronic length changes, immobilization, stroke, head injury, spinal cord injury, or cerebral palsy may be strongly affected by the amount and isoform of titin expressed in various muscles. Of course

the details of these relationships remain to be elucidated.

Taken together, these data should convince you of the tremendous importance of this intracellular cytoskeletal protein—not just in understanding basic muscle function but also with potentially profound clinical significance. To summarize, titin is a unique molecule for the following reasons:

1. Titin bears most of the passive load in muscle.
2. Titin is the largest protein ever discovered.
3. Titin's tremendous length (1.5 µm) allows it to play a potentially critical role in organizing the developing sarcomere.
4. Titin is ideally situated to serve as a "sensor" for altered muscle mechanical conditions such as chronic length change or chronic force change.
5. Titin is an intramuscular filament but, unlike actin, myosin or desmin, which are filaments composed of polymerized molecules, titin is a single molecule filament.

Therapist's Comments

Personally, I am glad that Dr. Lieber has provided this amount of detail on the novel protein, titin. Clearly, Dr. Lieber is being speculative when discussing the role of titin in the stiffness seen in neurological problems and joint contractures. It is possible that such stiffness changes, or even those associated with muscle hypertrophy or swelling after exercise would be difficult to pick up without specific measuring tools. I think that some clinicians can pick up slight changes in stiffness, so I think it is still a good example. The clinician must be sure that muscle stiffness changes are not confused with articular changes that may occur in joint contractures.

Because of the tremendous importance of passive tension in normal muscle function and the apparent differences in titin mechanical properties among muscles, there will be a great number of studies defining the plasticity of titin isoforms under many of the same conditions for which fiber type plasticity has been extensively studied (Chapters 4 and 5).

Force-Velocity Relationship: Isotonic Muscle Contraction

The length-tension relationship, explained above, describes a muscle's behavior at constant length (*i.e.*, under "isometric" conditions). However, much of the muscle use involves movement that is better described by the force-velocity relationship. Unlike the length-tension relationship, the force-velocity relationship does not have a precise, anatomically identifiable basis. The force-velocity relationship describes the force generated by a muscle as a function of velocity under conditions of constant load (*i.e.*, "isotonic" conditions). It can also be stated in the reverse, such that the velocity of muscle contraction depends on the force resisting the muscle. Historically, the force-velocity relationship was investigated to a much greater degree than the length-tension relationship because such mechanical studies were used to define the kinetic properties of the cross-bridges (Huxley, 1957). This was, in part, due to the technical limitations of the time, but also was based on the tremendous influence that enzyme kinetics had on muscle contraction theories of the time.

Experimental elucidation of the force-velocity relationship was first presented by Professors Hill (1938) and Katz (1939) in their classic papers, but the current description of the force-velocity relationship has been ascribed to the physiologist A.V. Hill. If you are interested in the conceptual basis for this relationship and would like to experience a "first hand" description of the scientific discovery process by an outstanding and very creative scientist, read A.V. Hill's "reflections" on this area

of study in his monograph entitled, *First and Last Experiments in Muscle Mechanics*, which he published near the end of his career (Hill, 1970). Hill, in his decades of important muscle studies, produced a general equation that describes the muscle force-velocity relationship in a form that is still used today. Sir Andrew Huxley, in 1957, developed a theory of isotonic muscle contraction based on specific cross-bridge properties, that yielded the actual force-velocity relationship developed by Hill and quantitatively explained the energy consumed by a muscle during contraction at different velocities (Hill, 1964; Huxley, 1957). The beauty of this theory was that it explained both mechanical and energetic data on a "molecular" level even before the molecules themselves were discovered (recall that Huxley had already done this in defining the molecular basis of the action potential using "ion channels" before they were even discovered). The general "truth" of this relationship is attested to by the fact that these results and concepts are still in widespread use after over four decades.

Experimentally, the force-velocity relationship, like the length-tension relationship, is a curve that represents the results of many experiments plotted on the same graph. Experimentally, a muscle is stimulated maximally and

---

Box 2-4. How Can You Make Muscles Stronger by Understanding the "Force-Velocity" Equation?

Muscles are strengthened based on the force placed across them during exercise. The force-velocity relationship of muscle indicates that high velocity movements correspond to low muscle force and that low velocity movements correspond to high muscle force. Since strengthening requires high force-producing exercises, the velocities must, necessarily be relatively low. High velocity movements may have other beneficial effects (*e.g.* improve muscle activation by the nervous system), but not at the muscle tissue level. The take home message—keep velocity low for strengthening.

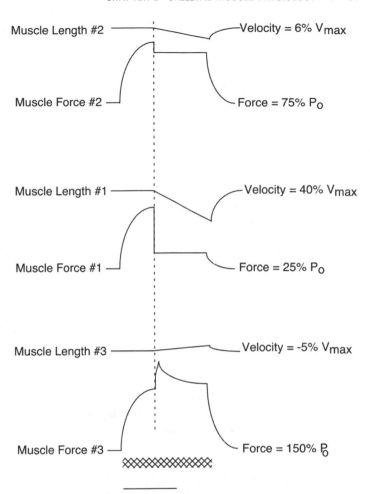

FIGURE 2-6. Individual isotonic contractions permit experimental determination of the force-velocity relationship. Each trace represents a schematic illustration of muscle length and muscle force vs. time records when muscles are maximally activated and permitted to shorten against various loads. Muscles are maximally activated and, initially, generate maximum isometric tension. After a delay force is dropped and the muscle is allowed to shorten. Each velocity of contraction at a given load for each contraction is plotted as a single data point to create the force-velocity curve plotted in Figure 2-7.

allowed to shorten (or lengthen) against a constant load (Fig. 2-6). The muscle velocity during shortening (or lengthening) is measured and plotted against the resistive force. The general form of this relationship is plotted in Figure 2-7. On the horizontal axis muscle velocity relative to maximum velocity (V_{max}) is plotted while on the vertical axis we have plotted muscle force relative to maximum force (P_o).

Concentric Contractions—Muscle Actively Shortening

When a muscle is activated and required to lift a load which is less than the maximum tetanic tension it can generate, the muscle begins to shorten. Contractions that permit the muscle to shorten are known in "muscle lingo" as concentric contractions. The word "concentric" in this context does not make much sense, but it is traditionally used to describe shortening contractions of muscle. In concentric contractions, the force generated by the muscle is always less than the muscle's maximum (P_o). As the load the muscle is required to lift decreases, contraction velocity increases. This occurs until the muscle finally reaches its maximum contraction velocity, V_{max}. V_{max} is a parameter used to characterize muscle, which is related to both fiber type distribution and architecture. The mathematical form of the force-velocity rela-

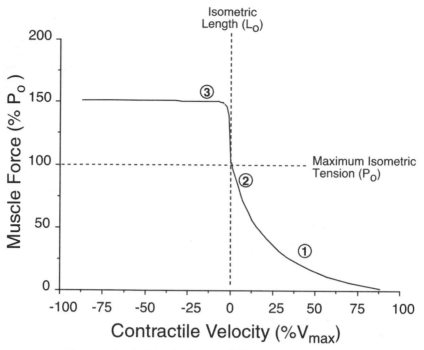

FIGURE 2-7. The muscle force-velocity curve for skeletal muscle obtained using sequential isotonic contractions such as those shown in Figure 2-6. The three-circled numbers represent the force and velocity data from the three corresponding contractions in Figure 2-6. Note that force increases dramatically upon forced muscle lengthening and drops precipitously upon muscle shortening.

tionship is a rectangular hyperbola and is given in Equation 2-1:

$$(P+a)\, v = b\, (P_o - P) \qquad \text{(Eq. 2-1)}$$

in which a and b are constants derived experimentally (usually about 0.25), P is muscle force, P_o is maximum tetanic tension, and v is muscle velocity. For this equation to work in terms of units, a must have units of force and b must have units of velocity. This equation can be used to determine the relative muscle force that occurs as a muscle is allowed to shorten. The equation can also be rearranged to provide an expression for maximum contraction velocity of a muscle based on its force-velocity properties. This is done by noting that, at V_{max}, muscle force is zero, substituting these values into Equation 2-1 and solving for V_{max} as shown below:

$$V_{max} = (b\, P_o)/a \qquad \text{(Eq. 2-2)}$$

It is important to note that the force-velocity relationship is a steep rectangular hyperbola. In other words, force drops off rapidly as velocity increases. For example, in a muscle that is shortening at only 1% of its maximum contraction velocity (extremely slow), tension drops by 5% relative to maximum isometric tension. Similarly, as contraction velocity increases to only 10% maximum (easily attainable physiologically), muscle force drops by 35%. Note that even when muscle force is 50% maximum, muscle velocity is only 17% V_{max}. Some of these values are presented below in Table 2-1. The take-home lesson is that as a muscle is allowed to shorten, force drops precipitously.

What is the physiologic basis of the force-velocity relationship? As mentioned above, a simply anatomical relationship cannot be invoked as an explanation, but rather the explanation is framed in the context of chemical reaction rates. It has been experimentally determined from biochemical studies (see below) that the cross-bridge connections between actin and myosin attach at a certain rate and detach at a certain rate. These rates are referred to as rate constants. At any point, the force generated by a muscle depends on the total number of cross-bridges attached. Obviously, this number represents the net balance between the number of cross-bridges attached versus detached. Because it takes a finite amount of time for cross-bridges to attach (based on the rate constant of attachment), as filaments slide past one another faster and faster (*i.e.*, as the muscle shortens with increasing velocity), force decreases because of the lower number of cross-bridges attached. Conversely, as the relative filament velocity decreases (*i.e.*, as muscle velocity decreases), more cross-bridges have time to attach and to generate force, and thus force increases. This discussion is not meant to provide a detailed description of the basis for the force-velocity relationship, only to provide insight as to how cross-bridge rate constants can affect muscle force generation as a function of velocity.

There are therapeutic implications of this relationship. Most of these will be discussed in Chapter 4 but note that muscles are strengthened based on the force placed across the muscle. Higher forces produce greater strength-

ening. Therefore, exercises performed with muscle activated in a way that allows them to contract at high velocities, necessarily imply that they are also contracting with relatively low force. This is intuitively obvious as you lift a light load compared to a heavy load—the light load can be moved much more quickly. However, these rapid movements would have small strengthening effects because the muscle forces are so low.

Eccentric Contractions—Muscle Actively Lengthening

As the load on the muscle increases, it finally reaches a point where the external force on the muscle is greater than the force that the muscle can generate. Thus, even though the muscle may be fully activated, it is forced to lengthen due to the high external load. This is referred to in "muscle lingo" as an eccentric contraction (remember that contraction in this context does not necessarily imply shortening. Also, note that there has been much debate in the literature about the use of this term to describe actively lengthening muscle and, although the term itself is not too descriptive, it is useful in communicating with the muscle world). There are two main features to note regarding eccentric contractions: First, the absolute tensions achieved are high relative to the muscle's maximum tetanic tension generating capacity and second, the absolute tension is relatively independent of lengthening velocity. This suggests that skeletal muscles are resistant to lengthening, a property which comes in handy for many normal movement patterns (Chapter 3). The basic mechanics of eccentric contractions are still a source of debate because the cross-bridge theory that so nicely describes concentric contractions is not as successful in describing eccentric contractions (Harry, Ward, Heglund, Morgan, & McMahon, 1990; Morgan, 1990).

Eccentric contractions are currently a popular area of study for three main reasons: First, much of a muscle's normal activity occurs while it is actively lengthening, so that eccentric contractions are physiologically common. Second, muscle injury and soreness are selectively asso-

TABLE 2-1	Relative Muscle Force at Various Muscle Velocities
Relative Force	**Velocity**
100% P_o	0% V_{max}
95% P_o	1% V_{max}
90% P_o	2.2% V_{max}
75% P_o	6.3% V_{max}
50% P_o	16.6% V_{max}
25% P_o	37.5% V_{max}
10% P_o	64.3% V_{max}
5% P_o	79.1% V_{max}
0% P_o	100% V_{max}

> **Box 2-5. Can You Make a Muscle Stronger by Lengthening it?**
>
> Eccentric contractions (*i.e.*, lengthening of an activated muscle), such as occurs as a dumbbell is lowered during a curl, result in high muscle forces and provide a potent stimulus to increase muscle strength. Eccentric contractions are also selectively associated with muscle injury. Taken together, these observations lead to the concept of "no pain-no gain" or " you have to break it down to build it up" that is so popular in weight-training these days. It is important to note that the basic biophysical properties of muscle (increased force during active lengthening) do support the concept of using eccentric contractions to build muscle strength.

---

ciated with eccentric contraction. Finally, muscle strengthening is greatest using exercises that involve eccentric contractions. Therefore, there are some fundamental structure-function questions that can be addressed using the eccentric contraction model and eccentric contractions have important applications therapeutically to strengthen muscle. These phenomena will be considered in more detail later in Chapters 4 and 6.

Length-Tension-Velocity Relationship

From the preceding discussion, it is apparent that muscle force changes because of changing length and/or due to changing velocity. However, both of these experimental relationships describe fairly unrealistic conditions—force generation at constant length or velocity of contraction at constant force—neither of which are common during normal activities. These conditions are studied primarily because of the ease of interpretation of the data under controlled conditions, but it has been shown that they do generalize fairly well to arbitrary changes of muscle length and velocity. Since muscle force changes with length and velocity

in a well-defined manner, it should not be surprising to suggest that when muscle length and muscle velocity change simultaneously, it is still possible to define the muscle force produced. This is because, conceptually, the length-tension experiment can be viewed simply as a series of length-force-velocity experiments performed at constant (zero) velocity. Similarly, the force-velocity relationship can be viewed as a series of length-force-velocity experiments performed at constant length (L_o). The point shared between the force-velocity and length-tension curves is the point of maximum isometric tension (L_o, at zero velocity, resulting in a tension of P_o). If both length and velocity simultaneously change, the result is the superposition of the two relationships.

The appearance of the length-tension-velocity relationship is shown in Figure 2-8. Do not let the three-dimensional nature of the relationship intimidate you. If the surface is viewed along one set of axes, it is simply a series of force-velocity curves at different lengths. When viewed along the other set of axes, it is simply a series of length-tension curves at different velocities. In this surface there are all possible combinations of muscle length and velocity and their resulting force for a muscle that is maximally activated. What can be concluded? For one thing, if muscle velocity is high, force will be low no matter the length. In other words, at high velocities, length is not that important. At low concentric velocities, muscle length becomes an important force modulator. At eccentric velocities, again muscle velocity dominates length as the determinant of force. This relationship is important in neuromotor control as we attempt to understand how muscle actions can be responsible for external movements observed. Although this relationship is fairly general, one could still argue that it is a bit artificial in that it is determined on a maximally activated muscle under steady-state conditions. It is known that, during normal activities of daily living, activation is usually submaximal and activation frequency, length, and velocity are changing. Studies have been performed that consider more physiological

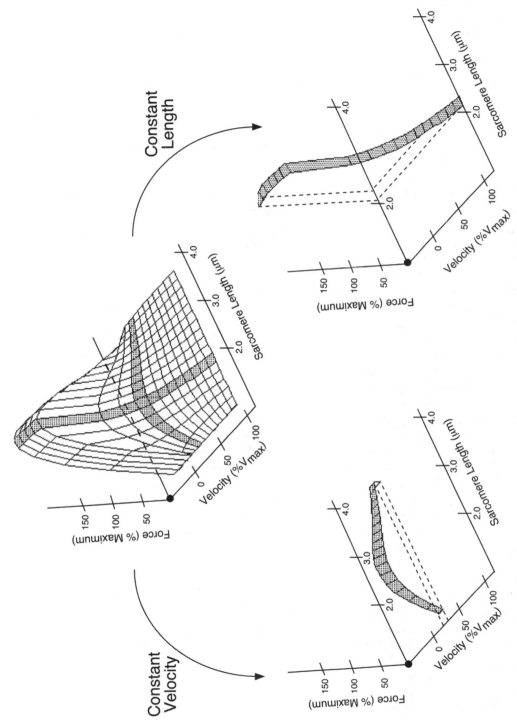

FIGURE 2-8. The hypothetical muscle length-force-velocity surface for skeletal muscle. Shaded regions represent a "slice" of the surface at either constant length or velocity. A "slice" of the surface at constant length is simply a force-velocity curve measured at that length (compare with Figure 2-7) while a "slice" of the surface at constant velocity is simply a length-tension curve measured at that velocity (compare with Figure 2-4). (Reprinted with permission from: Fridén, J., and Lieber, R. L. (1992). Structural and mechanical basis of exercise-induced muscle injury. *Medicine and Science in Sports and Exercise, 24,* 521–530.)

conditions but they are beyond the scope of this discussion (Baratta, Solomonow, Nguyen, & D'Ambrosia, 2000; Huijing, 1996; Rack & Westbury, 1969). More on this topic will be discussed in Chapter 3.

The Cross-Bridge Cycle

Cyclic interaction between actin and myosin has been alluded to in the structural discussion in Chapter 1 and in explaining the force-velocity curve above. How were such hypotheses generated? Much of our understanding of the mechanism of muscle contraction has come in large part from excellent biochemical studies performed from the 1950s to the mid-1970s (Webb & Trentham, 1983). It was during this period that methods for isolating specific muscle proteins were developed as well as the methods for measuring their physicochemical and biochemical properties. For example, if a muscle was homogenized in a blender and mixed with a concentrated salt solution (ionic strength of about 600 μM, well-above that observed physiologically), the high-ionic-strength solution caused individual myosin molecules to let go of their ionic interactions with one another within a filament and become soluble. Then this soluble portion was removed from the rest of the muscle debris, the ionic strength was slowly lowered to physiologic levels (about 120 μM), and myosin and actin filaments reformed and, in fact, formed a solid precipitate complex (Szent-Gyorgi, 1953). By simply adding ATP to this precipitate, it became clear again because ATP affected the relationship between actin and myosin (Maruyama & Gergely, 1962). Biochemists believed that by performing experiments such as these, they could investigate different steps of the cyclic interaction between muscle proteins. These types of experiments have become popular in recent muscle literature and have provided insights into muscle contraction as well as actin-myosin interaction in all eukaryotic cells. This provides another example of a relatively simple observation (acto-myosin precipitate becoming clear upon addition of ATP) having profound implications for all of biology. One of the most important traits of a successful scientist is the ability to appreciate the implications of an observation, not just in making observations. This is especially true when the experiment produces an unexpected result.

In its simplest form, based on experiments such as those presented above, the cross-bridge cycle can be envisioned as actin (A) combining with myosin (M) and ATP to produce force, adenosine diphosphate (ADP), and inorganic phosphate, P_i. This can be represented as a chemical reaction in the form

$$A + M + ATP \rightarrow A + M + ADP + P_i + Force \quad \text{(Eq. 2-3)}$$

However, it is also known that upon the death of a muscle, a rigor state is entered whereby actin and myosin interact to form a stiff connection. This can be represented as

$$A + M \rightarrow A \cdot M \text{ "rigor" complex} + Force \quad \text{(Eq. 2-4)}$$

If actin and myosin can interact by themselves to produce force, where is ATP involved in muscle contraction? As discussed in Chapter 1, the myosin molecule can be enzymatically split into its subfragments. Experiments that cleaved myosin into light meromyosin (LMM), subfragment 1 (S-1), and subfragment 2 (S-2) demonstrated that the myosin S-1 portion retained the ability to hydrolyze ATP into ADP and P_i although this reaction is fairly slow. In other words,

$$M + ATP \rightarrow M + ADP + P_i \quad \text{(Eq. 2-5)}$$

Based on these two observations, it was shown that ATP serves two main functions during skeletal muscle contraction: First, ATP disconnects actin from myosin, and second, ATP is hydrolyzed by the S-1 portion of the myosin molecule. Can you see the competition this creates? In contracting skeletal muscle, ATP binds to the actin-myosin complex, causing actin and myosin to dissociate. When it does, ATP is hydrolyzed by myosin into ADP and P_i, which then allows actin and myosin to reassociate.

Thus, Equation 2-3 (the simple cross-bridge cycle) can be combined with Equations 2-4 and 2-5 to yield the more detailed "two step" cross-bridge cycle shown below:

$$A + M \rightarrow A{\cdot}M \text{ "rigor" complex} \qquad \text{(Eq. 2-6)}$$
$$A{\cdot}M \text{ "rigor" complex} + ATP \rightarrow A + M + ADP + P_i + Force$$

This basic scheme has been expanded by many excellent works over the years, but the same basic idea remains: ATP is required to dissociate actin from myosin and is hydrolyzed by the S-1 portion of the myosin head. Several interesting experiments refined this concept to provide actual rate constants for the various reactions. For example, when myosin is alone in solution, it hydrolyzes ATP slowly. Thus, Equation 2-5 occurs only at a rate of about 0.1 second. However, an interesting observation is that when actin is added to a solution of S-1 and ATP, the previously slow hydrolysis rate increases about 200-fold! Thus actin acts as a catalyst for ATP hydrolysis by S-1. Modify the ATP hydrolysis mechanism to include two paths for hydrolysis—a path with and a path without actin. The path without actin is shown in Equation 2-8 and the path with actin shown in Equation 2-7:

$$A{\cdot}M + ATP \rightarrow A{\cdot}M{\cdot}ATP \rightarrow A + M + ADP + P_i \text{ (fast)} \quad \text{(Eq. 2-7)}$$

$$M + ATP \rightarrow M{\cdot}ATP \rightarrow M + ADP + P_i \text{ (slow)} \quad \text{(Eq. 2-8)}$$

It is also easy to interconnect these two schemes by adding a step whereby actin can dissociate from the A·M·ATP complex, and the scheme thus becomes

$$A{\cdot}M + ATP \rightarrow A{\cdot}M{\cdot}ATP \rightarrow A + M + ADP + P_i \text{ (fast)}$$
$$\text{ACTIN DISSOCIATES} \downarrow \uparrow \text{ACTIN ASSOCIATES} \quad \text{(Eq. 2-9)}$$
$$M + ATP \rightarrow M{\cdot}ATP \rightarrow M + ADP + P_i \text{ (slow)}$$

or, more simply,

$$A{\cdot}M + ATP \rightarrow A{\cdot}M{\cdot}ATP \rightarrow A + M + ADP + P_i$$
$$-A \downarrow \uparrow +A \qquad \text{(Eq. 2-10)}$$
$$M + ATP \rightarrow M{\cdot}ATP \rightarrow M + ADP + P_i$$

You can see that we have generated a reasonable approximation of cyclic interaction between actin, myosin, and ATP. The reactions with the fastest rate constants are shown in Equation 2-10 with bold arrows; they are the most likely to occur. This very simplified scheme actually explains a great deal of the experimental data and, conceptually, will allow you to understand many physiologic properties to be presented later in this chapter.

For those of you who are interested, there is an interesting caveat to the scheme of Equation 2-10. Experimental studies by Drs. Richard Lymn and Ed Taylor (Lymn & Taylor, 1971) demonstrated that, after formation of the A·M·ATP complex, the actin quickly dissociates, so that ATP hydrolysis occurs with the actin and myosin filaments separated. After the hydrolysis, the actin quickly reassociates with the M·ADP·P_i complex to cause dissociation of the hydrolysis products. The rate-limiting step of the entire sequence is the release of the reaction products from myosin, so that actin increases the ATP hydrolysis rate by speeding the release of hydrolysis products from myosin. The ATP hydrolysis scheme is therefore more accurately represented as

$$A{\cdot}M + ATP \rightarrow A{\cdot}M{\cdot}ATP \rightarrow A{\cdot}M{\cdot}ADP{\cdot}P_i \rightarrow A + M + ADP + P_i$$
$$-A \downarrow \qquad \uparrow +A \qquad \text{(Eq. 2-11)}$$
$$M + ATP \rightarrow M{\cdot}ATP \rightarrow M{\cdot}ADP{\cdot}P_i \rightarrow M + ADP + P_i$$

with the normal route of hydrolysis (that is, the fastest rate constants) shown with bold arrows. This sequence of biochemical steps is often referred to as the Lymn-Taylor actomyosin ATPase hydrolysis mechanism (1971).

The relationship between the Lymn-Taylor kinetic scheme and the mechanical cross-bridge cycle is not fully known. However, Lymn and Taylor proposed that their biochemical data could be incorporated into a four-step cross-bridge cycle that could be envisioned (Fig. 2-9):

1. The actin-myosin bridge very rapidly dissociates due to ATP binding.
2. The free myosin bridge moves into position to attach to actin, during which ATP is hydrolyzed.

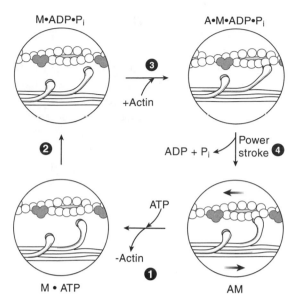

FIGURE 2-9. Schematic representation of the biochemical cross-bridge cycle along with the associated mechanical events. 1. ATP binds to actin-myosin (AM) complex, displacing actin. 2. ATP is hydrolyzed while on the M·ATP complex. 3. Actin reassociates with M·ADP·P$_i$ complex, causing release of P$_i$. 4. Attached cross-bridge generates force during power stroke. (Cross-bridge cycle based on report in: Lymn, R.W., Taylor, E.W. (1971). Mechanism of adenosine triphosphate hydrolysis by actomyosin. *Biochemistry, 10*, 4617–4624.)

3. The free myosin bridge along with its hydrolysis products rebinds to the actin filament.
4. The cross-bridge generates force, and actin displaces the reaction products (ADP and P$_i$) from the myosin cross-bridge. This is the rate-limiting step of contraction. The actin-myosin cross-bridge is now ready for the ATP binding of step 1.

It might be appreciated that confirmation of this mechanism would be difficult. In fact, a recent advance in biochemistry has allowed direct testing and manipulation of this scheme. The advance involves the development of "caged" compounds—compounds which are inactive in their caged form and become active when the cage is instantaneously removed by a pulse of high-energy laser light (McCray, Herbette,

Kihara, & Trentham, 1980). Using caged ATP, single muscle fibers have been subjected to experiments such as those described above and found to behave much as predicted based on the biochemical data (Goldman, 1987). These experiments, performed by Dr. Yale Goldman and his colleagues, are truly a case in which biochemistry and physiology have met head-on.

Molecular Mechanism of the Cross-Bridge Cycle

There is a great tradition in skeletal muscle physiology and biophysics of attempting to answer questions of structure-function relationships and mechanisms for muscle properties observed. Some of these were presented above in the context of the force-velocity and length-tension relationships. However, current studies continue to probe at the molecular mechanism of movement itself. In other words, how is chemical energy from ATP converted into the "motion" that is observed as muscle contraction? This is a question of tremendous fundamental significance because motion itself almost describes life. In fact, probing the molecular mechanism of movement in muscle has spawned an entirely new field of study that is described as "molecular motors" (Spudich, 1994). To date, there have been three proteins discovered that function as molecular motors: myosin (in muscle and other nonmuscle tissues such as brain and gut), kinesin (used to shuttle intracellular components throughout the nervous system) and dynein (used to move flagella). Obviously, a detailed explanation of the structure and function of each of these motor systems is beyond the scope of our discussion. However, the results of several fantastic studies of myosin structure and function at the molecular level should be presented because they bear directly on the discussion of the cross-bridge cycle presented above. This section can be skipped, moving directly to the discussion of muscle function of muscles with different architectures on page 72 without a loss of continuity, but it is encouraged that you retain the following studies to appreciate the sophistication and significance of such information. Also, such studies will become increasingly common as the molecular basis for many diseases is discovered.

X-RAY DIFFRACTION REVEALS THE STRUCTURE OF S-1

In what must be considered one of the most significant muscle publications of the last few decades, the structure of the S-1 subunit of chicken skeletal muscle was elucidated by Rayment and his colleagues (Rayment et al., 1993a, b) using X-ray crystallography, a powerful technique that can resolve structures at the atomic level. This report presented a number of structural features of myosin S-1 that have significant implications in understanding the cross-bridge mechanism described above (See Color Plate Section, Fig. C-3). The overall structure of S-1 was an elliptical molecule with dimensions of about 6 nm × 9 nm consisting of a globular "head" region attached to a long alpha-helical "neck" region. Interestingly, it turned out that the portion of the molecule that bound actin was on the opposite site of the globular head as the region that bound ATP and the two regions were "connected" by a long "cleft" through which communication could occur.

PROPOSED MOLECULAR MECHANISM OF THE CROSS-BRIDGE CYCLE:

Based on the crystallographic structure, S-1 was shown to be a "back door" enzyme (one in which the substrate [in this case, ATP] and catalyst [in this case, actin] bind on opposite sites of the molecule) and these observations provided a basis on which to propose a molecular mechanism by which ATP binding leads to actin dissociation (as noted above in Equation 2-10) and force generation. This represents a modification to the scheme presented above and is summarized as follows (Fig. 2-10):

1. In the initial configuration, when myosin and actin are tightly bound, the long cleft connecting the ATP to actin binding site is "closed." This "rigor" conformation is mutually exclusive with the presence of hydrolyzed ATP on the myosin molecule.

2. ATP binding to myosin changes the shape of the S-1, which is thought to be an "opening" of the cleft (Step #1, Fig. 2-10). Cleft opening disrupts the interaction between actin and myosin and thus, myosin "lets go" of the actin filament.

3. Hydrolysis of ATP into an intermediate state described as ADP-P_i is accompanied by a conformational change that represents the "cocking" of the cross-bridge while chemical energy from ATP is transferred to the myosin molecule (Step #2, Fig. 2-10). The molecular details of the cocking are not known.

4. Actin then rebinds to myosin, causing release of the terminal phosphate group of ATP which is believed to allow the myosin molecule to reverse the conformational change while bound to actin, thus providing the power stroke of muscle contraction (Step #3, Fig. 2-10).

This scheme represents the best synthesis of the available experimental data with the newly obtained structural data. It should be emphasized that a great deal of interpretation and literature synthesis is required to propose this dynamic scheme since only "snapshots" of the myosin-actin-nucleotide structure are available. Current experiments are being performed with "artificial" ATP molecules that "freeze" in a particular configuration (*e.g.,* just after hydrolysis but before inorganic phosphate release) to provide other "snapshots" of the process.

EXPERIMENTAL SUPPORT OF THE MOLECULAR MECHANISM OF THE CROSS-BRIDGE CYCLE

Molecular and biophysical experiments that test the mechanism proposed above represent state-of-the-art muscle biophysics. Many of these studies have been pioneered by Dr. Jim Spudich and his colleagues who have used a nonmuscle myosin system, *Dictyostelium discoideum* (slime mold) that is more amenable to

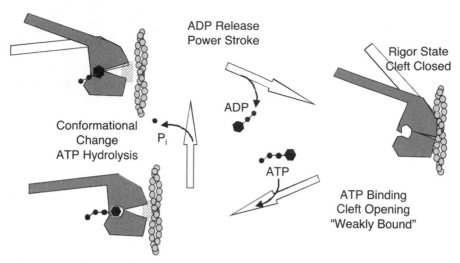

FIGURE 2-10. Cartoon diagram of the cross-bridge cycle based on the S-1 crystal structure shown in Color Plate Section, Figure C-2 as described in: Rayment, I., Holden, H. M., Whittaker, M., Yohn, C. B., Lorenz, M., Holmes, K. C., & Milligan, R. A. (1993). Structure of the actin-myosin complex and its implications for muscle contraction. *Science (Washington D.C.), 261,* 58–65. Abbreviations, ATP-adenosine triphosphate, P_i-inorganic phosphate.

molecular manipulation than more complicated mammalian systems. Spudich and colleagues altered the "neck" region of the S-1 molecule to test directly the hypothesis that rotation of the alpha-helical neck leads to filament translation during movement (Uyeda, Abramson, & Spudich, 1996). In this experiment, artificial molecules were generated that were composed of myosins with increased "neck" lengths of zero, one, two, or three "necks" long. Molecular translation velocity was measured under a microscope for each of these artificial molecules. What should the relationship between translation velocity and neck length be if molecular movement does indeed occur by the rotation of the S-1 "neck" region? Spudich and colleagues found a direct correlation between the length of the neck region and velocity, providing direct evidence that "neck rotation" was a fundamental event in muscle contraction (Fig. 2-11). This is one of the most direct forms of evidence for the cross-bridge movement that have been hypothesized to occur for over four decades. It would be interesting, given the capability for ultra-low force measurements (See below) to know if the neck length is inversely related to torque generated by the molecule, also predicted based on the fundamental model presented above.

One final experiment must be described based on its elegance and significance. Spudich collaborated with the eminent British scientist Dr. Robert Simmons to develop methods that actually measured the force and displacement produced by individual S-1 molecules (Finer, Simmons, & Spudich, 1994). They developed a "laser trap" (a device that uses the ultra-small forces generated by laser beams to hold onto molecules) that permitted precise control of position and measurement of force from S-1 molecules attached to a cover slip. It should be noted that previous high-resolution measurements of isolated single muscle fiber mechanical properties almost 30 years earlier had yielded estimates for the working distance of a single cross-bridge power stroke as well as the force produced by the molecule (Huxley & Simmons, 1971; Huxley, 1969). These esti-

FIGURE 2-11. Velocity of actin filament sliding as a function of "neck length" of myosin molecule created using artificial constructs. These experiments demonstrated that contraction velocity was directly proportional to "neck length" thus providing direct evidence for the α-helix portion of the S-1 molecule acting as a mechanical lever during muscle contraction. (Data from: Uyeda, T. Q., Abramson, P. D., & Spudich, J. A. (1996). The neck region of the myosin motor domain acts as a lever arm to generate movement. *Proceedings of the National Academy of Sciences of the United States of America, 93,* 4459–4464.)

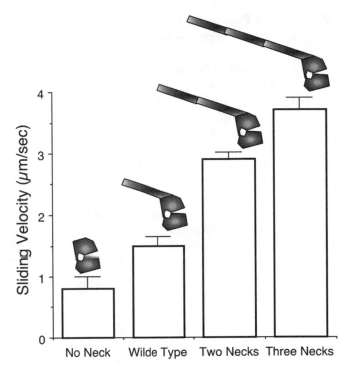

Box 2-6. How Can an Understanding of the Myosin Molecule Provide Relief for the Ailing Heart?

An understanding of the molecular mechanism of myosin movement has provided insights into diseases that result from mutations of the myosin molecule. The naturally occurring mutations studied to date result in relatively minor modifications to myosin function because mutations in the critical regions of the molecule (*e.g.* the actin or nucleotide binding domains) are lethal and therefore severely selected against. A significant myosin mutation currently under investigation is the one that causes the clinical manifestation of hypertrophic cardiomyopathy which results in ventricular wall thickening that decreases cardiac output and can lead to premature death or disability. Because one or a small number of amino acids is altered in this condition, there is hope that gene therapy can cure this disease.

mates, approximately 10 nm and 5 pN respectively turned out to be surprisingly close to the experimentally measured values of 11 nm and 4 pN respectively. This study, an experimental tour de force was viewed as some of the most powerful experimental evidence to date, for the molecular mechanism of actin-myosin cross-bridge interaction. Unfortunately, the story has turned out to be not as clear-cut as originally reported. For technical reasons, the spatial and temporal resolution of the laser trap experiments were probably insufficient to make reliable measurements as the resolutions required. Indeed, to their credit, these investigators have followed-up their original report with precise characterization of the experimental apparatus (Simmons, Finer, Chu, & Spudich, 1996) as well as technical modifications to the experimental protocol (Mehta, Finer, & Spudich, 1997). The numbers obtained with the technical and conceptual improvements on the experimental method still agree with the previously published values.

Mechanical Properties of Muscles with Different Architectures

Having completed a complex discussion of two of the most important mechanical properties of skeletal muscle, and the cross-bridge cycle, you are now in a position to understand the functional significance of muscle architecture that was introduced in Chapter 1. Even though the details of sarcomere structure and cross-bridge action might be understood, it is impossible to explain the force-generating property of a whole muscle without an understanding of muscle architecture. Architectural studies are not as popular as, for instance "fiber type" studies, but this is primarily because of the technical difficulties in obtaining accurate architectural information (review the detailed methods required in Chapter 1). The important point to remember regarding the functional significance of muscle architecture is that muscle force is proportional to physiologic cross-sectional area (PCSA), and muscle velocity is proportional to muscle fiber length. Note that by stating that velocity is proportional to fiber length, it is implicit that the total excursion (active range) of a muscle is also proportional to fiber length. Thus increased fiber length results in both increased muscle velocity and excursion. It is probably apparent to you, based on the discussion in Chapter 1, that neither fiber length nor PCSA can easily be deduced based on gross muscle inspection. The detailed methods of Chapter 1 are required for architectural determination. However, after determining these architectural properties, one can understand how much force the muscle generates and how fast it contracts (or how far it contracts). Consider two specific architectural examples and the way in which their structure directly leads to their length-tension and force-velocity relationships.

Comparison of Two Muscles with Different Physiologic Cross-Sectional Areas

Suppose that two muscles had identical fiber lengths and pennation angles, but one muscle had twice the mass (equivalent to saying that one muscle had twice the number of fibers and thus twice the PCSA). What would be the difference in their mechanical properties? How would the length-tension and force-velocity curves be affected?

The schematic in Figure 2-12A demonstrates that the only effect is to increase maximum tetanic tension so that the length-tension curve has the same basic shape but is amplified upward in the case of the stronger muscle. Similarly, the force-velocity curve changes the location of P_o, but the curve retains the same basic shape (Fig. 2-12B). Note that if both curves are plotted on relative scales (i.e., percent maximum tension instead of absolute tension), the two muscles of different architecture would appear to have identical properties. This demonstrates that although architectural properties profoundly affect the extrinsic muscle properties (i.e., the properties that vary with absolute muscle size, such as PCSA or mass), they have no affect on its intrinsic properties (i.e., the properties that are independent of absolute muscle size, such as fiber length/muscle length ratio).

Comparison of Two Muscles with Different Fiber Lengths

Consider the effects of architecture using an example of two muscles with identical PCSAs and pennation angles but different fiber lengths. Before reading ahead, try to predict the length-tension and force-velocity curves that variations in fiber length would produce.

As shown in Figure 2-12C, increasing fiber length increases the absolute muscle active range, but the peak absolute force of the length-tension curves is identical. That sounds much like active range of motion (ROM), a measurement that is important in clinical evaluation. In fact, it is directly related to ROM. This will be discussed in more detail in Chapter 3. For now, suffice it to say that ROM is a direct result of muscle architecture and the joint properties on which the muscle acts.

For the same reason that fiber length increases the active muscle range of the length-

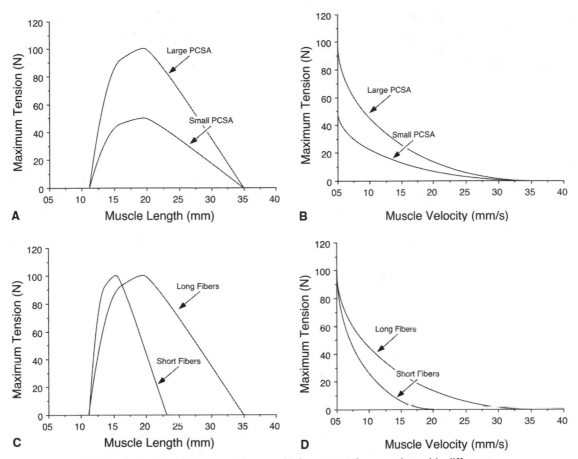

FIGURE 2-12. Schematic length-tension and force-velocity curves for muscles with different architectural properties. **(A)** Isometric length-tension curves for muscles with identical fiber lengths but different cross-sectional areas. **(B)** Isotonic force-velocity curves for muscles with identical fiber lengths but different cross-sectional areas. **(C)** Isometric length-tension curves for muscles with identical cross-sectional areas but different fiber lengths. **(D)** Isotonic force-velocity curves for muscles with identical cross-sectional areas but different fiber lengths.

tension relationship, it causes an increase in the muscle's absolute maximum contraction velocity (V_{max}, Fig. 2-12D). Again, although the fiber length increase causes an increase in these absolute properties (such as V_{max}), it has no effect on the intrinsic properties of the muscle.

Graphical representation of the functional effects of muscle architecture can be performed for any combination of PCSA and/or fiber length change. Try predicting force-velocity and length-tension curves for the case in which both architectural parameters are changed at the same time. Also try plotting these results on both absolute and relative scales. The results should demonstrate that muscle architectural changes cause variation in muscle absolute force, excursion and velocity, without changing the intrinsic shape of these relationships.

These are vivid examples of the profound influence of muscle architecture on functional properties. Return to the original discussion of architecture given in Chapter 1 and peruse Tables 1-3 and 1-4 to become more familiar with the architecture of several common muscles. Note that muscles with relatively long fibers (hamstrings, extensor carpi radialis longus, tibialis anterior) are muscles with high

---

Therapist's Comments

It helps me to understand the design of lower extremity muscles by summarizing major muscle groups as shown below in the two Tables constructed from the data in Table 1-4, page 30. These tables represent the average fiber length and the sum of the PCSAs for the muscles of the lower extremity. The quadriceps tend to have shorter fibers and larger PCSA compared with the hamstrings, demonstrating that the quadriceps muscles are designed for shorter excursion and higher force.

	Fiber length (cm)	PCSA (cm²)
Quadriceps	6.8	87.0
Hamstrings	11.2	35.4

· ·

In a similar comparison of the synergistic calf muscles, the medial and lateral gastrocnemius muscles have longer fibers and smaller PCSAs compared to the soleus. This is an interesting design that illustrates that synergistic muscles have very different architectures suggesting different functions. These functional differences among muscles may mean that exercise programs should be developed to meet the specific functional characteristics of the muscle by changing the range or strength over which a muscle is treated.

	Fiber length (cm)	PCSA (cm²)
Medial Gastrocnemius	3.5	23.0
Lateral Gastrocnemius	5.1	11.0
Soleus	2.0	58.0

---

contraction velocities and large excursions. Conversely, muscles with large PCSAs (quadriceps, flexor carpi ulnaris) generate large tensions. The architectural specialization observed in the numerous muscles has profound functional consequences. Muscles are able to perform a large range of tasks largely as a result of their intrinsic design rather than a specific set of command signals from the CNS. This design allows the CNS to act more as a coordinator of tasks rather than a definer of the particulars of the task. Interestingly, this is the same trend that is occurring in the microcomputer world regarding the tasks of computer central processing units (CPUs) and peripheral devices such as printers and video display terminals.

3 Muscle Fiber Types and Motor Units

Muscle Fiber Types

Historical View of Skeletal Muscle Fiber Types

Although it is true that all fiber types are created equal in terms of value, it is clearly not true in terms of properties. Some of the differences between fiber types have already been hinted at in the discussion of developmental anatomy. In fact, by understanding the anatomic differences between fiber types, insight is gained into the rationale for the anatomic features themselves. This is much the same approach that the comparative anatomist takes in understanding skeletal function by observing the same skeletal feature across a variety of species.

To retain the view that all muscle fibers are the same is an oversimplification in light of the overwhelming evidence that skeletal muscle fibers are heterogeneous. In the early 1800s it was observed that the gross appearance of different skeletal muscles ranged in color from pale white to deep red. In fact, one of the earliest classification schemes for muscle was based

TABLE 2-2[a]	Fiber Type Classification Schemes		
Basis for Scheme	**Fiber Type Spectrum**		**Authors**
Metabolic	SO	FOG	FG	Peter et al., 1972
Morphology and physiology	Slow red	Fast white	Fast white	Ranvier, 1873
Z-line width	Red	Intermediate	White	Gauthier, 1969
Histochemistry	III	II	I	Romanul, 1964
Histochemistry	Type 1	Type 2A	Type 2B	Brooke and Kaiser, 1972
Immunohistochemistry	Type 1	Types 2A and 2X	Type 2B	Schiaffino et al., 1989

[a] SO; slow oxidative
FOG; fast oxidative glycolytic
FG; fast glycolytic

on color, and thus muscles were classified as "red" or "white" (Table 2-2). However, as experimental methods became more sophisticated, it became clear that numerous other differences existed between muscles. For example, certain muscles contracted rapidly, whereas others contracted more slowly; certain ones could maintain force for a long period of time, whereas others fatigued rapidly, and certain muscles generated large forces, while others generated small forces. Thus, muscles were also classified as "fast" or "slow," and "fatigable" or "nonfatigable." In addition, with the advent of light microscopy and histochemistry, it was even possible to classify individual fibers based on their appearance following a particular staining protocol. Many of these schemes did not correlate simply with the muscle color. In fact, many of them did not correlate at all with one another. Table 2-2 presents a few of the classification schemes used historically and the bases for them. The main problem with fiber type classification schemes was that the classification only worked for one property but had no relationship to others. Therefore, although anatomists identified type 1 and type 2 fibers, physiologists spoke of "fast twitch" and "slow twitch" muscles. In addition, it was not clear whether muscle fibers were mutable over their life span.

Our current view of muscle fiber types is that skeletal muscle fibers possess a wide and nearly continuous spectrum of morphologic,

contractile, and metabolic properties. The appropriate view of any classification scheme, therefore, is that it is an artificial system superimposed on a continuum for our convenience. In my view, the most useful scheme is one that can be related to other types of measurements (*e.g.*, physiologic and biochemical) to understand more fully muscle's normal and adaptive properties. Luckily for us, most modern muscle fiber type classification schemes are based on some type of measurement of the myosin molecule. Thus, the lessons learned above about myosin structure and function will be useful in the discussion of muscle fiber types. To reiterate before beginning this discussion, in terms of functional importance, an understanding of muscle architecture is more important than the knowledge of muscle fiber types. Studies of muscle fiber types have been overperformed and overinterpreted.

Skeletal Muscle Metabolism

Before discussing the physiologic properties of the various fiber types and the experimental methods for fiber type identification, a brief review of cellular metabolism is presented. This is appropriate not only for our understanding, but because much of what is known about cellular metabolism was discovered in muscle tissue. In this section, the features of carbohydrate and lipid metabolism that are relevant to muscle function are presented. This overview of metabolism serves as the basis of a later discussion on muscle fiber types and fiber typing methods.

Muscle cells, like any other body cell, require energy to perform their normal function. In contrast to other cells that only have to generate enough energy to maintain normal cellular processes, muscle cells have the additional burden of providing energy for force generation. These metabolic pathways are important in determining a cell's ability to perform work under a variety of conditions (see pages 85–88).

The six-carbon carbohydrate molecule known as glucose serves as the major energy source of the cell. There are two main processes by which glucose can be oxidized to yield energy that is useable by the cell. Of these, one of them does not require oxygen (glycolysis) and one of them does (oxidative phosphorylation). Glycolysis occurs within the soluble cytoplasm of the cell, whereas oxidative phosphorylation occurs within the mitochondria (Fig. 2-13).

Glycolysis: Energy Without Oxygen

Glycolysis is the cellular process by which the glucose molecule is enzymatically broken down into two three carbon molecules known as pyruvate (Fig. 2-14A). The chemical reaction can be represented as

$$\text{Glucose} + 2\,\text{ADP} + 2\,\text{P}_i \rightarrow 2\,\text{Pyruvate} + 2\,\text{ATP} \quad \text{(Eq. 2-12)}$$

Glucose breakdown occurs as a series of chemical reactions that permits cellular control

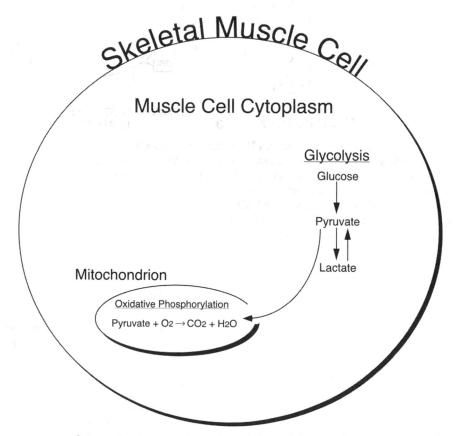

FIGURE 2-13. Schematic diagram of location of the cellular metabolic processes. Glycolysis and anaerobic glucose metabolism occurs in the cytoplasm while oxidative phosphorylation, which requires oxygen, occurs in the mitochondrion.

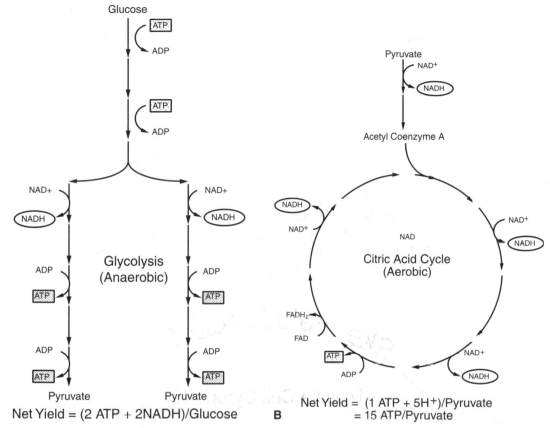

A Net Yield = (2 ATP + 2NADH)/Glucose

B Net Yield = (1 ATP + 5H$^+$)/Pyruvate
       = 15 ATP/Pyruvate

FIGURE 2-14. Summary of glucose metabolism. **(A)** Glycolysis represents the metabolism of glucose to 2 molecules of pyruvate. This process yields 2 ATP molecules and 2 NADH molecules (shown in shaded squares and ellipses), and occurs without oxygen. **(B)** The citric acid cycle represents the conversion of pyruvate into acetyl Coenzyme A, which then passes through various intermediates (not shown), and yields 1 molecule of ATP, 4 molecules of NADH and 1 molecule of FADH2. The NADH and FADH2 are available for further oxidation by the electron transport system, which yields much ATP. This process requires oxygen.

(continued)

of the rate and amount of glucose metabolized. Note that for every molecule of glucose metabolized, two ATP molecules are created. If the glycolytic process is to occur continuously without oxygen, several intermediate molecules must be regenerated by further oxidizing the pyruvate molecule to lactate:

$$\text{Pyruvate} + \text{NADH} \rightarrow \text{Lactate} + \text{NAD}^+ \quad \text{(Eq. 2-13)}$$

In which NADH and NAD$^+$ refer to the reduced and oxidized versions of nicotinamide adenine dinucleotide, a common reaction coenzyme.

ATP is the primary energy molecule used in the cross-bridge cycle. Although glycolysis can supply the energy needs of the cell, it not extremely efficient.

Oxidative Phosphorylation: Energy with Oxygen

Lactate buildup after anaerobic glycolysis within the cell has two main drawbacks: First, lactate is an acidic molecule, and accumulation can alter the intracellular pH, thus altering sub-

C

Oxidative Phosphorylation
(Aerobic)

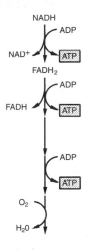

Net Yield = 3 ATP/NADH or 2 ATP/FADH
(2 ATP/NADH if NADH from cytoplasm)

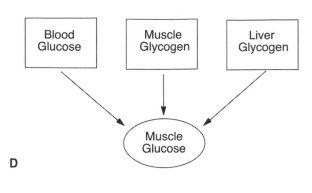

D

FIGURE 2-14. *(CONTINUED)* **(C)** Oxidative phosphorylation used to generate ATP from either NADH (3 molecules ATP per NADH) or FADH2 (2 molecules ATP per FADH2). If the NADH is derived from the cytoplasm via glycolysis, only 2 ATP are produced net, since one ATP is required to transport NADH into the mitochondrion. **(D)** Three sources of glucose that are available to skeletal muscle for metabolism.

sequent cellular contractile and metabolic activity. In addition, lactate clearance from the cell requires further bodily energy to transport it via the blood and further metabolizing elsewhere—for instance, in the liver. When oxygen is present, the preferable metabolic pathway for glucose metabolism is to completely oxidize glucose to pyruvate and then, within the mitochondria, to oxidize pyruvate further into CO_2 and H_2O, which are easily cleared from the cell via diffusion into the blood and exhaling of CO_2 via the lungs (Fig. 2-14B). Oxidative phosphorylation can thus be further represented as:

(Eq. 2-14)

$$\text{Pyruvate} + 15\ ADP + 15\ P_i + 4O_2 \rightarrow 3\ CO_2 + H_2O + 15\ ATP$$

Whereas anaerobic metabolism (glycolysis) of glucose yields 2 ATP per glucose molecule, oxidative metabolism yields 32 ATP per glucose molecule (15 ATP for each pyruvate and 2 ATP for glucose to pyruvate oxidation ([Fig. 2-14C and 2-15]). Thus, when oxygen is avail-

able, it is a much more energy efficient mechanism to generate cellular energy.

Fatty Acid Oxidation

Glucose is available from at least three sources: blood glucose, intracellular glucose, and muscle glycogen (Fig. 2-14D). Glycogen is a large polymer of chemically linked glucose molecules that are stored in muscle cells to provide energy under anaerobic conditions (seen as black "dots" on longitudinal electron micrographs of skeletal muscle; See Fig. 1-9 on page 23). However, another source of energy—fat— is also available to meet cellular needs. Fats, or more properly, fatty acids, are metabolized by a process called β-oxidation. β-Oxidation occurs in the mitochondria as with oxidative phosphorylation. From a simple 16-carbon chain of fatty acid (palmitate), two unit carbons are sequentially cleaved off to yield ATP:

(Eq. 2-15)

$$\text{Palmitate} + \text{Acetyl CoA} + 7O_2 \rightarrow 7\ CO_2 + 4\ H_2O + 129\ ATP$$

Notice that oxidative metabolism can yield great quantities of ATP from glucose and fatty acids, while metabolism under anaerobic conditions has a much lower energy yield. These concepts will come up again in the discussion of motor unit identification by glycogen depletion (pages 91–92) and muscle fatigue (page 102).

Methods for Typing Muscle Fibers

The Metabolic Classification Scheme

As mentioned above, many schemes were proposed to classify skeletal muscle histochemical, physiologic, and morphologic properties. To date, many agree that the so-called metabolic classification scheme is the most useful in terms of making a connection between "fiber type" and function. That is, the metabolic scheme allows one to switch back and forth between anatomic and physiologic studies and to understand one type of study based on the other. (Unfortunately, this scheme is not the one most widely used for study of human muscle.) This classification scheme was developed by Dr. V. Reggie Edgerton and colleagues in the late 1960s and early 1970s in an iterative fashion. For example, Edgerton and colleagues published early work describing the glycogen content of red and white muscle fibers (Gillespie, Simpson, & Edgerton, 1970). Later, based on theirs and others' physiologic observations that fast-contracting muscles were not always white, the scheme was expanded to include intermediate (in color) muscle fibers. Finally, again largely based on their work, along with that of Dr. James Peter, the metabolic classification scheme was developed (Peter, Barnard, Edgerton, Gillespie, & Stempel, 1972). The strength of this scheme is that physiologic, biochemical, and histochemical experiments were combined to develop a scheme consistent across methodologies.

Histochemical Methods—Visualizing Chemicals and Enzymes in Tissue

In the metabolic method, three fundamental muscle fiber properties are identified using histochemical methods. ("Histochemical" ["histo" = tissue] implies that the chemical reaction is occurring in the tissue itself, rather than in a test tube or other reaction vessel.) These histochemical methods rely on the fact that enzymes located in thin (6–8 μm) frozen sections of muscle fibers can be chemically reacted with certain products to visualize the activity of the enzyme. The most modern histochemical methods are actually able to quantify the activity of the enzymes in standard units (similar to in vitro biochemical studies) based only on measurements of optical density in frozen tissue sections (See Color Plate Section, Fig. C-4). Remember that a 6-μm section is still 2 to 4 sarcomeres thick so that there are a tremendous

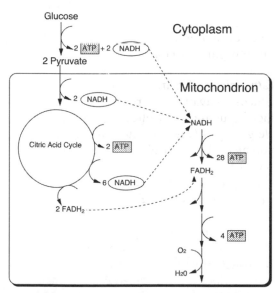

Summary of Glucose Metabolism

Aerobic: Glucose + 36 ADP + 3 O_2 → 6 CO_2 + 36 ATP + 6 H_2O
Anaerobic: Glucose + 2 ADP → 2 Pyruvate + 2 ATP

FIGURE 2-15. Summary of glucose metabolism under anaerobic or aerobic conditions. Note that only 2 ATP per glucose are produced anaerobically via glycolysis while 36 ATP per glucose are produced in the presence of oxygen.

number of proteins available that can participate in chemical reactions.

The basic requirement for a histochemical assay is similar, at least in principle, to the requirement for any biochemical assay. First, a substrate (fuel) is provided for the enzyme to be studied. Second, an energy source is provided that allows the enzyme to use the substrate. Finally, a reaction product is linked to another product that can be visualized microscopically (Dubowitz & Brooke, 1973). Of course, the entire reaction takes place in the tissue itself, not in a test tube. There are three histochemical assays typically used to determine muscle fiber types. These three assays are the myosin ATPase (MATPase) assay, the succinate dehydrogenase (SDH) assay, and the α-glycerophosphate dehydrogenase (α-GP) assay.

Myofibrillar ATPase—Identifying Fast and Slow Fibers

In a classic example of combined physiologic and biochemical experimentation, Dr. Michael Barany measured V_{max} in several skeletal muscles (Barany, 1967). He then biochemically isolated the myosin from these muscles and measured their myosin ATPase activities (an "activity" is a rate expressed for an enzyme in

---

Box 2-7. Does Lactic Acid Buildup Cause Muscle Pain?

There is no question that anaerobic exercise results in lactic acid buildup within skeletal muscle, that it is cleared by the microcirculation, and that it can be detected in the blood. Although changes in the exercise intensity at which lactic acid is detected (the so-called "lactic acid threshold") indicate improvement in the training condition of the individual, lactic acid itself has a very small direct effect on muscle—certainly it does not cause muscle soreness. Soreness results from damage to the tissue itself. The modest pH decrease resulting from lactic acid buildup may cause a slight decrease in the force produced by the myosin cross-bridge, but is not painful.

---

units of moles of product per unit mass per time interval—for example, millimoles per milligram protein per minute in the case of the myosin ATPase assay). Barany found that V_{max} and myosin ATPase activity were directly proportional. Barany demonstrated that the activity of the myosin molecule limited the rate of muscle contraction and thus provided an explanation by which myosin activity could be used to infer contractile speed. In other words, he provided the expected link that could be used to combine biochemical and physiologic studies in a seminal study that formed the basis for modern fiber typing schemes.

The histochemical assay for myofibrillar ATPase activity is used to distinguish between fast- and slow-contracting muscle fibers (although, strictly speaking, one should not histochemically type a fiber and call it fast or slow because the classification method does not actually measure speed but a histochemical appearance). Recall that the myosin molecule itself binds and hydrolyzes ATP during force generation. Because myosin ATPase activity is positively correlated with muscle contraction velocity, measures of ATPase activity can be interpreted in terms of contraction speed. The simplified cross-bridge cycle was presented as Equation 2-2. ATP is the reaction energy source and substrate, P_i is the reaction product, and myosin is the enzyme. Histochemically, P_i is invisible. Thus, the assay requires that P_i be chemically reacted with calcium (Ca) to produce $CaPO_4$ (limestone), a white precipitate. Subsequent steps in the process convert $CaPO_4$ into CoS_2, which is brownish-black, more easily viewable, and less soluble. Thus, effectively, as P_i is released, a brownish-black product is deposited on the section. Fast-contracting muscle fibers hydrolyze ATP faster than slow-contracting fibers. When given equivalent times, fast-contracting fibers appear dark histochemically, and slow-contracting fibers appear light (Color Plate Section, Fig. C-4D). In this manner, the myosin ATPase assay can be used to distinguish between fast- and slow-contracting muscle fibers.

Box 2-8. Do Fiber Types Make Sprinters Fast?

Statistically, athletes who are highly trained for sprinting tasks have a greater proportion of fast fibers in their vastus lateralis muscles compared with athletes who are highly trained for marathon running. However, such a fiber type difference probably has a negligible effect on their performance and is probably genetically determined rather than induced by training. Sprinters are fast based on their large, strong muscles that can accelerate their body mass rapidly. Most of the larger muscle fibers are also fast types. It is more appropriate to state that sprinters are so fast based on the large PCSA that results from their muscle architecture. In fact, as sprinters train for high speeds, their muscles become stronger, but intrinsically, actually become *slower*!

Succinate Dehydrogenase: Identifying Oxidative Potential

The histochemical assay for SDH is used to distinguish between oxidative and nonoxidative (actually, "less" oxidative) fibers. Recall that fibers with a high oxidative capacity generate ATP via oxidative phosphorylation. This sequence of reactions occurs in the mitochondria, which is one reason that highly oxidative fibers have a high volume fraction of mitochondria (Eisenberg, 1983). The SDH enzyme is located in the inner membrane of the mitochondrion, bound to the cristae. SDH is responsible for oxidizing succinate to fumarate in the citric acid cycle:

$$\text{Succinate} + \text{NAD}^+ \rightarrow \text{Fumarate} + \text{NADH} \quad \text{(Eq. 2-16)}$$

As this reaction proceeds, succinate is oxidized, and the reduced form of NADH is produced. Succinate is therefore the substrate, NADH is the reaction product (actually, a different electron acceptor is used for practical reasons), and SDH is the enzyme. The electron acceptor is chemically reacted in a second step with a purple tetrazolium salt to clearly visualize the location of the SDH enzyme. Similar to the ATPase assay, fibers rich in SDH (and thus rich in mitochondria) stain with a speckled pattern of the mitochondria, proportional to the number of mitochondria and the SDH activity within them (Color Plate Section, Fig. C-4F). Oxidative fibers have a relatively dense, purple speckled appearance, whereas nonoxidative fibers have only scattered purple speckles. Therefore, this histochemical assay reflects the relative oxidative potential of muscle fibers.

α-Glycerophosphate Dehydrogenase— Identifying Glycolytic Potential

The α-GP enzyme is used to distinguish among fibers based on their relative glycolytic potential. Recall that glycolysis is used to generate ATP in the absence of oxygen (anaerobically). The chemical reactions involved in glycolysis take place in the muscle cell cytoplasm (myoplasm). As such, the α-GP stain is not confined to a specific cellular organelle as is the SDH stain, and the appearance is much more continuous across the cell. The α-GP enzyme is not actually involved with direct steps in glycolysis. Rather, the α-GP enzyme is responsible for shuttling the NADH produced by glycolysis into the mitochondria where ATP can be produced. It is thus related to glycolytic activity in the sense that the more NADH that can be shuttled into the mitochondrion, the more energy that can be produced. It would be preferable to directly and selectively stain a rate-limiting glycolytic enzyme (such as phosphofructokinase [PFK], an important glycolysis regulatory enzyme), but technically, this is rather difficult to achieve. The α-GP enzyme is involved in the reaction

$$\text{reduced } \alpha\text{-GP} + \text{NADH} + \text{H}^+ \rightarrow \quad \text{(Eq. 2-17)}$$
$$\text{into mitochondrion} \rightarrow \text{NAD}^+ + \text{oxidized } \alpha\text{-GP}$$

As such, α-GP activity is directly related to the energy production of the glycolytic pathway. As with SDH, α-GP is an enzyme that "dehydrogenates" or oxidizes its substrate, glycerol-1-phosphate. The histochemical method is completely analogous to the SDH assay where the reaction product is linked to the purple tetrazolium salt. However, visually, the reaction appears more homogeneous across the entire cell since the α-GP enzyme is not organelle bound (Color Plate Section, Fig. C-4). This assay can thus distinguish between glycolytic and nonglycolytic fibers.

Fiber Type Classifications Using Histochemical Methods

In their most basic form, the three histochemical methods described above can classify muscle fibers into fast or slow, oxidative or nonoxidative, and glycolytic or nonglycolytic. Potentially, if a given muscle fiber is stained for all three properties, any of the eight (2^3) fiber types shown in Table 2-3 could be obtained. In reality (and fortunately), however, over 95% of normal muscle fibers can be classified into one of only three categories shown in Table 2-4.

A classification scheme has been created that fulfills the criteria set forth above: It can classify most muscle fibers, and it can be related to physiologic, biochemical, and morphologic measurements. Although classification schemes are, by definition, artificial, this one is less so in that it interleaves well with many different experimental methodologies.

TABLE 2-4	Actual Three Fiber Types Obtained By Histochemical Assay		
Fiber Type Designation	ATPase Activity (F or S)	SDH Activity (O)	α-GP Activity (G)
FG	High	Low	High
FOG	High	High	High
SO	Low	High	Low

Classification by Immunohistochemistry

Although histochemical fiber type identification can yield valuable insights into muscle function, it is limited in its ability to identify specific cellular proteins. For example, suppose two separate muscles were frozen, stained, and incubated for determination of myofibrillar ATPase activity. In both cases, suppose that light and dark fibers appeared, representing slow and fast fibers, respectively. Can we conclude that the fast fibers from one muscle are identical to fast fibers in the other muscle? Of course not, for the same reason that two individuals who run the same speed are not identical. Sometimes it is important to know exactly which type of protein is contained in the cell. For this purpose, we must use very specific identification methods that identify proteins with the same specificity that fingerprints have for humans.

With the advent of modern methods, and development of antibodies for protein identification, immunohistochemistry has become the "gold standard" for identification of muscle fiber types. As it turns out, muscle fibers are fairly easily classified using immunohistochemistry since different forms of the myosin heavy chain (MHC) molecule (different isoforms) are expressed within the different fiber types. However, it is important to point out that the MHC isoform itself does not actually correlate exactly with the physiological properties measured as oxidative and glycolytic capacities. Thus, one fiber-typing scheme may not correlate exactly with another. However, because

TABLE 2-3	Eight Potential Fiber Types Based on Histochemical Assay		
Potential Fiber Type Designation	ATPase Activity (F or S)	SDH Activity (O)	α-GP Activity (G)
F	High	Low	Low
FO	High	High	Low
FG	High	Low	High
FOG	High	High	High
S	Low	Low	Low
SO	Low	High	Low
SG	Low	Low	High
SOG	Low	High	High

MHC isoform is highly correlated with many metabolic processes, fiber type identification of normal cells using MHC antibodies is extremely informative. The most complete set of MHC isoforms have been developed on rat skeletal muscle and these sets have been applied to other mammalian systems. Thus, the fiber typing scheme developed for rat skeletal muscle will be discussed in some detail.

Mammalian Fiber Types Based on MHC Isoform

Using modern immunohistochemical methodology, Dr. Stefano Schiaffino and his colleagues generated a collection of monoclonal antibodies that react against the MHC. The monoclonal antibodies were generated to react against only a single portion of the MHC molecule. When sections of muscle were incubated with the monoclonal antibodies, most of the different clones reacted with all of the fibers within the section. In other words, even though there were differences in MHC isoform between fiber types, most of the MHC molecules are extremely similar and reacted identically with most monoclonal antibodies against MHC. However, fortunately, Schiaffino and colleagues (Schiaffino, et al., 1989) were able to identify a collection of antibodies that demonstrated selective reactivity between fiber types and they attempted to correlate the pattern of reactivity with the traditional fiber-typing scheme using ATPase activity. It would have been nice if they had found a specific clone that reacted with each of the MHC isoforms, but this was not the case. It was only possible to identify MHC isoforms within muscle fiber types by a process of elimination based on examination of many serial sections of muscle labeled with various antibody sets. The result of these studies was to generate a set of monoclonal antibodies that could identify four major fiber types in adult rat skeletal muscle tissue. Of these four fiber types, one was clearly a "slow" fiber type and three fiber types corresponded to "fast" isoforms. Since this scheme is widely used today, and because the antibodies are readily available from the

community hybridoma bank (ATCC) and since the scheme applies to human skeletal muscle, it will be reviewed here. The most surprising result was that the antibody panel clearly identified three different fast fiber isoforms. Previous classification schemes had identified two major types 2A and type 2B fibers (or with the metabolic schemed, FG and FOG fibers) and many had alluded to an additional "type" that was considered a "transitional" type and was named type 2C. Yet, Schiaffino and colleagues clearly identified a fairly prevalent third isoform, distinct from types 2A and 2B, which they termed type "2X" because they thought it might be a transitional form in between 2A and 2B.

Overall, Schiaffino and colleagues identified 7 different monoclonal antibodies that could be used to distinguish between the four major fiber types (Table 2-5). Type 1 fibers were selectively identified using two different antibodies, BAD5, which labeled only type 1 fibers, or SC75, which labeled everything but type 1 fibers. Type 2A fibers were identified using the SC71 antibody and type 2B fibers with the BFF3 antibody. There was no antibody that selectively labeled the type 2X fiber type, but antibody BF35 labeled all fiber types except type 2X, which rendered it useful for identification by elimination. In practice, fiber types within a histological section are identified by labeling successive sections with all of the relevant antibodies. These "serial section" studies assume that MHC isoform is constant along the fiber length sectioned (Color Plate Section, Fig. C-4E).

Even though type BAD5 antibody is considered a specific antibody that provides definitive identification of type 1 fibers in rat skeletal muscle, the tissue source is critical. It is not possible, without extensive testing, to state that this same BAD5 antibody will identify a type 1 fiber in any other species. In fact, a recent study in frog muscle demonstrated that this was absolutely not the case (Lutz, Cuizon, Ryan, & Lieber, 1998).

Regarding these antibodies used on human muscle, in a subsequent study, these authors demonstrated, using in situ hybridization (a

TABLE 2-5	Monoclonal Antibodies Used to Identify Myosin Heavy Chain Isoforms in Rat Skeletal Muscle[a]
Antibody	**Fiber Type Labeled**
SC75	All types but type 1
BAD5	Type 1 fibers
BF32	Types 1 and 2A
BFF3	Type 2B fibers
BF35	All types except type 2X
RTD9	Types 2X and 2B
SC71	Type 2A

a-Based on the work described in: Schiaffino, S., Gorza, L., Sartore, S., Saggin, L., Vianello, M., Gundersen, K., Lømo, T. (1989). Three myosin heavy chain isoforms in type 2 skeletal muscle fibers. *Journal of Muscle Research and Cell Motility, 10,* 197–205.

method where specific cDNA probes are used to label specific mRNA sequences within the cell), showed that the muscle fibers that had been identified as type 2B were actually expressing mRNA transcripts of the type 2X isoform (Smerdu, Karsch-Mizrachi, Campione, Leinwand, & Schiaffino, 1994). This type of study demonstrates that, just because a fiber type is "named," for example, type 2B, this is merely a placeholder name until definitive identification of the protein product is made using modern molecular methods. Hopefully, this discussion has made it clear that these types of studies can be complex to perform and interpret. Clearly, a number of studies in the literature are confounded by the fact that the investigators do not understand the limitations of interpretation of results from histochemical or immunohistochemical studies.

Other Muscle Fiber Classification Schemes

Before leaving the topic of muscle fiber classification schemes, and having laid the foundation for the most widely used scheme, it is time to take a closer look at some of the other schemes that were developed but proved to be less useful.

The "red" and "white" classification scheme, as mentioned earlier, was one of the earliest developed. The earliest observations were that muscles had a red appearance contracted slowly while muscles with a paler, white appearance contracted rapidly. It was thus concluded that "red" was the same as "slow contracting" and "white" was the same as "fast contracting." However, it was soon determined that many red muscles were indeed fast contracting when measured physiologically. Thus, although "red" and "white" were distinctions that could be applied to most muscles, they did not uniquely correlate with other measured muscle properties and thus were not useful in describing muscle (aside from color, of course). The red appearance many muscles have is due to their high muscle blood supply and myoglobin content. Since high capillary density is correlated with muscle oxidative capacity, muscles composed of either slow oxidative (SO) fibers or fast oxidative glycolytic (FOG) fibers can possess a reddish appearance. Obviously, SO fibers are slow contracting and FOG are fast contracting, which explains the observed discrepancy.

A second scheme used often in human muscle pathology and even in animal experiments is the so-called ATPase-based classification scheme (Brooke & Kaiser, 1970). In this scheme, several repetitions of the ATPase assay mentioned above are carried out on serial sections of muscle (serial sections are consecutive 6–8-μm sections in which the same fiber can be identified on one section and then the next, etc.) However, although the routine ATPase assay is carried out under alkaline conditions (pH, 9.4), in the ATPase-based classification scheme, several other assays are performed under increasingly acidic conditions (around pH of 4), and optical density is measured. Thus the assay determines the sensitivity of the ATPase enzyme to the pH of the medium. It turns out (for reasons that are not clear) that fast muscle myosin has a different pH sensitivity than slow muscle myosin. Thus at acid pH, slow fibers stain more darkly than fast fibers, while at alkaline pH the opposite is true. In fact, the scheme takes this differential pH sensitivity a step further. It turns out that fast fibers themselves can be subdivided based on differential pH sensitivity over the range of pH 4.3–4.6. This classification scheme can thus differentiate between fast fibers (termed type 2) and slow fibers (termed type 1), and between (at least) two fast fiber subtypes (termed type 2A and type 2B). Table 2-6 presents the definitions of type 1, 2A, and 2B fibers based on the ATPase scheme. Note that this technique must be fine tuned to accurately and repeatedly obtain valid results on various tissues. The values presented are those obtained by Brooke and Kaiser for human muscle (Brooke and Kaiser, 1970).

It has been indirectly concluded that type 2A fibers have a greater oxidative capacity than type 2B fibers, and therefore, many equate them (incorrectly) with type FOG fibers. A number of studies have directly demonstrated that the metabolic scheme does not correlate well with the ATPase-based scheme. This should not be surprising based on an understanding of what the two schemes measure. Why should the pH sensitivity of the ATPase molecule be related to the oxidative or glycolytic capacity of the cell? A relationship may exist in general, as most cellular metabolic processes are complimentary. However, the relationships may not hold following a perturbation of the cellular environment and, therefore, must be used with great caution. It seems most prudent to measure directly the property of interest (*e.g.,* oxidative capacity) rather than relying on an indirect measure associated with the property of interest.

Physiologic Properties of Muscle Fiber Types

What are the differences between muscle fibers in terms of their physiologic properties? This is a difficult question to answer because it is currently not technically possible to perform all of the interesting physiologic measurements on isolated, intact mammalian skeletal muscle fibers in the way in which they were performed by Gordon, Huxley, and Julian on frog muscle fibers since the large amount of interfibrillar connective tissue precludes single fiber isolation. The best information comes either from physiologic experiments on muscles composed mainly of one fiber type or on single "skinned" muscle fibers whose type is determined immunohistochemically. The problem with the whole muscle approach is that it assumes that a muscle's properties are simply the sum of all the available fibers in the muscle and that each fiber exerts the same relative influence. This approach also assumes that, for example, an SO fiber from a muscle with several fiber types (a "mixed" muscle) is the same as an SO fiber from a muscle composed entirely of SO fibers (a "homogeneous" muscle). Therefore, we proceed in our discussion of fiber type-specific properties obtained from whole muscle studies with the understanding that we may have to qualify the results to some extent as more data become available. The single fiber studies are more specific in that only a single muscle fiber is examined, but interpretation of these data is also not without some degree of ambiguity (see below).

Maximum Contraction Velocity of Different Muscle Fiber Types
The force-velocity relationship described previously provides a convenient tool for muscle fiber type-specific characterization of "speed." The parameter V_{max} can be compared between

TABLE 2-6	Human Fiber Types Definition Using the ATPase Assay[a]		
Preincubation pH	Type 1	Type 2A	Type 2B
9.4	Light	Dark	Dark
4.6	Dark	Light	Medium
4.3	Dark	Light	Medium

[a]Based on the work in: Brooke and Kaiser, (1970). Muscle fiber types: how many and what kind? Archives of Neurology 23, 369–379.

muscles that have large differences in fiber type distribution to measure fiber type-specific values for V_{max}. As we have seen, muscle architecture has a profound influence on absolute contraction velocity, and therefore, all absolute velocities measured experimentally must be expressed in terms of a normalized velocity such as fiber lengths per second or sarcomere lengths per second to determine the intrinsic value of V_{max} for a fiber. Again comparison between muscles of different fiber types without correcting for architectural differences can lead to (and has led to) grossly errant conclusions.

Assuming that the correct type of experiment is performed, you will find that fast-contracting muscle fibers shorten two to three times faster than slow-contracting fibers at V_{max} (Close, 1972). This is actually not a large difference, and, as will be discussed in the next chapter, probably has little influence on performance in sports or in rehabilitation. In spite of the popular discussion of fiber type distribution, it probably has little to do with performance.

Architectural uncertainties and uncertainty due to variability between fiber types is almost completely eliminated by studying isolated single muscle fibers. Unfortunately, for technical reasons, isolation of single intact single fibers is not possible from rat skeletal muscle, the species on which fiber types are most completely understood (Schiaffino & Reggiani, 1996). However, it is possible to perform contractile experiments on pieces of rat muscle fibers that are isolated from intact muscles. These types of preparation are referred to as "skinned" muscle fiber preparations (Hellam & Podolsky, 1969). They are called skinned because the fiber membrane is rendered permeable by either using a mild detergent treatment ("chemical skinning") or by direct dissection of the sarcolemma from the surface of the cell ("mechanical skinning"). Chemical skinning is much more common because it is technically easier, but both methods have been used to provide insights into muscle fiber function.

Schiaffino and colleagues (Schiaffino, et al.,

1991) measured V_{max} on single skinned muscle fiber segments and also identified the MHC isoform within the single fiber at the end of the experiment. V_{max} measured in terms of fiber lengths/sec, was found to be in the order type 2B > type 2X > type 2A >> type 1. Thus, a large difference was observed between the fast isoforms and slow isoforms (not surprising) whereas a more subtle difference was seen between the fast isoforms (Bottinelli, Schiaffino, & Reggiani, 1991). There was a tremendous variation in V_{max} within the type 2B subtype and these same authors later demonstrated an additional significant effect of the light chains that were placed on the heavy chains (Bottinelli, Betto, Schiaffino, & Reggiani, 1994). The ratio of light chain 3 to light chain 1 provided about as much modulation to type 2B isoform V_{max} as did a complete subtype change to type 2A. This certainly complicates the interpretation of contractile data as a function of fiber type. Light chains can alter the contractile properties of the MHC isoforms, but the relative importance of light and heavy chains on contractile function has not been definitively determined. Currently, most studies of contractile properties as a function of fiber type consider the heavy chain to be the major determinant of contractile function.

Maximum Tension Generated by Different Muscle Fiber Types

In a manner similar to that used for measurement of V_{max}, maximum tetanic tension ($P_{o,}$) can be measured in muscles of different fiber type distributions. Again, one must account for differences in architecture to attribute differences in force to fiber type differences and not to architectural differences (i.e., PCSA). This value is then normalized to the PCSA of the muscle studied, to yield the value known as "specific tension," or force of contraction per unit area of muscle.

This is a controversial area of current muscle physiology; therefore, it is likely that this discussion will require modification as more data are obtained. However, in measuring the specific tension of whole skeletal muscle, most investigators find that muscles composed mainly of fast fibers have a greater specific tension than muscles composed mainly of slow fibers. The typical value for specific tension of fast muscle is approximately 22 N/cm^2 (250 kPa in SI units) while that for slow muscle is 10-15 N/cm^2 (~125 kPa in SI units). The common interpretation of these whole-muscle experiments has been that fast muscle fibers have a greater specific tension than slow muscle fibers. Of course the problem with this interpretation is that it assumes that a muscle fiber from a mixed muscle has the same properties as a muscle fiber of the same type that is in a homogeneous muscle. This assumption may not be untrue.

The best estimates of specific tension come from isometric contractile experiments of single motor units (discussed below). These experiments will be discussed in more detail later in the chapter, but will hint at the results because they are relevant to the present topic. Muscle fibers within a motor unit can be classified histochemically and it turns out that they are generally the same fiber type. Thus, if the force generated by a motor unit is measured, and the motor unit PCSA is determined, specific tension of different motor unit types (and therefore muscle fiber types) can be calculated. The advantage of this method is that the contractile properties are all measured from the same fiber type. The problem with this scenario is that measurement of motor unit PCSA is technically difficult. Generally, methods used for motor PCSA determination are extremely indirect, relying on a series of questionable assumptions (see motor unit section). In only one experiment have all of the fibers belonging to a motor unit been identified and summed to yield PCSA. These experiments, performed in Edgerton's laboratory, showed that fast muscle fibers develop just slightly more tension than slow muscle fibers (Bodine, Roy, Eldred, & Edgerton, 1987). This is the best information available to date.

Specific tension of isolated, skinned mammalian muscle fibers has been determined. However, it is so difficult to estimate cross-sectional area of a single fiber and the experimental methods themselves have such potential problems that these measurements probably add little to the discussion already presented.

Endurance of Different Muscle Fiber Types

The endurance (or its opposite, fatigue) of muscle fibers is even more difficult to precisely define than speed or strength. This is because endurance depends on the type of work the muscle is required to perform. For example, if the workload is extremely light, there is almost no difference between fiber types. If the workload is extremely heavy, the muscle fibers themselves do not fatigue; rather, the neuromuscular junction fatigues, and again, there is no difference between types. Because excitation-contraction coupling involves a chain of events, it is possible to produce fatigue by interrupting any point in the chain. Thus, a danger exists in simply ascribing a drop in force to muscle fiber fatigue without understanding the basis for the drop. The currently used method for fatigue measurement was developed for classification of single motor units and will thus be deferred until the motor unit presentation. Suffice it to say that the endurance of the various motor units (and muscle fiber types) differs considerably. However, it is difficult to give a quantitative difference unless the work conditions are known. Generally, SO fibers have the greatest endurance, followed by FOG fibers, and, lastly FG fibers. This is not surprising in that FG fibers have a very low oxidative capacity.

Morphologic Properties of Different Muscle Fiber Types

If we understand the histochemical and physiologic differences between muscle fiber types, presented above, structural differences between the various fiber types generally follow logically (Table 2-7).

Contractile Protein Differences between Fiber Types

Myosin differs considerably between fast and slow muscle fibers. Although this difference is profound functionally, there is really not a large structural difference between the different myosins as determined by electron microscopy and X-ray diffraction (Haselgrove, 1983). In fact, in terms of sarcomere force-generating components, while the proteins have very different functional properties, structurally they are quite similar. Fast and slow myosin have approximately the same mass and shape. Muscles composed of either fast or slow sarcomeres have approximately the same filament spacing and cross-bridge density (Zappe & Maeda, 1985).

Metabolic Differences Between Fiber Types

Clearly, the large difference in oxidative and glycolytic capacity is represented in the cell as large differences in the concentration of the metabolic enzymes. For example, in the fast fibers, the cytoplasm has a much higher concentration of all of the glycolytic intermediates. Similarly, all of the oxidative fibers (FOG and SO) have a much higher concentration of oxidative enzymes. Since oxidative phosphorylation occurs in the mitochondria, oxidative fibers have a higher mitochondrial density than nonoxidative fibers. In a detailed quantitative study of the ultrastructure of the various fiber types, Brenda Eisenberg confirmed that highly oxidative fibers have a high concentration of mitochondria (up to 25%!) and may contain twice the volume fraction of lipid (Eisenberg, 1983). This alone is one reason why it is difficult to compare the specific tension of the various fiber types even if we were able to isolate intact single fibers. Not all of the space within the fiber is contractile material, and the difference between the fibers in the amount that is contractile material is type specific. A method for quantifying SDH activity within single muscle fibers and between various fiber types was developed by Edgerton and colleagues (Martin, Bodine-Fowler, Roy, Eldred, & Edgerton, et al., 1985; Martin, Vailas, Durivage, Edgerton, & Castleman, 1988) and provided a general correlation between fiber type, oxidative activity and fiber size. The general trend was as follows and best appreciated by inspecting a graph of fiber size versus SDH activity (Fig. 2-16). These data demonstrate that the smallest muscle fibers in the typical "mixed fiber type" muscle were type 1 fibers with high SDH activity (open circles, Fig. 2-16). The largest fibers (which, based on the skinned fiber studies described above, are also the fastest) also have the lowest SDH activity and are the type 2B subtype (open squares, Fig. 2-16). Intermediate in size and oxidative capacity between these two extremes are the type 2X and type 2A fibers. While the type 1-type 2B extremes appear to be consistent between species, in some species type 2A fibers have a greater oxidative capacity compared with type 2X fibers while, in other species, the opposite is true.

Membrane Differences Between Fiber Types

Recall that the T-system and SR are involved in the excitation portion of excitation-contraction coupling. It makes sense that muscles that are required to respond rapidly (fast fibers) would have a well-developed membranous activation system. This is exactly what Eisenberg showed in her quantitative studies (Eisenberg, 1983). The SR and T-system of fast fibers may occupy two to three times more volume in fast fibers than slow fibers. Thus differences in speed between fast and slow fibers result from

TABLE 2-7	Differences between Fiber Types		
Parameter	SO	FOG	FG
T/SR system quantity	Little	Much	Much
Z-disk width	Wide	Intermediate	Narrow
Contractile speed	Slow	Fast	Fast
Mitochondrial density	High	Moderate	Low
Lipid droplets	Many	Few	None
Glycogen granules	Few	Many	Many
Endurance	High	Moderate	Low

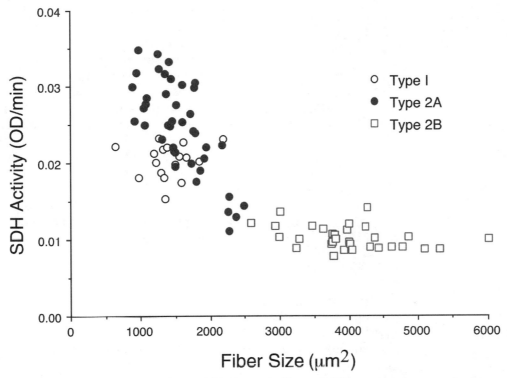

FIGURE 2-16. Oxidative capacity of individual muscle fibers of different types measured using quantitative histochemistry. Fiber types were identified using the monoclonal antibody panel shown in Table 2-5. Note that the largest fibers are the fastest (type 2B) with the lowest oxidative capacity. The smallest fibers are type 1 with a high oxidative capacity. This "parabolic" relationship, ranging from small highly oxidative to large low oxidative capacity is fairly typical for mammalian skeletal muscle. However, the relative oxidative capacity of type 2A and type 1 fibers can be reversed.

differences in cross-bridge cycling rates and differences in activation speed (Gonzalez-Serratos, 1971).

Other Structural Differences Between Fiber Types

A final interesting structural difference between fiber types that is useful but poorly understood is the difference between muscle fiber type Z-disk thickness. Again, in her pioneering work, Eisenberg (1983) showed that FG fibers have the most narrow Z-disks (60 nm) while SO fibers have the widest Z-disks (150 nm). The thickness of the Z-disk in FOG fibers is intermediate (80 nm). As stated, the reason for this difference is not clear, but it is interesting

to note that in eccentric contraction-induced muscle injury, the Z-disk appears to be the weak link that is most susceptible to injury (see Chapter 6 for more details).

In their excellent anatomic ultrastructural studies, Drs. Lars-Eric Thornell and Michael Sjöstrom (Sjöstrom et al., 1982; Thornell, Sjöstrom, & Ringqvist, 1976) have demonstrated differences between fiber types in their M-band structure. The M-band of type 1 fibers has five distinct bridges, whereas that from the 2B fiber has only three bridges (Fig. 2-17). The 2A fiber M-band has three prominent central bridges and two faint outer bridges. Although both of these ultrastructural differences hold true generally, there is a continuum of Z-disk

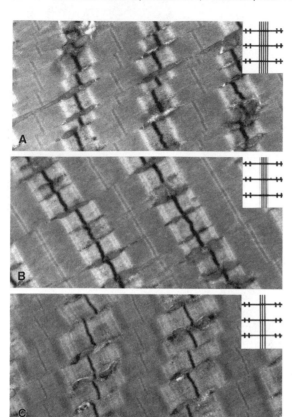

FIGURE 2-17. Ultrastructural fiber type classification scheme based on M-band morphology. Fibers with M-bands (magnification X20,000), showing all five M-bridges with equal density, are classified as type 1 fibers **(A)**. All other fibers are termed type 2. Of these fibers, those with M-band with the three middle M-bridges clearly visible but the two outer ones relatively less distinct are termed type 2A fibers **(B)**. Fibers with only the three middle M-bridges clearly visible are allocated to type 2B **(C)**. (Reprinted with permission from: Sjöström, M., Ängquist, K. A., Bylund, A. C., Fridén, J., Gustavsson, L., and Schersten, T. (1982). Morphometric analysis of human muscle fibre types. *Muscle and Nerve, 5,* 538–553. (Micrographs courtesy of Dr. Jan Fridén, Göteborg University, Sweden).

widths and M-band bridging pattern, so that it is not a simple task to measure a Z-disk width or observe an M-band and then to unambiguously type the fiber. It appears that in about 80% of the fibers, M-band width provides a good indication of fiber type.

The Motor Unit

Introduction

To this point, the properties of whole skeletal muscles and their composite muscle fibers have been discussed. However, during normal activities, muscle fibers are activated by their composite nerves. What determines the distribution of muscle fibers that are normally activated during a particular task? How does the nervous system determine the force generated by a particular muscle? How are muscle fiber properties tailored to the task at hand? The answer to all of these questions requires an understanding of the anatomy and physiology of the motor unit (Burke, 1981).

Motor Unit Anatomy

Although the functional unit of force generation is the sarcomere (actually, the half-sarcomere due to sarcomere symmetry), the functional unit of movement is the motor unit. A motor unit is defined as an α-motoneuron plus the muscle fibers it innervates. Motoneurons have their cell bodies in the ventral root of the spinal cord. The cell body is responsible for synthesis of the various nutrients responsible for maintenance of neuronal integrity. The long projection that extends from the cell body is known as the axon. Each cell body projects one axon through the ventral root, and this axon extends, along with many other axons projecting from other cell bodies (together these axons are known as a peripheral nerve), to innervate a particular muscle. As the axon (or neuron) approaches the muscle, it branches many times (from just a few to hundreds of branches), and normally each small terminal branch innervates a single muscle fiber (see Chapter 1 for a description of the way in which this anatomic arrangement arises).

Thus a whole muscle contains many motor units, each of which contains a single motoneuron and its composite muscle fibers. The number of muscle fibers belonging to a motor unit (*i.e.*, the innervation ratio) and the number of motor units within a whole muscle vary. The significance of innervation ratio and motor unit number will be discussed in the next section.

One might guess that all of the muscle fibers within a motor unit might be located in a cluster within the muscle. This is not the case and actually would represent a pathologic condition. Although muscle fibers belonging to a particular motor unit are scattered over subregions of the muscle, fibers from one motor unit are interspersed among fibers of other motor units. The functional consequence of this dispersion is that the forces generated by a unit will be spread over a larger tissue area. This may minimize mechanical stress in focal regions within the muscle.

Identification of Muscle Fibers Belonging to a Motor Unit

A prerequisite to any discussion of motor unit properties is a general understanding of the methods used for identification of muscle fibers within a motor unit. Currently, it is not possible to stain for fibers belonging to the same motor unit in the same way that is done for muscle fibers. Motor unit identification methods must identify muscle fibers that are all innervated by the same α-motoneuron. Thus one logical place to begin identifying motor units is the ventral root of the spinal cord, where the motoneurons exit.

Experimentally, the spinal cord can be surgically exposed, and the many motoneurons that exit the ventral root can be delicately teased apart. These dissected ventral root filaments (motor neuron axons) are then activated individually to stimulate only the muscle fibers belonging to that particular motor unit. If the entire peripheral nerve is stimulated, many units and fibers are activated. Even when isolating ventral root filaments, it is possible to isolate, for example, two small axons that appear to be the same axon. Thus, certain tests are performed to ensure that, indeed, a single axon has been isolated. The main test is to stimulate the filament and record the tension generated by the fibers in that unit. If a single axon were isolated, all muscle fibers belonging to the unit would contract at a single stimulation intensity.

If the intensity is increased, and muscle force increases, then more than one axon has been isolated. This is because different axons have different thresholds for activation (see below). This criterion is known as the all-or-none response. If a unit demonstrates an all-or-none response, it is assumed that all of the fibers belong to a single motor unit. In an alternate method, the motoneuron cell body can be impaled by a microelectrode and stimulated to activate all terminal axon branches along with the motor unit muscle fibers.

Now that it is certain that a single axon and its composite fibers have been isolated, how are those fibers identified? The ideal method would be to somehow "see" fibers that were actively contracting and ignore those that were not. Presently, this is not possible. However, the active fibers can be tricked into making themselves visible by stimulating them in a certain way. Active fibers can't be seen, but the results of what active fibers do can sometimes be seen. For example, as a muscle fiber is repetitively stimulated in a way that forces it to generate force anaerobically, it uses intracellular glycogen preferentially as a fuel source. It is a straightforward procedure to stain a muscle cross-section for glycogen. Thus, if muscle fibers are forced to perform anaerobic metabolism, glycogen will be depleted from the activated fibers and will remain in the nonactivated fibers. This "glycogen depletion" method for isolating motor units was pioneered by Edstrom and Kugelberg (Edstrom & Kugelberg, 1968) and has been of critical importance in current motor unit studies.

It is clear that the glycogen depletion method is not without ambiguity. The most obvious problem is developing stimulation protocols that force those muscle fibers that have a choice of aerobic or anaerobic metabolism to choose anaerobic metabolism. Thus, the method itself tends to select for the easily identified fibers (the FG fibers) and select against identification of the highly oxidative fibers, which have little anaerobic capacity (the SO fibers). This has implications in determining, by glycogen depletion, how many fibers belong to a motor unit. Values for innervation ratio obtained by glycogen depletion would tend to overestimate the number of FG fibers and underestimate the number of SO fibers.

As a side note, an alternative method is to "feed" radioactive glucose to the muscle and then stimulate it repetitively. The active cells transport the glucose into the cell, thereby labeling them. This method has the advantage that it is not necessary to selectively activate the glycolytic pathway.

Motor Unit Physiological Properties

Many of the classic motor unit physiology experiments were performed in the late 1960s and early 1970s. The work often cited is that of Bob Burke and his colleagues (Burke, 1967; Burke, Levine, Zajac, Tsairis, & Engel, 1971). These investigators isolated single cat hindlimb motor units (using intracellular motoneuron stimulation) and measured numerous electrophysiological properties of the motoneuron and mechanical properties of the motor units within the whole muscle. Interestingly (and fortuitously), they found that motor units could generally be classified into three categories based on several physiologic properties of the contracting fibers (Fig. 2-18). In other words, motor units were most easily classified based on the physiologic properties of their muscle fibers. These physiologic properties were (a) the motor unit twitch tension, (b) the fatigability of the unit in response to a specific stimulation protocol, and (c) the behavior of the tetanic tension record at an intermediate stimulation frequency. These will be discussed sequentially.

Motor Unit Twitch Tension

Early motor unit studies revealed that in response to a single electrical impulse, some units developed high twitch tensions whereas others developed relatively low twitch tensions and still others generated intermediate tensions. The exact basis for this difference was not clear. However, the units with low twitch tensions also tended to have slow contraction times while those with higher tensions tended to have fast contractions. This provided some of the first evidence that the different properties of motor units might have profound physiologic significance (Fig. 2-18).

Motor Unit Fatigue Index

A second functional property used to distinguish between the various motor units was their "fatigue index," or how much the muscle tension declined upon repetitive stimulation. It was important in these early studies to choose a stimulation frequency that fatigued the muscle fibers themselves. As mentioned, the long chain of events in excitation-contraction coupling can be interrupted at any point, resulting in a force decrease. If the purpose is to identify muscle fibers of a motor unit, it must be certain that the fatigue measured is muscle fiber fatigue and not fatigue, for instance, of the nerve or neuromuscular junction. Experimentally, the electrical activity of the muscle fibers was measured during repetitive stimulation to guarantee that the activation pulses were reaching the muscle fibers. The fatigue index test required stimulation of the motor unit at approximately 40 Hz (generating about half-maximum tension) for one-third of a second, allowing the muscle to relax for two-thirds of a second, and then repeating the sequence. Therefore every second, the motor unit received a burst of 40-Hz pulses. This sequence has been slightly modified by other investigators but is still basically used by many to identify the fatigue index of muscles and motor units. The stimulation protocol was continued for 2 minutes and the muscle tension measured. If the motor unit was highly fatigable, the tension dropped significantly compared to the initial tension. If the unit was not fatigable, the tension dropped only slightly or not at all. Using this approach, it was observed that units could be classified as highly fatigable (defined as units that generated less than 25% of the initial tension after 2 minutes), fatigue resistant (units that generated over 75% of the initial tension after 2 minutes), and fatigue intermediate (units that generated

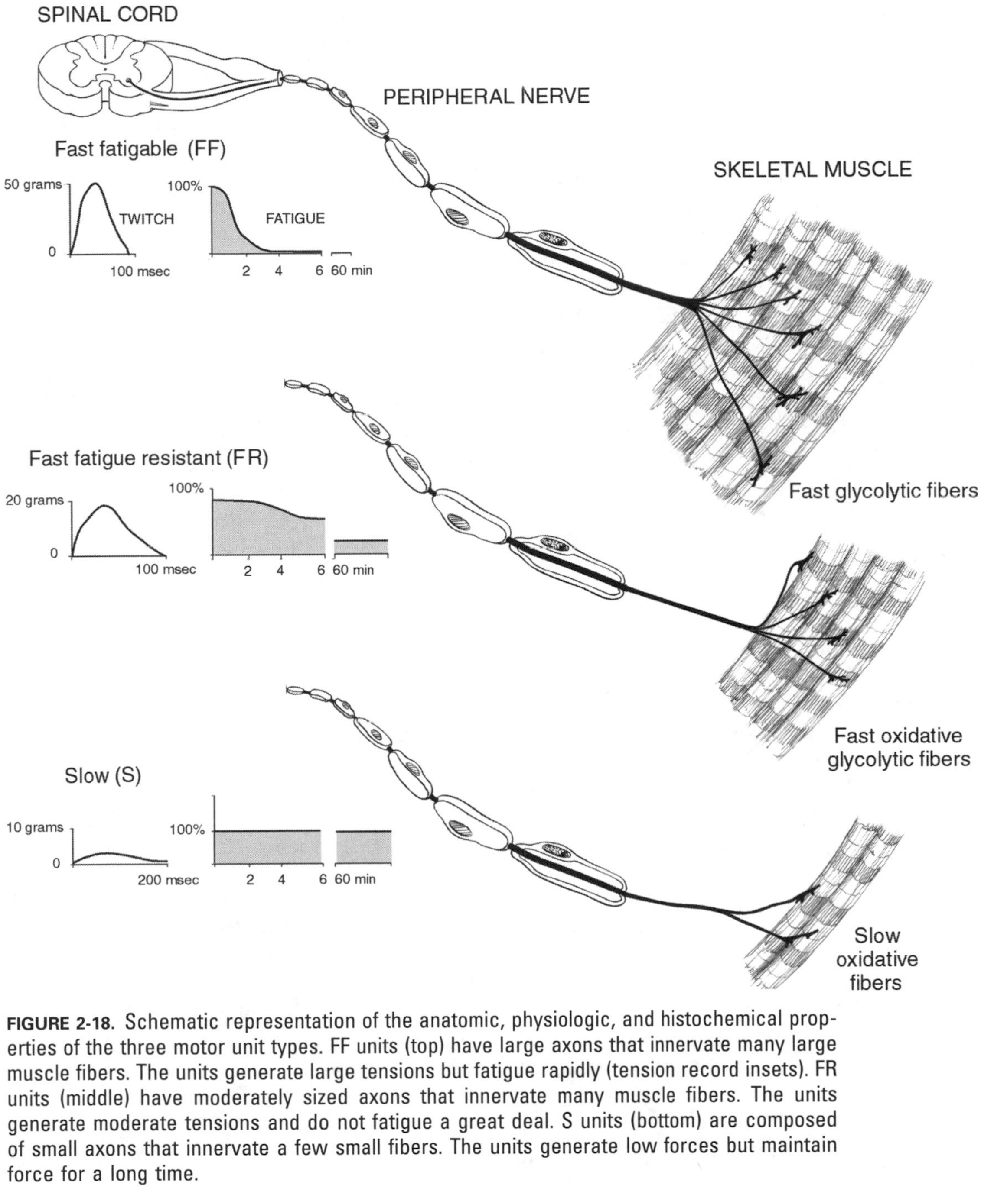

FIGURE 2-18. Schematic representation of the anatomic, physiologic, and histochemical properties of the three motor unit types. FF units (top) have large axons that innervate many large muscle fibers. The units generate large tensions but fatigue rapidly (tension record insets). FR units (middle) have moderately sized axons that innervate many muscle fibers. The units generate moderate tensions and do not fatigue a great deal. S units (bottom) are composed of small axons that innervate a few small fibers. The units generate low forces but maintain force for a long time.

between 25% and 75% of the initial tension after 2 minutes; (Fig. 2-18)).

Motor Unit "Sag" Property

At this point, there are two classification criteria for motor units: twitch tension and fatigue index. A final and less well understood criterion for motor unit classification is based on the nature of the tension record in response to an unfused tetanic contraction. In some units, the tension was observed to increase smoothly, whereas in other units, the tension record first increased, and then decreased or "sagged" slightly. The presence or absence of "sag," although not clearly understood at the time, became the final classification criterion (Fig. 2-18). In a manner completely analogous to muscle fiber type classification, these three properties when measured in motor units result in eight potential motor unit types. However, again in a manner analogous to muscle fiber types, only three types of motor units were commonly observed. A summary of these types is shown in Table 2-8.

As was demonstrated with muscle fiber types, motor units also come only in three flavors: Those that have a fast contraction time, a low fatigue index, and sag are known as fast fatigable units (abbreviated FF). Those that have a fast contraction time, a high fatigue index, and demonstrate sag are known as fast fatigue resistant units (abbreviated FR). Finally, those with slow contraction times, a high fatigue index, and no sag are known as slow units (abbreviated S).

Motor Unit Histochemistry

The alert student may already have an idea of what is to come. The issue to be addressed at this point is, what determines the physiologic properties of the motor units? (Hint: Compare Tables 2-4 and 2-8). Using the glycogen depletion method, Burke and his colleagues identified the muscle fibers belonging to various motor units using the histochemical procedures previously described (Fig. 2-18). It was determined that motor units of different types were composed of muscle fibers of different types. The correspondence between motor units and muscle fibers was, as would be expected, based on their physiologic properties. The FF motor units were composed of FG muscle fibers, the FR motor units were composed of FOG muscle fibers, and the S units were composed of SO muscle fibers (Table 2-9). A warning will be added following this discussion. It is often stated in the motor unit literature that muscle fibers within a motor unit are exactly the same. Although it is true that they are the same fiber type, it is known that all fibers of a given type are not exactly the same. Recent quantitative studies of the oxidative capacity of different muscle fibers within the same unit reveal a surprising degree of variability between fibers (Martin, et al., 1988). These data suggest that although the α-motoneuron certainly influences motor unit properties, it does not absolutely determine them. This result has significant implications in studies of muscle plasticity (adaptation), which will be discussed in Chapters 4 and 5.

Determinants of Motor Unit Tension

As previously described, different motor unit types develop different tensions. Generally, fast motor units develop higher tensions than the slow motor units. Why is this? You might presume that because fast motor units are com-

TABLE 2-8	Three Motor Unit Types Obtained Using Physiologic Measurements			
Motor Unit Designation	Twitch Tension	Twitch Contraction Time	Fatigue Index	"Sag" Present?
FF	High	Fast	Low	Yes
FR	Moderate	Fast	Moderate	Yes
S	Low	Slow	High	No

TABLE 2-9	Correspondence Between Motor Unit and Muscle Fiber Types
Motor Unit Designation	**Muscle Fiber Type in the Motor Unit**
Fast fatigable (FF)	Fast glycolytic (FG)
Fast fatigue-resistant (FR)	Fast oxidative glycolytic (FOG)
Slow (S)	Slow oxidative (SO)

posed of fast muscle fibers that fast muscle fibers generate more tension than slow muscle fibers. On the other hand, perhaps fast and slow fibers generate the same tension, but fast units simply have a greater number of fibers than slow units. Perhaps still, fast and slow units have the same number of fibers of equal intrinsic strength, but the fast fibers are larger and therefore generate more tension. Which (if any) of these possibilities is the reason for the differences in muscle tension?

As you might imagine, determination of the number of fibers belonging to a motor unit (innervation ratio) is difficult experimentally. It was mentioned that experimental identification of muscle fibers belonging to a unit requires the glycogen depletion method, which tends to select for FG fibers (FF units) and against SO fibers (S units). This is the first problem. However, even after these fibers have been glycogen depleted, it is technically difficult to find them all within the muscle, especially if the muscle has a pennated architecture. Burke and others used a series of indirect calculations that attempt to account for the various anatomic features (innervation ratio, specific tension, and fiber size). They concluded that fast muscle fibers within a motor unit have a much larger specific tension than slow muscle fibers and have a somewhat higher innervation ratio (Burke, 1981). However, using a different approach, Edgerton's laboratory, directly measured innervation ratio in a muscle with longitudinally oriented fibers (the cat tibialis anterior) and, using a stepwise regression model, demonstrated that the major reason that motor units generate different tensions is that high-tension motor units have a greater number of fibers (Bodine, Roy, Eldred, & Edgerton, 1987). In addition, these high-tension units tend to have larger fibers within them (Fig. 2-18). These two factors taken together suggest that motor unit tension is determined primarily by the number and size of the fibers within the unit and not as much by intrinsic differences (specific tension) between the fibers themselves.

The final chapter in this story has not yet been written. The take-home lesson is that the best evidence to date is that fast and slow muscle fibers within a motor unit have about the same specific tension, but that fiber size and innervation ratio differ significantly between motor unit types.

Fiber Arrangement Within Motor Units

Detailed measurements of muscle fiber length within intact whole muscles have revealed the seemingly paradoxical result that, in many muscles, fibers do not extend from one tendon plate to the other (Loeb, Pratt, Chanaud, & Richmond, 1987; Ounjian et al., 1991). This immediately suggests that the previous discussion of muscle architecture was probably oversimplified because muscle fibers may not extend between tendons. The idea that series-fibered muscles exist (i.e., muscles contain fibers that are arranged end-to-end, in series within a fascicle) is not new but the concept was revived with the report of Loeb et al. (Loeb, Pratt, Chanaud, & Richmond, 1987) who documented this arrangement in the cat sartorius

---

Therapist's Comments

Students may be interested in the observation that, exceptions to the orderly recruitment of motor units occurs with rapid muscular eccentric contractions (Nardone, Romano, & Schieppati, 1989). It is thus, apparently, possible to alter this recruitment order under extraordinary circumstances.

muscle. They argued that the extreme length of the sartorius muscle (approximately 10 cm) necessitated such an arrangement because the conduction velocity along muscle fibers was not fast enough to activate the entire fiber simultaneously. Although the applicability of such an argument is debatable, clearly a mechanical inefficiency would result if contracting sarcomeres were permitted to shorten rapidly against adjacent, compliant, inactivated sarcomeres. One can posit a rationale for such a series-fibered arrangement if the fibers so arranged are members of the same motor unit. In this way, multiple axons could innervate and simultaneously activate many fibers in series, which would, in effect, behave as a single fiber. To test this idea, Edgerton and colleagues (Ounjian et al., 1991) measured the length and distribution of muscle fibers within motor units using the glycogen depletion method. They demonstrated that not only did some of the fibers within a single unit not extend the entire fascicle length, but also many units had their origin or insertion completely in the center of the muscle belly (Fig. 1-13 page 36). How could muscle fiber contractile force be transmitted to the tendon if the fiber did not even terminate in the tendon? These and other studies have now laid to rest the oversimplified concept that all muscle fibers are arranged in bundles and transmit force along their length to the end regions where they insert onto major tendon plates. Despite the fact that muscle fiber insertion sites are highly specialized with respect to geometry and protein composition (Tidball & Daniel, 1986; Trotter, Corbett, & Avner, 1981; Trotter, Eberhard, & Samora, 1983), the finding that many muscle fibers taper into almost a pointed end precludes force from being transmitted only at their tips because the stress concentration at the small tapered fiber tip would be tremendous.

LATERAL FORCE TRANSMISSION AMONG MUSCLE FIBERS

How else might muscle fibers transmit tension to the "outside world?" A creative experiment by Dr. Sybil Street showed that muscle force could be transmitted laterally between muscle fibers (Street, 1983). She dissected a single frog muscle fiber from one end of the muscle and left the surrounding fibers intact on the other end. Although securing the bare end of the single muscle fiber and using a carefully placed electrode that activated only the single fiber, she measured the force generated by the single fiber (Fig. 2-19A). She then released the bare end of the single fiber and secured the remaining muscle fibers adjacent to the single fiber at the opposite end (Fig. 2-19B). It is important to note that at this point the single fiber was completely free at the isolated end. Again, she activated the bare single fiber and measured an isometric force nearly equivalent to that measured when the bare end of the single fiber was secured. Note that this force was measured in spite of the fact that the bare single fiber was free to shorten. How could such tension be generated when the bare fiber end was totally free? The interpretation of this experiment was that the physical interaction between adjacent fibers was sufficient so that the activated single fiber transmitted its force radially to adjacent fibers that were secured and that force was transmitted to the force-measuring end via these adjacent fibers. This experiment demonstrates the significant degree to which muscle fiber force can be transmitted outside of the fiber itself to neighboring muscle fibers. Note that this result was obtained in amphibian muscle, which has a relatively poorly developed endomysial connection tissue network. The situation for mammalian muscle would undoubtedly be more impressive where the endomysial connective tissue matrix is even more highly developed.

These results suggest a model of force transmission in whole muscle in which force is generated by the myofibrils and transmitted along and between myofibrils until it ultimately reaches the outside world by specialized adhesion receptors along the muscle length and at the fiber ends. In this model, there is no problem with muscle fibers that taper or with fibers that terminate within the muscle itself because force is transmitted all along the fiber length to

FIGURE 2-19. Schematic arrangement of experimental measurements on frog muscle to determine magnitude of force transmitted laterally between fibers. Experimental condition is shown on left and tetanic tension resulting from single fiber stimulation shown at right. **(A)** Isolated fiber is secured at bare end and at end still containing surrounding fibers. **(B)** Isolated fiber secured only at end containing surrounding fibers. The surrounding fibers themselves are secured to the measuring device. Only the single fiber is activated in both cases and isometric force generation is essentially identical. This demonstrates that force can be transmitted between fibers as well as directly at the fiber ends. (Experiments reported in: Street, S. F. (1983). Lateral transmission of tension in frog myofibers: a myofibrillar network and transverse cytoskeletal connections are possible transmitters. *Journal of Cellular Physiology, 114,* 346–364.)

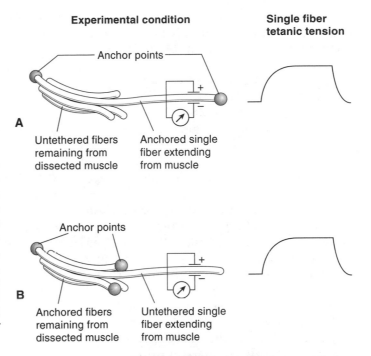

the well-developed endomysial connective tissue matrix described by Dr. John Trotter (Trotter, 1990; Trotter & Purslow, 1992). These striking pictures of the intramuscular connective tissue matrix are reminiscent of the well-defined endoneurial tubes that guide, nourish, and protect single axons (Fig. 2-20).

It may be strategic to have a mechanically redundant muscle fiber force generating system (*i.e.,* one with numerous series and parallel connections) in the same way that is observed within the fiber in which mechanical redundancy is present so that sarcomeres can transmit force serially or radially. Lateral force transmission obviates the need for mechanical continuity along the fiber length for force generation to occur. Thus, if a fiber experiences focal injury, remaining fiber segments may still transmit tension to the outside world, effectively bypassing the injured region (See complete discussion in Chapter 6). Thus, force generation in muscle would result from a "volume" of myofibrils that generate and transmit force along multiple complex pathways and via a va-

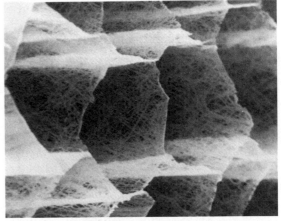

FIGURE 2-20. High power scanning electron micrograph of the endomysial connective tissue within skeletal muscle. This image was generated by scanning electron microscopy of a muscle whose fibers were removed by acid digestion. Note the fibrous appearance of the endomysial "fabric" surrounding the muscle fibers. (Original micrograph kindly provided by John Trotter (University of New Mexico) and reprinted with permission from: Trotter, J. A., & Purslow, P. P. (1992). Functional morphology of the endomysium in series fibered muscles. *Journal of Morphology, 212,* 109–122.)

riety of filamentous systems. Future studies are required to define the pathway for force transmission within and between muscle fibers.

PHYSIOLOGICAL SIGNIFICANCE OF VARYING MUSCLE FIBER LENGTH

Several physiological and mechanical studies have been published that may represent manifestations of the significant variability in muscle fiber length that occurs within a muscle and even between motor units of different types within a muscle. For example, significant differences between fast and slow motor unit stiffness was reported for the cat peroneus tertius muscle (Petit, Filippi, Emonet-Dénand, Hunt, & Laporte, 1990a; Petit, Filippi, Gioux, Hunt, & Laporte, 1990b). Numerous other studies of motor units had been performed in which contractile properties were measured under isometric conditions (Bodine, Roy, Eldred, & Edgerton, 1987; Burke, Levine, Tsairis, & Zajac, 1971; Gordon, Thomas, Stein, & Erdebil, 1988). It was previously shown that fast-contracting units (type FR and FF units) developed a higher tension and had lower endurance than slow units (type S units) within the same muscles. However, Petit et al. (Petit, et al., 1990) applied small rapid stretches to the activated motor units and measured motor unit stiffness rather than isometric tension. Stiffness was calculated as the change in force divided by the change in length. They found that, although the fast units generated higher absolute isometric forces compared with slow units, the slow units had a stiffness that was over twice that of the faster units. They subsequently demonstrated that the stiffness difference was indeed due to cross-bridge properties by applying a second stretch to the stable population of cross-bridges formed after the stretch (Petit et al., 1990b). Alternatively, it is possible that the stiffness difference between units is a manifestation of shorter fibers within slow units that would appear to be stiffer because they would undergo a greater strain for a given muscle deformation. In either case, the physiological effect of increased stiffness would be to provide increased

stability against small positional perturbations. Huijing and Baan (1992) measured the length-tension properties of motor unit populations recruited at different thresholds. They found that the width of the length-tension curves (which should be directly proportional to average fiber length) varied between low threshold and high threshold units again suggesting that motor units of different types may be composed of muscle fibers of different lengths. (The possibility exists that this phenomenon was confounded by alterations in stimulation frequency that can occur with the type of activation method used). Clearly, sophisticated mechanical studies of motor units are required to unravel the answers to such questions. These types of provocative results warrant further study and presents a considerable challenge to those who are currently generating biomechanical models of muscle. This is because whole muscles may have a level of organization that is much more complicated than presented in classic anatomy and physiology texts. Although molecular studies of muscle are justifiably increasing in popularity, excellent physiological studies of whole muscles are also necessary to clarify many of the issues raised above.

Motor Unit Recruitment

In the discussion of temporal summation, it was mentioned that the nervous system can vary muscle force output by varying the stimulation frequency to the muscle fibers. This phenomenon is termed temporal summation. However, muscle force can also be varied by changing the number of motor units that are active at a given time. For relatively low-force contractions, few motor units are activated, whereas for higher force contractions, more units are activated. The process by which motor units are added as muscle force increases is known as recruitment. What factors determine the point during a contraction that a motor unit is recruited?

FIGURE 2-21. Demonstration of orderly recruitment according to the size principle. As the muscle is passively stretched, axons of various sizes (labeled 1 to 5) are recruited. Continuous line across each trace represents muscle passive tension. As tension decreases (bottom panel) units drop out in the reverse order of recruitment. (Modified with permission from: Henneman, E., Somjen, G., & Carpenter, D. O. (1965). Functional significance of cell size in spinal motorneurons. *Journal of Neurophysiology, 28,* 560–580.)

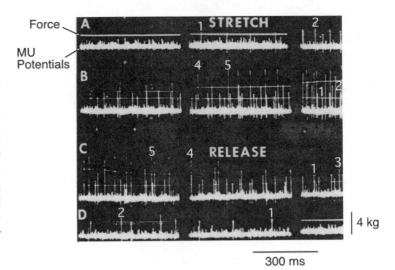

A classic study was performed in the 1960s by Dr. Elwood Henneman and colleagues (Henneman, Somjen, & Carpenter, 1965) whereby motoneuron electrical activity was measured as a muscle was slowly stretched, and therefore tension slowly increased. The increase in passive tension applied to a muscle caused more motor units to be recruited as shown in Figure 2-21 (Binder & Mendell, 1990). Henneman et al. found that, at very low forces, electrical spikes were observed on the nerve, which were very low in amplitude. (It was already known at the time that the amplitude of the spike is related to the size of the axon). As muscle force increased, the size of the spikes also increased in an orderly fashion. In other words, as force continued to increase, the units recruited always had increasingly larger spikes. The entire process was reversed as force decreased. Henneman and colleagues interpreted this result to mean that at low muscle force levels motor units with small axons were first recruited, and, as force increased, increasingly larger axons were recruited. This became known as the "size principle" and provided an anatomic basis for the orderly recruitment of motor units to produce a smooth contraction. Based on other studies, it was determined that generally, small motor axons innervated slow

motor units and larger motor axons innervated fast motor units. In fact, the FF units had the largest axons of all.

Human Voluntary Motor Unit Recruitment

Essentially all of the data presented above were obtained from animal studies of isolated motor units. What evidence is there that human motor unit properties and recruitment patterns are similar? Obviously, it is not possible to perform the identical surgical isolation of ventral roots for experiments in humans. However, one method has been developed to study human motor unit properties that have validated many of the results from animal studies.

In the early 1970s, Milner-Brown and his colleagues (Milner-Brown, Stein, & Yemm, 1973) developed an ingenious method for measuring the contractile properties of human motor units The experimental apparatus consisted of small needle electrodes placed in the muscle of interest, a force transducer placed on the joint of interest, and surface electrodes to measure muscle electrical activity (Fig. 2-22).

After placing the small electrodes in the muscle of interest, Milner-Brown et al., asked the subject to attempt to activate voluntarily a single motor unit! With a little practice and feedback, this task can be performed. During these low-level voluntary activations, motor unit spike trains were recorded from the intramuscular electrodes. As voluntary activation level increased, the size of the motor unit spikes also increased. However, the really slick part of the experiment was the manner in which the investigators "measured" motor unit tension. At very low contraction levels, the force recorded was a noisy force record—

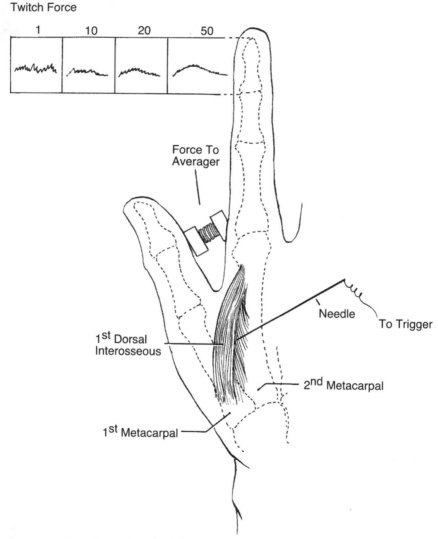

FIGURE 2-22. Experimental method for demonstration of human motor unit properties according to the spike-triggered averaging method. A needle is placed into the first dorsal interosseous muscle to record motor unit spikes and connect to a trigger. After each spike, finger abduction force is recorded. Many records are recorded and averaged (upper panels), which decrease background noise and reveal motor unit twitch tension. Number above each box represents number of traces averaged (from 1–50) to reveal twitch force.

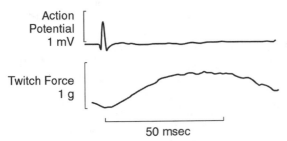

FIGURE 2-23. Single twitch recorded from human first dorsal interosseous muscle using spike-triggered averaging. Top record is the action potential and bottom record is averaged twitch record. Note that this twitch looks very much like that obtained from isolated muscle (c.f., bottom panel of Figure 2-2). (Reprinted with permission from: Milner-Brown, H. S., Stein, R. B., & Yemm, R. (1973). The contractile properties of human motor units during voluntary isometric contraction. *Journal of Physiology (London), 228,* 285–306.)

nothing like the smooth twitches recorded from animal motor units. Milner-Brown et al., thus synchronized the force recording with the intramuscular electrical spikes recorded. Thus each time a spike of a particular size was recorded, they triggered their force recording equipment to measure tension. As more and more spikes triggered the recording equipment, the force records were averaged to yield records that looked like muscle twitches (Fig. 2-23). This technique was named spike-triggered averaging for obvious reasons. Using this technique, it has also been shown that at low levels of voluntary effort, slow contracting motor units with low tensions are recruited. As effort increases, faster motor units with higher tensions are recruited (Fig. 2-24). Numerous subsequent experiments on a variety of muscles have essentially verified these initial studies. Thus, it appears that the size principle is applicable to human as well as animal subjects.

Using all of this information, the following scheme was proposed for the manner in which motor units are recruited voluntarily (Fig. 2-25): At very low exertion levels, the smallest axons (which have the lowest threshold to activation) are first activated. Most of these

small axons innervate SO muscle fibers within S units. As voluntary effort increases, most of the next-larger axons are recruited, which activates the FOG fibers belonging to FR units. Finally, during maximal efforts, the largest axons

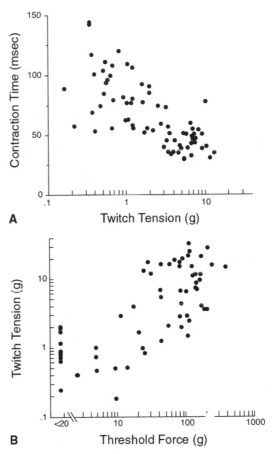

FIGURE 2-24. (A) Human motor unit twitch contraction time as a function of twitch tension recorded by spike-triggered averaging. Note that as contractile tension increases, contraction time decreases. This suggests that the motor units with larger tension have faster contractile speed, as predicted by the size principle. **(B)** Human motor unit twitch tension as a function of threshold voltage. As threshold increases, larger units are recruited, as predicted by the size principle. (Data from: Milner-Brown, H. S., Stein, R. B., & Yemm, R. (1973). The contractile properties of human motor units during voluntary isometric contraction. *Journal of Physiology (London), 228,* 285–306.)

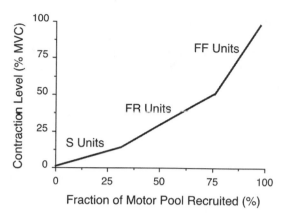

FIGURE 2-25. Schematic demonstration of predicted orderly recruitment of motor units during voluntary activity as a function of contractile force. At lower forces S units are recruited, while as force increases FR and FF units are recruited. Change in slope for each motor unit type represents the fact that different motor unit types generate different forces. (Redrawn from: Edgerton, V. R., Roy, R. R., Bodine, S. C., and Sacks, R. D. (1983). *The matching of neuronal and muscular physiology* (pp. 51–69) in: *Human Muscle Power.* Illiniois: Human Kinetics Publishers.

are activated, most of which innervate FG fibers and make up FF units. An appealing aspect of this hypothesis is that the units most often activated (S units) are those with the greatest endurance. The FF units, which are rarely activated, have the lowest endurance. In addition, the S units develop the lowest tension, and thus as contractions begin, low tensions are generated. This provides a mechanism for smoothly increasing tension as first S, then FR, and then FF units are recruited. This exquisite interrelationship of anatomic specialization and physiologic function is just one more structure-function relationship, which is the hallmark of the neuromuscular system.

Physiologic Basis of Fatigue

Nearly everyone is familiar with the feeling of muscle fatigue following prolonged exercise. However, a strict definition of fatigue has been more difficult to establish. This is due, in part,

to the complex nature of voluntary contractions themselves. At least three major components are involved in the production of voluntary contractions (Fig. 2-26): the CNS, the peripheral nerve and neuromuscular junction, and the skeletal muscles. A priori any one of these systems might be involved in the fatigue process. Several of the classic fatigue studies that add to your current understanding of muscle fatigue will be examined.

Intuitively, it is obvious that low forces can be maintained longer than high forces. In fact, this relationship was quantified for several human muscles (Rohmert, 1960). Subjects were asked to maintain a target force ranging from 5 to 100% of their maximum voluntary contraction (MVC) level. For contraction levels less than 15% MVC, subjects could maintain the target level indefinitely (>45 minutes). However, as the target force increased, endurance time rapidly decreased (Fig. 2-27). How can these changes in endurance time be ex-

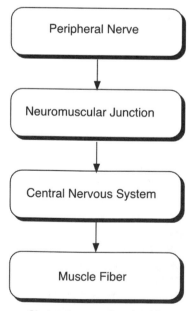

FIGURE 2-26. Chain of events involved in normal contraction and potential sites for fatigue. Contractile force can decrease if any portion of this chain, from the peripheral nerve to the muscle fiber is interrupted.

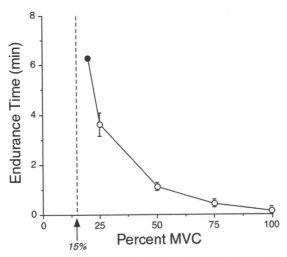

FIGURE 2-27. Relationship between endurance time and contraction intensity (% MVC). Note that forces lower than approximately 15% MVC can be maintained indefinitely (here defined as >45 min). As force increases, endurance time rapidly decreases. (Data replotted from: Rohmert, W. (1960). Ermittung von Erholung-spausen für statische Arbeit des Menschen. *Physiologist, 18*, 123–130.)

plained? Why does muscle force decrease? Which of the different systems (Fig. 2-26) changes in response to prolonged contraction?

Substrate Depletion in Fatigue

ATP is the immediate energy source for force generation in muscle. However, under normal conditions, skeletal muscle only contains enough ATP to fuel two or three maximal contractions! What happens as ATP levels suddenly drop following contraction? An ATP regenerating system is present in muscle that is composed of the high-energy molecule creatine phosphate and the enzyme creatine phosphokinase (CK). Immediately after ATP depletion begins, it is replenished according to the reaction

$$\text{Creatine Phosphate} + \text{ADP} \rightarrow \text{Creatine} + \text{ATP} \quad \text{(Eq. 2-18)}$$

which is catalyzed by CK. As contraction proceeds, ATP levels remain relatively constant while creatine phosphate levels steadily drop (Bergstrom, 1967). The greater the workload, the greater the decrease in creatine phosphate.

As cellular ATP levels continue to drop, cellular glycogen and fat are mobilized to replenish energy stores. The relative degree of glycogen and fat mobilized depends largely on the intensity of the exercise and the capability of the muscle fiber.

In an experimental investigation of glycogen metabolism, the Scandinavian physician Dr. Eric Hultman measured glycogen content in muscle biopsies obtained from the vastus lateralis muscles of cross-country skiers (Hultman, 1967). Hultman found, as expected, that as exercise proceeded, muscle glycogen levels dropped dramatically. In fact, the amount of time these skiers could pedal a bicycle ergometer at an intense level was directly related to the amount of glycogen in their muscles (Fig. 2-28A). He also found that, following glycogen depletion, if the subjects were fed a high-carbohydrate diet, the amount of glycogen restored in the muscle actually exceeded the original amount. This overshoot was not seen if subjects were fed a high fat and protein diet following glycogen depletion (Fig. 2-28B). The overshoot was also not seen in the contralateral leg, which indicates that the "control" of glycogen storage was at the level of the muscle and not something that would affect all muscles in the body. In intense anaerobic exercise, substrate availability can thus limit performance.

Fatigue Mechanisms

However, when muscle force declines, how can you be sure that the central drive from the CNS has not decreased? In a now classic study, Merton measured muscle force decline during fatiguing contractions (Merton, 1954). He was interested in addressing this question of whether muscle force declined because of a decrease in drive or intensity from the CNS (*i.e.*, CNS fatigue). To answer this question, periodically during the person's voluntary effort, Merton superimposed a massive electrical stimulation onto the voluntary contraction. He hypothesized that if muscle force decreased because of CNS fatigue, that electrical stimulation superimposed on the voluntary contraction

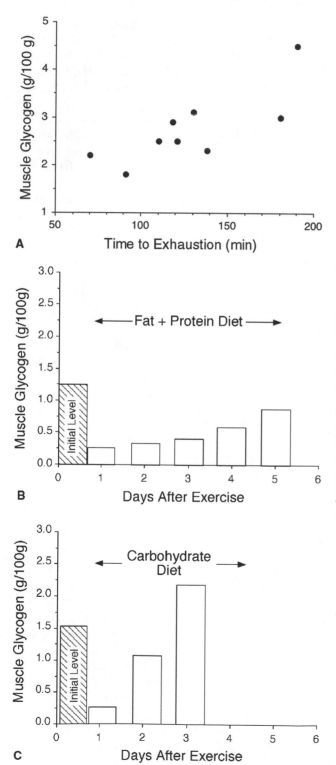

FIGURE 2-28. (A) Relationship between muscle glycogen content and endurance time for intense bicycle ergometry. Increased muscle glycogen enables greater exercise time before exhaustion occurs. **(B)** Muscle glycogen content before exercise (hatched bar) and after exercise following a fat with protein diet (open bar). **(C)** Muscle glycogen content before exercise (hatched bar) and after exercise following a carbohydrate only diet (open bar). Note that after exercise and a high carbohydrate diet, muscles store more glycogen than prior to exercise while a fat + protein diet results in glycogen levels below the original level even for six days. (Modified from: Hultman, E. (1967). Physiological role of muscle glycogen in man, with special reference to exercise. *Circulation Research, 21*, I99–I112.)

would increase muscle force. In fact, no force increase was observed, and Merton concluded that CNS fatigue was not the cause for the muscle fatigue. This type of experiment has been confirmed by others, and it is generally agreed that muscle fatigue in highly motivated, trained subjects is not due to CNS fatigue.

Similar experiments have been performed to determine whether fatigue of the neuromuscular junction or sarcolemma occurs during muscle fatigue. In these experiments, during fatiguing MVCs, electrical stimuli were again superimposed and the muscle mass action potential measured (i.e., the M-wave). Brenda Bigland-Ritchie and her colleagues (Bigland-Ritchie, Kukulka, Lippold, & Woods, 1982) demonstrated that almost no change in the M-wave occurred in spite of the force decrease. These data suggested that the weak link in fatigue was also not the neuromuscular junction or muscle sarcolemma. A subsequent experimental and theoretical study has provided even stronger support for this assertion (Fuglevand, Zackowski, Huey, & Enoka, 1993). Finally, it should be noted that yet another report performed in a different muscle group did not support the original report (Macefield, Fuglevand, Howell, & Bigland-Ritchie, 2000). Thus, this might not be a general fatigue property of all muscles.

Fatigue in Isolated Nerve-Muscle Preparations

In contrast to human studies, many investigators have studied the behavior of the muscle action potential and muscle force during repetitive electrical stimulation to the point of fatigue in isolated nerve-muscle preparations (Pagala, Namba, & Grob, 1984). Experimentally, muscles are indirectly stimulated via the motor nerve and muscle force and action potential are measured. Several investigators have shown that during muscular fatigue, force and M-wave changes do not follow the same time course. For example, at moderate stimulation frequencies (e.g., 30 Hz), muscle force declines faster than the action potential, which

suggests that both excitation and contraction can be altered during fatigue (refer to the above discussion of excitation-contraction coupling). However, it is not clear that these same mechanisms are functionally significant during voluntary activity in humans. These studies do emphasize that the fatigue process may involve several different links in the neuromotor chain.

Neuromotor Control and Muscle Fatigue

Recently, Bigland-Ritchie and her colleagues (Bigland-Ritchie, Johansson, Lippold, & Woods, 1983a; Bigland-Ritchie, Johansson, Lippold, Smith, & Woods, 1983b) succeeded in measuring single muscle fiber action potentials in human adductor pollicis longus muscles (Table 1-1) during MVCs. They found that as muscle force declined during the MVC, the average motor unit firing rate decreased from approximately 30 Hz to approximately 15 Hz (Fig. 2-29). However, based on the previous discussion of temporal summation (See page 50), will decreased firing frequency result in decreased muscle force? Interestingly, these investigators hypothesized a reasonable neuromotor control strategy for such a frequency decrease. By measuring the time course of the muscle twitch during fatigue, they found that the muscle contracted and relaxed more slowly, with the time-to-peak tension (TPT) and half-relaxation time (HRT) dramatically increasing. What would be the effect of muscle slowing? Slower muscles generate higher forces at lower frequencies because the muscle is not able to keep up with the incoming impulses, much as a slow-contracting muscle shows tetanic fusion at lower frequencies than a fast muscle. Therefore, if firing rate decreased and TPT and HRT increased, the net effect would be to maintain approximately the same degree of fusion in the contractile record. It is as if the nervous system has a feedback system that senses the muscle speed and drives it with the appropriate stimulation frequency. Support for this idea was obtained by comparing the average firing rate of fast muscles (e.g., biceps brachii) to

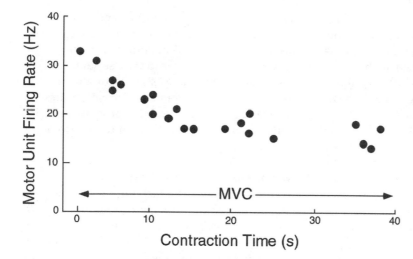

FIGURE 2-29. Motor unit firing frequency during maximal voluntary activation of the adductor pollicis longus muscle. As fatigue occurs, firing rate decreases. (Modified from: Bigland-Ritchie, B., Johansson, R., Loppold, O., Smith, S., & Woods, J. (1983). Changes in motoneurone firing rates during sustained maximal voluntary contractions. *Journal of Physiology (London), 340,* 335–346.)

slow muscles (*e.g.,* soleus). They found that although the biceps muscle motor unit firing rate was approximately 31 Hz, the soleus firing rate was only about 10 Hz. These firing rates varied in proportion to the relative speeds of the two muscles, providing support for the idea that firing rates are tailored to muscle contractile properties.

The Electromyogram

The Electromyogram—An Electrical Activation Signal

At this point, you might be wondering how these various neuromuscular components function in daily activities, not simply involuntary isometric contractions under experimental conditions. Before moving onto that exciting topic, you should first understand a measurement often made from muscles to understand their normal function. This measurement is the electromyogram (EMG).

Recall from the discussion of excitation-contraction coupling that each time a muscle fiber is activated, an action potential is conducted from the nerve, along the muscle and into the fiber. Thus an electrical signal is emitted by the muscle fiber during each activation. If a suitable receiver is placed near the fiber (for example, an EMG electrode), this electrical ac-

tivity can be measured (Fig. 2-30A). This receiver is usually a small needle electrode that acts as an antenna to record local electrical activity. As such, the raw EMG signal is useful to determine when a particular muscle is active. In fact, one of the best uses for the EMG is to determine the relative timing of muscle activation during gait (discussed in Chapter 3). Some have taken the measurement of EMG a step further—EMG quantification.

Quantifying the EMG

If the raw EMG signal is observed, it is difficult to quantify the activity of the muscle. Theoretically at least, the EMG contains electrical signals from every muscle fiber in the vicinity of the EMG electrode. Can this be counted? Again, theoretically, it has been shown that it is reasonable to process the EMG signal into a "rectified, integrated" signal that is more easily managed than the raw signal. The rectification step converts the EMG record into one that contains only positive voltages (Fig. 2-30B). The integration step electrically "adds up" all of these separate spikes to yield a number proportional to all of the spikes generated (Fig. 2-30B). Recently, Drs. Carl Gans and Jerry Loeb (Loeb & Gans, 1986) have presented an excellent discussion of practical EMG measurement methods. In addition, Drs. John Basmajian and Carlo DeLuca (Basmajian &

DeLuca, 1985) have provided a comprehensive review of the electrical activity of different muscles during various movements as well as many theoretical aspects of EMG measurement. Most of these discussions are a compromise between experimental and theoretical considerations.

EMG-Force Relationship

Much has been written about the predictability and reliability of the EMG-force relationship. There is general agreement on the utility of the EMG as an indicator of the activation pattern for a motor pool. However, it should be recognized that the EMG cannot be uniquely related

> ### Box 2-9. Can EMG Measure Muscle Force?
>
> The electromyogram (EMG) provides only an "interferogram" that represents the summated electrical activation pattern of the muscle near the electrode. Since muscle force is highly dependent on length (due to the length-tension property) and velocity (due to the force-velocity property), electrical activity alone cannot possibly provide an accurate measurement of muscle force. In addition, since the EMG summates in a way that does not uniquely represent all of the motor units activated, EMG measurements that are used to infer force are *highly* suspect.

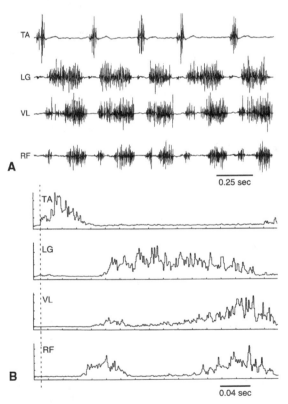

FIGURE 2-30. **(A)** Raw electromyograms obtained from rat leg muscles at a slow walking speed. Note that muscles fire cyclically and relatively regularly during these five cycles. **(B)** Data from panel **(A)** rectified and averaged over the five cycles. This processed EMG permits description of the "typical" muscle activation signal. (Experimental records courtesy of Dr. Roland R. Roy, University of California, Los Angeles).

to muscle force. For example, suppose the EMG is measured from a muscle that is shortening at 5% V_{max}. The force generated by this muscle will be approximately 75% P_o. However, the EMG from the same muscle might be measured under conditions in which it is shortening at only 1% V_{max}. In this case, much more tension will be generated (90% P_o versus 75% P_o) because of the slower contraction velocity, but the EMG signal will be the same. The take-home lesson is, an EMG can give you information regarding muscle activation patterns but be careful when interpreting an EMG record in terms of muscle force. In isometric or perfectly eccentric or concentric conditions, forces might be estimated, but otherwise, correlating EMG with muscle forces is difficult.

One especially clear demonstration of potential problems of EMG interpretation was presented in a theoretical model by Dr. Roger Enoka and colleagues (Yao, Fuglevand, & Enoka, 2000). In their study, the EMG interference pattern was created mathematically by summation of the electrical activity of ten hypothetical motor units. One parameter that they investigated was the level of synchrony that occurred between the motor units. In their model, high synchrony occurred when two motor units were activated at the same time and low synchrony occurred when two motor units were activated at random times. They

---

Therapist's Comments

One common application of EMG used is in the context of biofeedback. In this case, the EMG is simply used as an indicator that a certain muscle has been "fired." Small, commercially available device permit visual or auditory feedback so that the patient can "relearn" to activate a muscle after disease or disuse. One common application of the EMG for biofeedback is the relearning of activation in the vastus medialis obliques after anterior cruciate ligament surgery. The EMG that is discussed in this chapter is the kinesiological EMG and is primarily used as a research tool.

---

their physiologic properties. Motor units are recruited generally in an orderly fashion according to Henneman's size principle. Although the size of a unit can be estimated in several ways, the order of recruitment seems to be closely matched with the unit's maximum tetanic tension. The next chapter will synthesize much of this information in a form relevant to normal movement.

found that when synchrony was high, EMG signal was high because most of the electrical signals added (Fig. 2-31). However, when synchrony was low, the EMG signal was lower due to cancellation of the individual action potentials. Degree of synchrony had a small effect on force production magnitude. This simulation is just one more example of why EMG measurements must be made carefully and interpreted appropriately to gain insight into muscle function.

■ Chapter Summary

Skeletal muscle is activated sequentially by the process known as excitation-contraction coupling. Muscle force is generated by the cyclic interaction between actin and myosin, using ATP as the direct energy source. Isometric muscle force varies with length as explained by the length-tension curve. The force-velocity relationship describes isotonic behavior, muscle contraction velocity at constant load. Muscle fiber types and motor units come in three general types that can be characterized physiologically and histochemically. The properties of the fibers that make up the various motor unit types generally follow logically from knowledge of

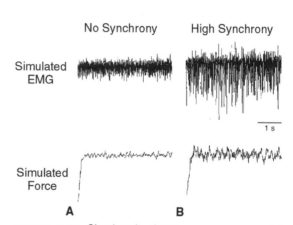

FIGURE 2-31. Simulated electromyograms created based on assumptions regarding motor unit homogeneity and synchronization of action potentials between units. **(A)** Electromyogram (EMG, upper panel) based on the assumption that motor units fire completely independently along with calculated force (lower panel). In this case, action potentials tend to cancel one another out and the summated EMG is smaller compared to the case when units are synchronized. **(B)** Electromyogram (EMG, upper panel) based on the assumption that motor units fire synchronously 20–30% of the time independently along with calculated force (lower panel). In this case, action potentials tend to summate and the summated EMG is larger compared to the case when units fire completely randomly relative to one another. Modified from: Yao, W., Fugelvand, R.J., Enoka, R.M. (2000). Motor unit synchronization increases EMG amplitude and decreases force steadiness of simulated contractions. *Journal of Neurophysiology 83,* 441–452.

REFERENCES

American Type Culture Collection (ATCC), Manassas, VA 20110.

Barany, M. (1967). ATPase activity of myosin correlated with speed of muscle shortening. *Journal of General Physiology, 50,* 197–216.

Baratta, R.V., Solomonow, M., Nguyen, G., D'Ambrosia, R. (2000). Characterization of load-length-velocity relationships of nine different skeletal muscles. *Journal of Biomechanics, 33,* 381–385.

Basmajian, J.V., DeLuca, C.J., (1985). *Muscles Alive. Their Functions Revealed by Electromyography.* Baltimore, MD: Williams & Wilkins.

Bergstrom, J. (1967). Local changes of ATP and phosphorylcreatine in human muscle tissue in connection with exercise. *Circulation Research, 21,* 191–198.

Bigland-Ritchie, B., Johansson, R., Lippold, O., Woods, J.J. (1983). Contractile speed and EMG changes during fatigue of sustained maximal voluntary contractions. *Journal of Neurophysiology, 50,* 313–324.

Bigland-Ritchie, B., Johansson, R., Lippold, O., Smith, S., Woods, J. (1983). Changes in motoneurone firing rates during sustained maximal voluntary contractions. *Journal of Physiology (London), 340,* 335–346.

Bigland-Ritchie, B., Kukulka, C.G., Lippold, C.J., Woods, J.J. (1982). The absence of neuromuscular transmission failure in sustained maximal voluntary contractions. *Journal of Physiology (London), 330,* 265–278.

Binder, M.D., Mendell, L.M. (1990). *The segmental motor system.* New York, NY: Oxford University Press.

Bodine, S.C., Roy, R.R., Eldred, E., Edgerton, V.R. (1987). Maximal force as a function of anatomical features of motor units in the cat tibialis anterior. *Journal of Neurophysiology, 6,* 1730–1745.

Bottinelli, R., Betto, R., Schiaffino, S., Reggiani, C. (1994). Unloaded shortening velocity and myosin heavy chain and alkali light chain isoform composition in rat skeletal muscle fibres. *Journal of Physiology (London), 478,* 341–349.

Bottinelli, R., Schiaffino, S., Reggiani, C. (1991). Force-velocity relations and myosin heavy chain isoform compositions of skinned fibres from rat skeletal muscle. *Journal of Physiology (London), 437,* 655–672.

Brooke, M.H., Kaiser, K.K. (1970). Muscle fiber types: how many and what kind? *Archives of Neurology, 23,* 369–379.

Burke, R.E. (1967). Motor unit types of cat triceps surae muscle. *Journal of Physiology (London), 193,* 141–160.

Burke, R.E. (1981). Motor units: anatomy, physiology, and functional organization. In L. D. Peachey (Ed.) *Handbook of physiology* (pp. 345–422). Bethesda, MD: American Physiology Society.

Burke, R.E., Levine, D.N., Tsairis, P., Zajac, F.E. (1973). Physiological types and histochemical profiles in motor units of the cat gastrocnemius. *Journal of Physiology (London), 234,* 723–748.

Burke, R.E., Levine, D.N., Zajac, F.E., Tsairis, P., Engel, W.K. (1971). Mammalian motor units: physiological-histochemical correlation in three types in cat gastrocnemius. *Science, 174,* 709–712.

Close, R.I. (1972). Dynamic properties of mammalian skeletal muscles. *Physiological Reviews, 52,* 129–197.

Dubowitz, V., Brooke, M.H. (1973). *Muscle Biopsy: A Modern Approach.* Philadelphia: W.B. Saunders.

Ebashi, S., Maruyama, K., Endo, M. (1980). Muscle contraction: Its regulatory mechanisms. New York: Springer Verlag

Edman, K. (1966). The relation between sarcomere length and active tension in isolated semitendinosus fibres of the frog. *Journal of Physiology (London), 183,* 407–417.

Edstrom, L., Kugelberg, E. (1968). Histochemical composition, distribution of fibers and fatigability of single motor units. *Journal of Neurology, Neurosurgery, and Psychiatry, 31,* 424–433.

Eisenberg, B.R. (1983). Quantitative ultrastructure of mammalian skeletal muscle. In L. D. Peachey, Adrian, R.H., and Geiger, S.R., (Ed.). *Skeletal Muscle. Vol. 10* (pp. 73–112). Baltimore, MD: American Physiological Society.

Entman, M.L., Van Winkle, W.B. (1986). *Sarcoplasmic Reticulum in Muscle Physiology.* Boca Raton, FL: C.R.C.Press.

Finer, J.T., Simmons, R.M., Spudich, J.A. (1994). Single myosin molecule mechanics: piconewton forces and nanometre steps. *Nature, 368,* 113–119.

Fuglevand, A.J., Zackowski, K.M., Huey, K.A., Enoka, R.M. (1993). Impairment of neuromuscular propagation during human fatiguing contractions at submaximal forces. *Journal of Physiology (London), 460,* 549–572.

Gillespie, C.A., Simpson, D.R., Edgerton, V.R. (1970). High glycogen content of red as opposed to white skeletal muscle fibers of guinea pigs. *Journal of Histochemistry and Cytochemistry, 18,* 552–558.

Goldman, Y.E. (1987). Kinetics of the actomyosin ATPase in muscle fibers. *Annual Review of Physiology, 49,* 637–654.

Gonzalez-Serratos, H. (1971). Inward spread of activation in vertebrate muscle fibers. *Journal of Physiology (London), 212,* 777–799.

Gordon, A.M., Huxley, A.F., Julian, F.J. (1966). Tension development in highly stretched vertebrate muscle fibres. *Journal of Physiology (London), 184,* 143–169.

Gordon, A.M., Huxley, A.F., Julian, F.J. (1966). The variation in isometric tension with sarcomere length in vertebrate muscle fibres. *Journal of Physiology (London), 184,* 170–192.

Gordon, T., Thomas, C.K., Stein, R.B., Erdebil, S. (1988). Comparison of physiological and histochemical properties of motor units after cross-reinnervation of antagonistic muscles in the cat hindlimb. *Journal of Neurophysiology, 60,* 365–378.

Harry, J.D., Ward, A.W., Heglund, N.C., Morgan, D.L., McMahon, T.A. (1990). Cross-bridge cycling theories cannot explain high-speed lengthening behavior in frog muscle. *Biophysical Journal, 57,* 201–208.

Haselgrove, J.C. (1983). Structure of vertebrate striated muscle as determined by x-ray-diffraction studies. In *Handbook of physiology* (pp. 143–171). Bethesda, MD: American Physiological Society.

Hellam, D.C., Podolsky, R.J. (1969). Force measurements in skinned muscle fibres. *Journal of Physiology (London), 200,* 807-819.

Henneman, E., Somjen, G., Carpenter, D.O. (1965). Functional significance of cell size in spinal motorneurons. *Journal of Neurophysiology, 28,* 560–580.

Hill, A.V. (1938). The heat of shortening and the dynamic constants of muscle. Proceedings of the Royal Society of London Series B: *Biological Sciences (London), 126,* 136–195.

Hill, A.V. (1964). The effect of load on the heat of shortening of muscle. Proceedings of the Royal Society of London Series B: *Biological Sciences (London), 159,* 297–318.

Hill, A.V. (1970). First and Last Experiments in Muscle Mechanics. New York, NY: Cambridge University Press.

Hoffer, J.A., Loeb, G.E., Marks, W.B., O'donovan, M.J., Pratt, C.A., Sugano, N. (1987). Cat hindlimb motoneurons during locomotion. I. destination, axonal conduction velocity, and recruitment threshold. *Journal of Neurophysiology, 57,* 510–573.

Hoffer, J.A., O'donovan, M.J., Pratt, C.A, Loeb, G.E. (1981). Discharge patterns of hindlimb motorneurons during normal cat locomotion. *Science, 213,* 466–468.

Horowits, R. (1999). The physiological role of titin in striated muscle. *Reviews of Physiology, Biochemistry, and Pharmacology, 138,* 57–96.

Horowits, R., Kempner, E.S., Bisher, M.E., Podolsky, R.J. (1986). A physiological role for titin and nebulin in skeletal muscle. *Nature, 323,* 160–164.

Huijing, P.A. (1996). Important experimental factors for skeletal muscle modelling: non- linear changes of muscle length force characteristics as a function of degree of activity. *European Journal of Morphology, 34,* 47–54.

Huijing, P.A., Baan, G.C. (1992). Stimulation level-dependent length-force and architectural characteristics of rat gastrocnemius muscle. *Journal of Electromyography and Kinesiology, 2,* 112–120.

Hultman, E. (1967). Physiological role of muscle glycogen in man, with special reference to exercise. *Circulation Research, 21,* I199–I112.

Huxley, A.F. (1957). Muscle structure and theories of contraction. *Progress in Biophysics and Molecular Biology, 7,* 255–318.

Huxley, A.F., Simmons, R.M. (1971). Proposed mechanism of force generation in vertebrate striated muscle. *Nature, 233,* 533–538.

Huxley, H.E. (1969). The mechanism of muscular contraction. *Science (Washington DC), 164,* 1356–1366.

Katz B. (1939). The relation between force and speed in muscular contraction. *Journal of Physiology (London), 96,* 45–64.

Labeit, S., Kolmerer, B. (1995). Titins: Giant proteins in charge of muscle ultrastructure and elasticity. *Science, 270,* 293–296.

Lieber, R.L., Raab, R., Kashin, S., Edgerton, V.R. (1992). Sarcomere length changes during fish swimming. *Journal of Experimental Biology, 169,* 251–254.

Loeb, G.E., Gans, C. (1986). Electromyography for experimentalists. Chicago: University of Chicago Press.

Loeb, G.E., Pratt, C.A., Chanaud, C.M., Richmond, F.J.R. (1987). Distribution and innervation of short, interdigitated muscle fibers in parallel-fibered muscles of the cat hindlimb. *Journal of Morphology, 191,* 1–15.

Lutz, G.J., Cuizon, D.B., Ryan, A.F., Lieber, R.L. (1998). Four novel myosin heavy chain transcripts in Rana pipiens single muscle fibres define a molecular basis for muscle fibre types in the frog. *Journal of Physiology (London), 508,* 667–680.

Lymn, R.W., Taylor, E.W. (1971). Mechanism of adenosine triphosphate hydrolysis by actomyosin. *Biochemistry, 10,* 4617–4624.

Macefield, V.G., Fuglevand, A.J., Howell, J.N., Bigland-Ritchie, B. (2000). Discharge behaviour of single motor units during maximal voluntary contractions of a human toe extensor. *Journal of Physiology (London), 528,* 227–234.

Magid, A., Law, D.J. (1985). Myofibrils bear most of the resting tension in frog skeletal muscle. *Science, 230,* 1280–1282.

Martin, T.P., Bodine-Fowler, S., Roy, R.R., Eldred, E., Edgerton, V.R. (1988). Metabolic and fiber size properties of cat tibialis anterior motor units. *American Journal of Physiology, 255,* C43–C50.

Martin, T.P., Vailas, A.C., Durivage, J.B., Edgerton, V.R., Castleman, K.R. (1985). Quantitative histochemical determination of muscle enzymes: biochemical verification. *Journal of Histochemistry and Cytochemistry, 33,* 1053–1059.

Maruyama, K., Gergely, J.(1962) Interaction of actomyosin with adenosine triphosphate at low ionic strength: dissociation of actomyosin during the clear phase. *Journal of Biological Chemistry, 237,* 1095–1099.

McCray, J.A., Herbette, L., Kihara, T., Trentham, D.R. (1980). A new approach to time-resolved studies of ATP-requiring biological systems: laser flash photolysis of caged ATP. *Proceeding of the National Academy of Sciences of the United States of America, 77,* 7237–7241.

Mehta, A.D., Finer, J.T., Spudich, J.A. (1997). Detection of single-molecule interactions using correlated thermal diffusion. *Proceedings of the National Academy of Sciences of the United States of America, 94,* 7927–7931.

Merton, P.A. (1954). Voluntary strength and fatigue. *Journal of Physiology, 123,* 553–564.

Milner-Brown, H.S., Stein, R.B., Yemm, R.(1973). The contractile properties of human motor units during voluntary isometric contraction. *Journal of Physiology (London), 228,* 285–306.

Morgan, D.L. (1990). New insights into the behavior of muscle during active lengthening. *Biophysical Journal, 57,* 209–221.

Moss, R.L. (1979). Sarcomere length-tension relations of frog skinned muscle fibers during calcium activation at short lengths. *Journal of Physiology (London), 292,* 177–192.

Nardone, A., Romano, C., Schieppati, M. (1989). Selective recruitment of high-threshold human motor units during voluntary isotonic lengthening of active muscles. *Journal of Physiology (London), 409,* 451–471.

Ounjian, M., Roy, R.R., Eldred, E., Garfinkel, A., Payne, J.R., Armstrong, A., Toga, A.W., Edgerton, V.R. (1991). Physiological and developmental implications of motor unit anatomy. *Journal of Neurobiology, 22,* 517–559.

Pagala, M., Namba, T., Grob, D. (1984). Failure of neuromuscular transmission and contractility during muscle fatigue. *Muscle and Nerve, 7,* 454–464.

Peachey, L.D., Franzini-Armstrong, C. (1983). Structure and function of membrane systems of skeletal muscle cells. In *Handbook of Physiology* (pp. 23–73). Baltimore, MD: American Physiological Society.

Peter, J.B., Barnard, R.J., Edgerton, V.R., Gillespie, C.A., Stempel, K.E. (1972). Metabolic profiles on three fiber types of skeletal muscle in guinea pigs and rabbits. *Biochemistry, 11,* 2627–2733.

Petit, J., Filippi, G.M., Emonet-Dènand, C., Hunt, C.C., Laporte, Y. (1990). Changes in muscle stiffness produced by motor units of different types in peroneus longus muscles of cat. *Journal of Neurophysiology, 63,* 190–197.

Petit, J., Filippi, G.M., Gioux, C., Hunt, C.C., Laporte, Y. (1990). Effects of tetanic contraction of motor units of similar type on the initial stiffness to ramp stretch of the cat peroneus longus muscle. *Journal of Neurophysiology, 64,* 1724–1731.

Podolsky, R.J., Shoenberg, M. (1983). Force generation and shortening in skeletal muscle. In *Handbook of physiology* (pp. 173–187). Baltimore, MD: American Physiological Society.

Rack, P.M.H., Westbury, D.R. (1969). The effects of length and stimulus rate on tension in the isometric cat soleus muscle. *Journal of Physiology (London), 204,* 443–460.

Ramsey, R.W., Street, S.F. (1940). The isometric length-tension diagram of isolated skeletal muscle fibers of the frog. *Journal of Cell and Comparative Physiology, 15,* 11–34.

Rayment, I., Holden, H.M., Whittaker, M., Yohn, C.B., Lorenz, M., Holmes, K.C., Milligan, R.A. (1993a). Structure of the actin-myosin complex and its implications for muscle contraction. *Science, 261,* 58–65.

Rayment, I., Rypniewski, W.R., Schmidt-Base, K., Smith, R., Tomchick, D.R., Benning M.M., Winkelmann, D.A., Wesenberg, G., Holden, H.M. (1993b). Three-dimensional structure of myosin subfragment-1: a molecular motor. *Science, 261,* 50–58.

Rohmert, W. (1960). Ermittlung von Erholungspausen für statische Arbeit des Menschen. *Physiologist, 18,* 123–130.

Rome, L.C., Klimov, A.A. (2000). Superfast contractions without superfast energetics: ATP usage by SR- Ca2+ pumps and crossbridges in toadfish swimbladder muscle. *Journal of Physiology (London), 526,* 279–286.

Rome, L.C., Swank, D., Corda, D. (1993). How fish power swimming. *Science, 261,* 340–343.

Schiaffino, S., Gorza, L., Sartore, S., Saggin, L., Vianello, M., Gundersen. K., Lømo, T. (1989). Three myosin heavy chain isoforms in type 2 skeletal muscle fibers. *Journal of Muscle Research and Cell Motility, 10,* 197–205.

Schiaffino, S., Reggiani, C. (1996). Molecular diversity of myofibrillar proteins: gene regulation and functional significance. *Physiological Reviews, 76,* 371–423.

Simmons, R.M., Finer, J..T, Chu, S., Spudich, J.A. (1996). Quantitative measurements of force and displacement using an optical trap. *Biophysical Journal, 70,* 1813–1822.

Sjöström, M., Ängquist, K.A., Bylund, A.C., Fridén, J., Gustavsson, L., Schersten, T. (1982). Morphometric analysis of human muscle fibre types. *Muscle and Nerve, 5,* 538–553.

Smerdu, V., Karsch-Mizrachi, I., Campione, M., Leinwand, L., Schiaffino, S. (1994). Type IIx myosin heavy chain transcripts are expressed in type IIb fibers of human skeletal muscle. *American Journal of Physiology, 267,* C1723–C1728.

Spudich, J.A. (1994). How molecular motors work. *Nature, 372,* 515–518.

Street, SF. (1983) Lateral transmission of tension in frog myofibers: a myofibrillar network and transverse cytoskeletal connections are possible transmitters. *Journal of Cellular Physiology, 114,* 346–364.

Szent-Gyorgi, A.G. (1953). Meromyosins, the subunits of myosin. *Archives of Biochemistry and Biophysics, 42,* 305–320.

Taylor, S.R., Rüdel, R. (1970). Striated muscle fibers: inactivation of contraction induced by shortening. *Science, 167,* 882–884.

Thornell LE, Sjöström M, Ringqvist M. (1976). Attempts to correlate histochemical and ultrastructural features of individual skeletal muscle fibers. *Journal of Ultrastructural Research, 57,* 224–224.

Tidball, J.G., Daniel, T.L. (1986). Myotendinous junctions of tonic muscle cells: structure and loading. *Cell and Tissue Research, 245,* 315–322.

Trotter, J.A. (1990). Interfiber tension transmission in series-fibered muscles of the cat hindlimb. *Journal of Morphology, 206,* 351–361.

Trotter, J.A., Corbett, K., Avner, B.P. (1981). Structure and function of the murine muscle-tendon junction. *Anatomical Record, 201,* 293–302.

Trotter, J.A., Eberhard, S., Samora, A. (1983). Structural connections of the muscle-tendon junction. *Cell Motility and the Cytoskeleton, 3,* 431–438.

Trotter, J.A., Purslow, P.P. (1992). Functional morphology of the endomysium in series fibered muscles. *Journal of Morphology, 212,* 109–122.

Uyeda, T.Q., Abramson, P.D., Spudich, J.A. (1996). The neck region of the myosin motor domain acts as a lever arm to generate movement. *Proceedings of the National Academy of Sciences of the United States of America, 93,* 4459–4464.

Wang, K., McCarter, R., Wright, J., Beverly, J., Ramirez-Mitchell, R. (1993). Viscoelasticity of the sarcomere matrix of skeletal muscles. The titin-myosin composite filament is a dual-stage molecular spring. *Biophysical Journal, 64,* 1161–1177.

Webb, M.R., Trentham, D.R.(1983). Chemical mechanism of myosin-catalyzed ATP hydrolysis. In L.D. Peachey (Ed.). *Handbook of physiology* (pp. 237–255). Baltimore, MD: American Physiological Society.

Yao, W., Fuglevand, R.J., Enoka, R.M. (2000). Motor-unit synchronization increases EMG amplitude and decreases force steadiness of simulated contractions. *Journal of Neurophysiology, 83,* 441–452.

Zappe, H.A., Maeda, Y. (1985). X-ray diffraction study of fast and slow mammalian skeletal muscle in the live relaxed state. *Journal of Molecular Biology, 185,* 211–214.

CHAPTER 3

The Production of Movement

Chapter Overview

In this chapter, the anatomy and physiology of nerves and muscles that were presented in the previous two chapters come alive. You will see how these systems, along with tendons and bones, produce movement. This chapter will begin with a discussion of the basic components of the movement generating system: the muscles, skeleton, and tendons. Then these components are pieced together to describe how movement is produced. One of the lessons of this section is that the interaction between muscles, tendons, and joints is complex. This lesson is relevant to the determination of strength and range of motion and has implications for physical examination and therapy. This is the home stretch of the basic science portion of the text and is also probably the most unique chapter of the text.

Educational Objectives

- To be able to define stress and strain as it applies to biological tissues.
- To be able to define torque in terms of force and moment arm.
- To be able to define the relationship between anatomical structures and the joint moment.
- To be able to define and distinguish between the terms strength, torque, force, and moment.
- To be able to define and state the significance of muscle-tendon interaction.
- To be able to define and state the significance of muscle-joint interaction.
- To be able to name the major "design" param-

eters of the musculoskeletal system and the functional parameter that they affect.

Introduction

In the preceding two chapters, a description of the structure and function of the pieces that make up the motors that drive the human movement machine was provided. You now have a great deal of knowledge about skeletal muscle anatomy and physiology as well as some idea of the relationship between the nervous system and the muscles (motors) that it controls. The way that muscle force is regulated by either altering activation frequency or altering the number of activated motor units has been discussed. This is precisely the position in which many students find themselves after a good neuromuscular physiology course. These courses are taken by undergraduate and graduate students, medical students, trainers, and therapists who need to apply this information to the real world of weak or injured patients and elite or injured athletes. Does this basic information apply to the real world of patients and athletes? Can this newfound information be used to the benefit of the patient? The answer is, yes. However, certain definitions, which are needed to describe the action of muscles located in the real-world environment, must be given. It is not possible to simply speak of isometric or isotonic muscle contractions in the real world because muscle activation is never truly maximal, nor is it performed at a constant length or under a constant load nor is it ever directly measured. In fact, before discussing movement per se, the muscle-tendon motors and the joints on which they act to produce movement should be discussed further. After this introduction, these ideas will be applied to the musculoskeletal system.

Muscle-Tendon Interaction

Most anatomy texts teach that tendons function only to connect skeletal muscles to bones. However, tendons should not be considered simply as rigid linkage structures. It is well-known that tendons are relatively compliant (stretchy) tissues and they also have just the "right amount" of compliance to affect in a positive way, the overall function of the muscle-tendon unit.

Tendon Structure and Composition

The connective tissue that surrounds muscle fibers and muscle fascicles has been discussed in previous chapters. These tissues converge and exit the muscle belly to become the tendon which is white, glossy, and smooth upon gross inspection. Some tendons are enclosed in a connective tissue sheath to facilitate sliding (such as the digital flexor tendons) whereas others slide relative to adjacent tissues and skin (such as the Achilles tendon). Some tendons wrap around connective tissue "pulleys" that function to increase functional excursion (such as the dorsiflexor retinaculum of the ankle) whereas others pull in a direct line directly from muscle to bone (such as the triceps brachii tendon). All in all, tendons are exquisitely designed to perform their job: transmit muscle force and slide during movement.

Tendons are composed primarily of the structural protein, collagen. The smallest unit of collagen is made up of polypeptide chains that are composed primarily of three amino acids arranged in series: glycine (~30%), proline (~10%), and hydroxyproline (~10%; Fig. 3-1A) (Amiel, Frank, Harwood, Fronek, & Akeson, 1984). These chains, due to the three-dimensional nature of the repeating amino acid structure, polymerize in groups of three to cre-

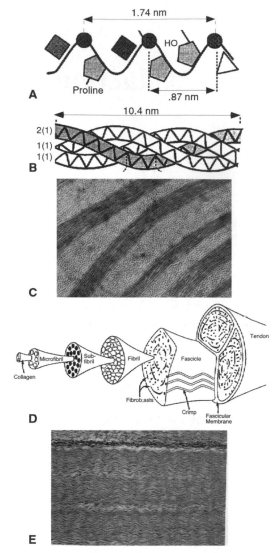

FIGURE 3-1. Schematic structure of tendons. **(A)** Primary structure of polypeptide chain of collagen, the major structural protein within tendons. Most of the amino acids in collagen are glycine, proline, and hydroxyproline, illustrated by different shapes. **(B)** Collagen molecule composed of three polypeptide chains. In fact, different isoforms of collagen can result in many different collagen types. **(C)** Collagen fibril, formed by a staggered arrangement of collagen molecules. **(D)** Structural hierarchy of collagen tissue based on bundling of collagen fibrils. **(E)** Longitudinal light micrograph of tendon showing the wavy appearance of the collagen fibers along with occasional fibroblasts interspersed in the interfibrillar space.

ate the collagen molecule (Fig 3-1B). There are numerous types of chains and thus, collagen itself may exist in one of many isoforms or types. Currently, there are 20 known types of collagen (Myllyharju & Kivirikko, 2001). To accurately specify the type, the structure of the three component chains must be identified. Adult tendons are composed primarily of type I and type III collagen. Incidentally, the hydroxyproline amino acid within collagen molecules is specifically made within tendon fibroblasts by modifying the amino acid proline. Thus, hydroxyproline serves as a biochemical "marker" for tendon material.

Collagen molecules are arranged in a staggered pattern that creates a collagen "fibril" with a banding pattern that roughly resembles muscle (Fig. 3-1C). Here is another structural hierarchy: fibrils are bundled into fascicles that are bundled into whole tendons (Fig. 3-1D). Under simple light microscopy, the dominant feature of tendons is the wavy appearance of the collagen fibers with sparse fibroblasts interspersed within the interfibrillar space (Fig. 3-1E). This wavy appearance disappears when the tendon is placed under load and thus, some of the elasticity of tendons appears to result directly from the wavy structure of the collagen fibers. This wavy pattern of collagen fiber undulation has been termed the "crimp" pattern. Other extracellular matrix proteins are present in tendons that give it some of its viscoelastic properties. These materials include highly charged gylcosaminoglycans that attract water and elastin that provides some of the elasticity of normal tendons (Kannus, 2000; Myllyharju & Kivirikko, 2001).

Compared with many tissues, tendons are relatively acellular with a poorly developed blood supply. As a result, it may not be surprising that, in some cases, it is difficult to get tendons to heal fully after laceration or rupture.

Tendon Mechanical Properties

Numerous experimental measurements of isolated tendons have revealed fairly consistent mechanical properties among different tendons (however, see the specializations described later in this section). To determine these properties, a tendon is physically connected to a force transducer and stretched. Then, the lengthening of the tendon material is measured at the same time as the applied tendon force. Change in tendon length can be measured in absolute units (*e.g.,* mm), but it is more useful to express the lengthening in relative terms to account for the fact that tendons come in a variety of lengths. The most common manner of expressing relative length is as tendon "strain" (ε) which is defined in Equation 3-1 as the following:

$$\varepsilon = \frac{l-l_o}{l_o} \qquad \text{(Eq. 3-1)}$$

in which l is the tendon length, l_o is the initial length, and ε is strain. Strain is, therefore, the change in tendon length relative to its starting length and is a convenient method for expressing the "stretchiness" or, more correctly, compliance of materials. When a tendon is loaded and strain measured, a curve such as that shown in Figure 3-2A is obtained. Because tendons also come in a variety of thicknesses, it is convenient to express force in relative terms as well. To normalize tendon force, divide by the tendon cross-sectional area which yields tendon "stress," (σ) defined in Equation 3-2 as the following:

$$\sigma = \frac{F}{A} \qquad \text{(Eq. 3-2)}$$

in which F is the tendon load (in Newtons of load or force), A is the tendon cross-sectional area (in area units such as m^2), and σ is stress (in units of N/m^2, which are abbreviated as Pascals or Pa). By expressing load in terms of stress (which is normalized) and deformation in terms of strain (which is also normalized), it is possible to compare the properties of materials of different sizes and shapes independent of the absolute size of the material. Thus, stress and strain can provide measures of the intrinsic material properties of a tendon. An interesting parameter that can be derived from these mea-

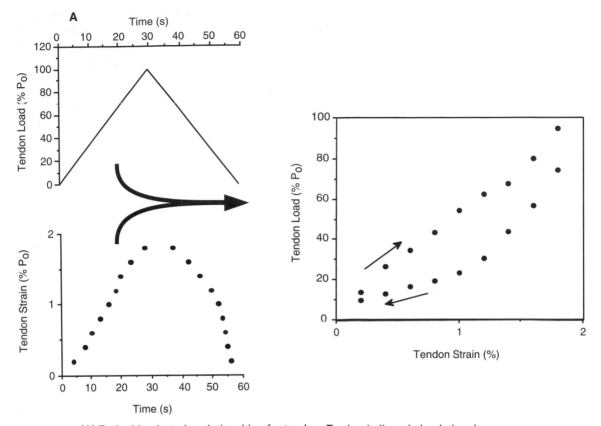

FIGURE 3-2. (A) Typical load-strain relationship of a tendon. Tendon is linearly loaded and unloaded over time. Strain is measured in tendon during loading and unloading phases. Load and strain at corresponding time points are plotted to yield the load-strain relationship. Note that, at low loads, the tendon elongates (strains) a great deal for a given change in load. However, at higher loads, the tendon is stiffer and, therefore, elongates less for a given change in load. Shown in the figure are the loading and unloading portions of the curve (arrows). **(B)** Strain measured in the insertion tendons of the five prime movers of the wrist when loaded to a force equivalent to the maximum tetanic tension of the muscle to which that tendon was attached. Maximum tetanic tension was estimated based on the architectural determination of physiological cross-sectional area. Note that strain varies significantly among the tendons from about 1.5% to 3.5%. (Data from: Loren, G.J., Lieber, R.L. (1995). Tendon biomechanical properties enhance human wrist muscle specialization. *Journal of Biomechanics, 28*, 791–799.) **(C)** Relationship between tendon strain measured under a load equivalent to muscle P_O (abscissa) and tendon length: fiber length ratio (ordinate). Note the significant positive correlation between the two parameters suggesting that material properties actually accentuate the muscle tendon design. Note also that the flexors (open circles) strain to a greater extent than the extensors (filled circles). *(continued)*

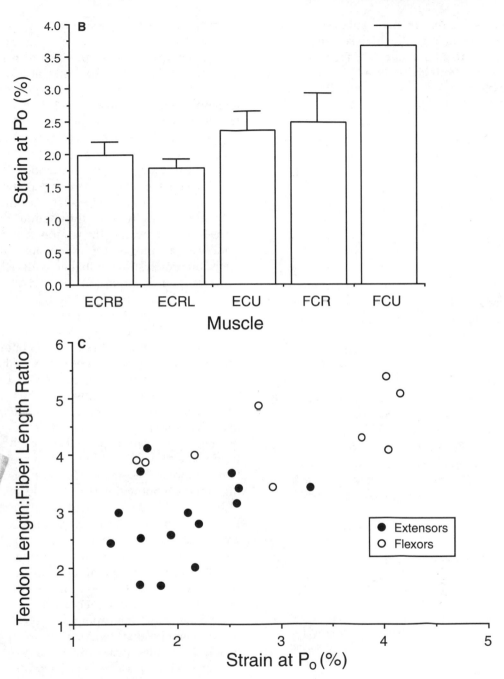

FIGURE 3-2. *(CONTINUED)*

surements is the relative stiffness (Young's modulus) of a material, which is defined as the change in stress for a given change in strain. In other words, Young's modulus (E) is calculated as shown in Equation 3-3 as the following:

$$E = \frac{\sigma}{\varepsilon} \qquad \text{(Eq. 3-3)}$$

Since strain has no units, the units of modulus are the same as those for stress, namely, Pascals. Stress, strain, and modulus values are characteristic for certain materials and it is interesting to compare common materials with biological materials as a point of reference. The easiest way to do this is to compare the Young's modulus among materials. Note that the Young's modulus for tendon (1 GPa or 1000 kPa) is about the same as the Young's modulus for a soft wood such as pine (0.6 GPa). The Young's modulus for a passive muscle being stretched (10 kPa) is about the same as the Young's modulus for rubber (20 kPa). Finally, the Young's modulus for bone (20 GPa) is about the same as that of a hardwood such as walnut (15 GPa). From these values, it is clear that bone is the stiffest and muscle the least stiff of the connective tissues.

Inspection of the shape of the stress-strain relationship in a soft tissue such as tendon (although similar comments could be made for almost any biological tissue such as skin, liga-

ment, mesentery, or passive muscle) provides insight into the unique properties of most soft tissues compared with traditional materials such as steel or wood. Note that, at low loads, relatively large tendon strain is associated with a relatively small change in load (Fig. 3-2A). In this low-load region, the tendon is thus very compliant, and this region is known as the "toe" region (Butler, Grood, Noyes, & Zernicke, 1978). It is believed that, as a tendon is elongated in this toe region, the crimp pattern, described above, disappears. As load continues to increase, the stiffness of the tendon also increases so that, overall, the tendon behaves in a nonlinear manner—very compliant at low loads, but much stiffer at higher loads. How are these properties important to in vivo tendon function? Unfortunately, although numerous measurements of tendon stress-strain properties were made historically (Woo et al., 1981), few were made under physiological conditions, i.e., under loading conditions that would be expected based on the force that could be produced by the attached muscles. Thus, the in vivo tendon properties are more difficult to estimate than the simple material properties of tendon tested in isolation. Several approaches have been taken to define tendon in vivo properties. In one approach, estimates of tendon strain during muscle contraction were made by Zajac (1989) based on a synthesis of literature values. He concluded that tendons nominally strain about 3% during muscle contraction. Direct measurement of tendon strain during passive loading of a muscle-tendon unit (Lieber, Leonard, Brown, & Trestik, 1991) and during muscle contraction (Lieber, Leonard, & Brown-Maupin, 2000) yielded approximately the same result, namely, that tendons strain approximately 3% at muscle maximum tetanic tension.

For obvious reasons, tendon properties of human tendons under physiological conditions are much more difficult to obtain. It is not difficult to obtain human tendon specimens, but it is difficult to measure their properties either during muscle contraction or at loads simulating muscle contraction. To try to measure

---

Box 3-1. Does "Stretching Out" Prevent Muscle Injury?

Although there is no question that tendons and muscles can be passively stretched in a way that causes passive force to decrease, there is almost no scientific evidence that stretching programs affect muscle injury. The best studies to date demonstrate that an aggressive stretching program increases range of motion significantly. However, interestingly, the increased range of motion appears to be because of increased tolerance to the high forces rather than a change in the properties of either the muscle or tendon.

tendon properties under loads to which they would normally be exposed, the relationship between muscle physiological cross-sectional area (PCSA) and maximum tetanic tension (P_o) was exploited. In the prime movers of the wrist, architectural analysis was first performed on each muscle-tendon unit, obtained from cadaveric specimens, to obtain PCSA. Then, each tendon was loaded to the P_o predicted from PCSA for that muscle (Loren & Lieber, 1995). Interestingly, for the five prime wrist movers—extensors carpi radialis brevis (ECRB), extensor carpi radialis longus (ECRL), extensor carpi ulnaris (ECU), flexor carpi radials (FCR), flexor carpi ulnaris (FCU), loading the tendons to P_o resulted in significantly different strain among tendons (p<0.01, Fig. 3-2B). Average strain across the five tendons was 2.8±0.5% with the largest strain observed in the FCU (3.78±0.31%) and the smallest strain observed in the ECRL (1.88±0.14%). This implied a certain level of specialization between tendons that was not observed using traditional elongation-to-failure methods on the same specimens.

Physiological Significance of Tendon Compliance

What is the physiological significance of the tendon compliance measured? In Chapter 2, recall that muscle force generation is length and even more velocity sensitive (Chapter 2, pages 51–66). Therefore, think about what might occur during muscle contraction if tendon compliance was significantly high or very low. Intuitively, if a compliant tendon is considered as a "spring," then as a muscle is activated and develops force, the tendon will strain, allowing the muscle to shorten further (Fig. 3-3A). The process is iterative in the sense that muscles will always generate force based on their length-tension and force-velocity properties, causing tendon deformation (Fig. 3-3B). The magnitude of tendon deformation will depend on its own stress-strain properties. This process will continue (muscle force generation and tendon deformation) until both muscle and tendon ve-

locity are zero. Therefore, muscle activation, even a fixed joint angle will never produce a truly isometric muscle contraction. In addition, as a joint is permitted to move, even though the muscle-tendon unit may shorten at a constant velocity, that velocity is not necessarily either the muscle velocity or the tendon velocity. A vivid example of such a phenomenon was presented by Griffiths and Hoffer et al. (Griffiths, 1991; Hoffer, Caputi, Pose, & Griffiths, 1989) who surgically implanted a length measuring device along the muscle fascicles of the medial gastrocnemius in the cat. Muscle fascicle length was measured during locomotion and a most interesting phenomenon occurred (Fig. 3-4). As the cat planted its paw (recall that cats are digigrade, walking on their toes), the triceps surae complex was stretched (vertical line in Fig. 3-4). The muscle was highly active as indicated by high EMG activity. In spite of the increase in length of the muscle tendon unit during paw strike, the medial gastrocnemius muscle actually decreased in length during this time. Although this may not be a general phenomenon across all muscle-tendon units, it illustrates the complexity of the muscle-tendon unit compared with the isolated properties of muscles or tendons alone.

Muscle fiber shortening and rotation during "isometric" human muscle contraction has recently been illustrated using ultrasonic imaging of tendon. The Japanese sport scientist Dr. Tetsuo Fukunaga (Ikai & Fukunaga, 1968; Fukunaga et al., 1992; Fukunaga et al., 1996; Fukunaga, Ichinose, Ito, Kawakami, & Fukashiro, 1997; Kuno & Fukunaga, 1995) has pioneered the use of ultrasound to measure both muscle and tendon properties in humans during various activities. In one study, he and his colleagues measured the orientation and length of tibialis anterior (TA) muscle fascicles during dorsiflexion. Subjects' ankles were secured to a dynamometer in about 20° of plantarflexion and asked to gradually increase isometric dorsiflexion torque up to their maximal effort (Ito, Kawakami, Ichinose, Fukashiro, & Fukunaga, 1998).

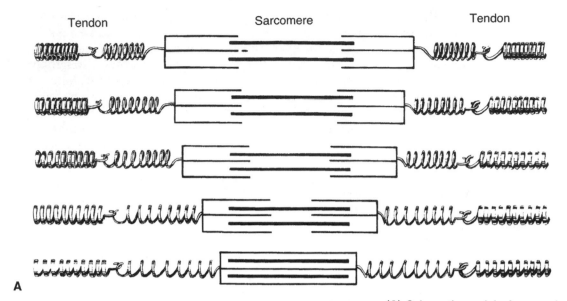

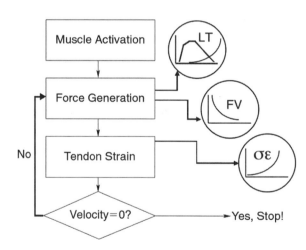

FIGURE 3-3. **(A)** Schematic model of a muscle "isometrically" contracting while in series with a tendon. The muscle (schematically represented by a sarcomere) shortens at the expense of tendon lengthening (schematically represented by springs). The springs may strain to different extents due to differences in intrinsic compliance at the fiber-tendon or tendon-bone junctions. **(B)** Flowchart representing the interaction between muscles and tendons during contraction. Muscles generate force based on their length-tension and force-velocity properties. Based on the tendon's stress-strain properties, tendons will deform under the force of muscle contraction. This process continues until both muscle and tendon velocity are zero.

Fascicle length and orientation were measured and images similar to that shown in Figure 1-12 were generated. As relative torque was increased, TA fiber length decreased from ~88 mm to ~78 mm (Fig. 3-5A) and pennation angle increased from 9.8° to almost 12° (Fig. 3-5B). Finally, they were able to generate a stress-strain curve for the tendon which ended up looking similar to those seen in other experimental studies of isolated tendons (Fig. 3-5C).

The encouraging result from these in vivo human studies is that the lessons learned from animal experiments are completely consistent with and seem to explain fully, the human results. This is encouraging because, in spite of the great pains that investigators go to simulate physiological conditions, there is always the possibility that, when including the complex motor unit activation patterns that occur normally (which are difficult to simulate), some new principle might emerge. In the case of tendon compliance, a great deal of agreement exists between animal and human studies.

There is another significant functional effect of tendon compliance that goes beyond the simple "disconnect" between the length of the tendon or muscle and length of the muscle-tendon unit. Tendon compliance results in a systematic change in the width and the shape of the muscle-length tension curve. Stated another way, the muscle-tendon unit length-tension curve is not simply the muscle's length-tension curve with some added tendon length. The fact that sarcomeres are allowed to shorten at the expense of tendon elongation results in a rightward shift of that muscle-tendon unit's length-tension relationship (Fig. 3-6A). The magnitude of this distortion of the length-tension relationship depends on the amount of tendon in series with the muscle fibers. The greater the length of tendon, the more distorted this relationship becomes (Fig. 3-6B).

Because of tendon compliance, not only is the intrinsic shape of the length-tension curve distorted, the over length-tension property of the muscle-tendon unit will also be altered. In fact, the muscle along with its compliant ten-

dons will have an increased operating range relative to the range attributed to muscle fibers alone (Fig. 3-7). This is because some of the length change that would be required to be taken up by muscle fibers is taken up by tendons instead. This phenomenon is simulated in Figure 3-7 in which the length-tension relation of a muscle is presented along with two different length-tension curves of muscle-tendon units. Figure 3-7A shows a muscle's length-tension curve with a total width of approximately 10 cm. This is a direct result of the muscle's fiber length (10 cm) within this fictitious muscle. In Figure 3-7B, the simulated length-tension curve of a muscle-tendon unit that has 5 cm of additional tendon attached on either end (but the tendons are perfectly stiff) is plotted—they simply act as rigid linkages, connecting the muscle to the bone. The result of this "simulation" of the muscle-tendon unit is a simple offset of the absolute length over which

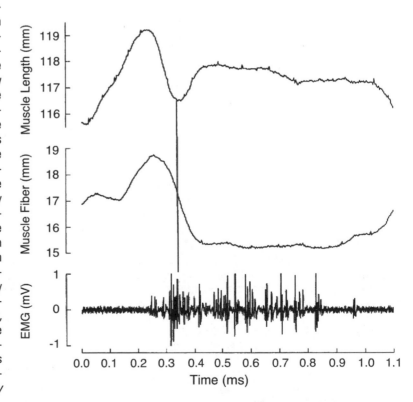

FIGURE 3-4. Time course of muscle fiber length, muscle-tendon unit length, and electromyographic activity during locomotion in the cat hindlimb. Notice that, as the cat plants its paw (vertical line) and dorsiflexes the ankle (indicated by rapid increase in muscle length), the muscle-tendon unit elongates (upper record), but the muscle fibers continue to shorten (middle record) because the muscle is highly active, as evidence by a high EMG activity (lower record). This result highlights the important differences between muscles and muscle-tendon units and demonstrates that tendon compliance can significantly modify muscle mechanical behavior. (Modified from: Griffiths, R.I. (1991). Shortening of muscle fibres during stretch of the active cat medial gastrocnemius muscle: The role of tendon compliance. *Journal of Physiology (London), 436*, 219–236.)

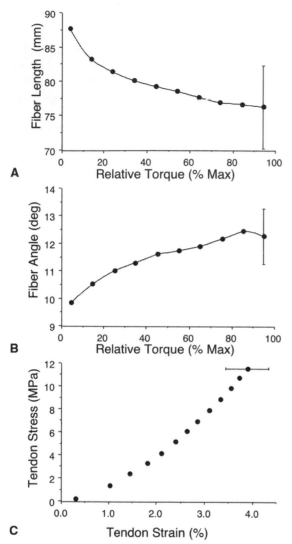

FIGURE 3-5. Ultrasonic measurement of muscle fiber shortening and tendon lengthening measured during an "isometric" dorsiflexion of the tibialis anterior. **(A)** Muscle fiber shortening in the tibialis anterior during "isometric" dorsiflexion. **(B)** Muscle fiber rotation in the tibialis anterior during "isometric" dorsiflexion. **(C)** Tendon stress-strain curve obtained during measurement of isometric joint torque. (Data from: Ito, M., Kawakami, Y., Ichinose, Y., Fukashiro, S., Fukunaga, T. (1998). Nonisometric behavior of fascicles during isometric contractions of a human muscle. *Journal of Applied Physiology, 85,* 1230–1235.)

the muscle-tendon unit operates by 5 mm, but there is no real change in either the shape of the curve or its width. Add 5 lengths of a "real" tendon, with a compliance equal to about 3% at P_O and another difference emerges (Fig. 3-7C). This is a typical amount of tendon present in many muscle-tendon units and was shown to produce modest changes in the sarcomere length-tension curve (Fig. 3-6B). Yet this "modest" change at the micro level produces significant changes at the macro level. First, there is an increase in the absolute range over which the muscle-tendon unit curve operates of about 50% so that the overall range over which this muscle-tendon unit is increased simply by having a "stretchy" tendon in series with the muscle. In addition, the tendon has just the "right" amount of compliance to produce such a change—any more and the muscle would shorten to nothing, any less and the increased range would not be obtained. The second more subtle change is a change in the basic shape of the curve so that P_O is now achieved at a relatively longer length. This is a manifestation of the shift in optimal sarcomere length previously seen (Fig. 3-6B). These two phenomena—increased operating range and shift in optimal length—are both a result of sarcomere shortening at the expense of tendon lengthening.

Sarcomere shortening at the expense of tendon lengthening has been explicitly modeled in an animal system, the frog, for which muscle and tendon properties could be directly measured (Lieber, Brown, & Trestik, 1992). This model permitted simulation of sarcomere shortening during a "fixed-end" contraction (*i.e.*, one in which the muscle-tendon unit length was held constant). From this simulation, it can be seen that, as sarcomeres generate force, they are also permitted to shorten. However, the magnitude of their shortening depends on their initial length (Fig. 3-8). Shorter sarcomeres, on the ascending limb of the length-tension curve shorten against a compliant tendon because the passive force is nearly zero at the initiation of contraction. Longer sar-

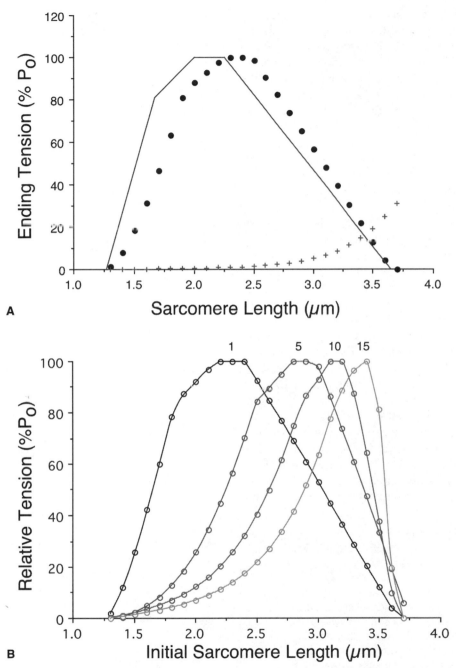

FIGURE 3-6. **(A)** Change in the shape muscle length-tension relationship due to tendon compliance in the frog semitendinosus model system. The effect of tendon compliance is to skew sarcomere length-tension curve (dotted line) relative to a muscle with no extremely stiff tendons (solid line). **(B)** Theoretical calculation of the progressive distortion in the length-tension relationship obtained by adding more tendon in series with the muscle fibers. The number above each curve represents the tendon length:fiber length ratio of the simulated muscle-tendon unit. (From: Lieber, R.L., Brown, C.G., Trestik, C.L. (1992). Model of muscle-tendon interaction during frog semitendinosus fixed-end contractions. *Journal of Biomechanics, 25*, 421–428.)

comeres, on the descending limb of the length-tension curve are shortening against a stiffer tendon because of the high passive force at long lengths. The net result is a differential degree of sarcomere shortening depending on the initial length, which provides the explanation for the change in shape of the muscle-tendon unit length-tension curve compared with the muscle length-tension curve alone. This differential sarcomere shortening has also received experimental support (Kawakami & Lieber, 2000).

Does this amount of change apply to all muscle-tendon units? Or, stated differently, can this information be applied to a specific muscle-tendon unit? Of course, appropriate application of this information depends on knowing two things: the compliance of the tendon to which the muscle is attached and the length of the tendon in series with the muscle. By increasing the length of the tendon, this effectively increases the amount of sarcomere shortening that occurs at the expense of tendon lengthening. Therefore, it would be more proper to state that the important parameter that determines the degree of sarcomere shortening is the length of tendon in series with the length of muscle fiber; in other words the tendon length: fiber length ratio—the longer the tendon relative to the fiber, the greater the overall effect of tendon compliance on the muscle-tendon unit. If you return to the previous exam-

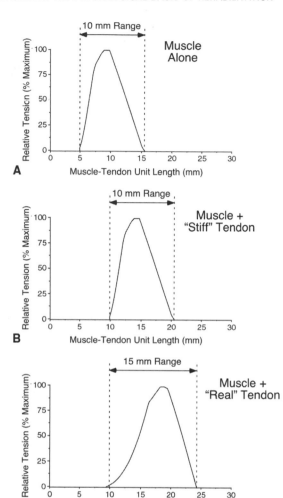

FIGURE 3-7. Simulation of the overall length-tension properties of muscles and muscle-tendon units. **(A)** Length-tension property of a muscle with fibers of length ~10 mm. Overall width of the length-tension curve is about 10 mm. **(B)** Length-tension property of a muscle with fibers of length 10 mm and infinitely stiff tendons of length 5 mm. Overall width is still 10 mm but absolute lengths are shifted by 5 mm. **(C)** Length-tension property of a muscle with fibers of length 10 mm in series with 5 lengths of a "normally" compliant tendon of length 5 mm. Note that the width of the length-tension relationship increases by ~50% (increased range) and the optimal length has shifted to longer lengths as a function of initial sarcomere length.

Box 3-2. Can a Tendon Lengthen While a Muscle Shortens?

Amazingly, yes! Tendons are fairly compliant tissues. Under conditions where a muscle is highly active and the entire muscle-tendon unit is forced to lengthen rapidly (for example, hopping on toes, when your toes hit the ground), much of the length increase caused by ankle dorsiflexion can be all taken up by the tendon while muscle fibers continue to shorten! This has been directly demonstrated in walking cats using sophisticated implanted length transducers.

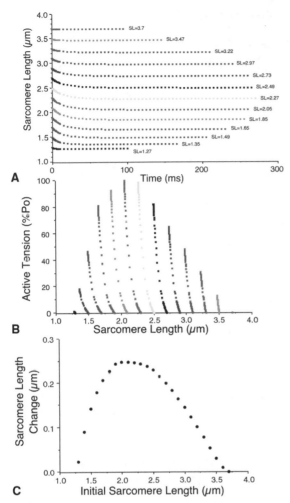

FIGURE 3-8. (A) Simulated sarcomere shortening as a function of time after activation. **(B)** Sarcomere length versus tension during isometric activation. Note that sarcomeres shorten until they reach the appropriate portion of the length-tension curve. **(C)** Summary relationship between initial sarcomere length and change in sarcomere length for this system. (Data From: Lieber, R.L., Brown, C.G., Trestik, C.L. (1992). Model of muscle-tendon interaction during frog semi-tendinosus fixed-end contractions. *Journal of Biomechanics, 25*, 421–428.)

ple and double the length of the tendon in series with our muscle, the overall length range of the muscle-tendon unit increases even further and that the length at which muscle force peaks also

continues to shift (Fig. 3-7). Why not keep increasing tendon length to increase MTU operating range? The answer is that with an extremely long tendon, sarcomere shortening would be so great as to allow the sarcomeres to shorten to the point in which no force was generated at all. Clearly, there are positive and negative aspects to high tendon length and high tendon compliance (Loren & Lieber, 1995).

After this discussion about the positive aspects of tendon compliance, it should be mentioned that there is another "down side" to tendon compliance. Recall that the purpose of muscles is to move the trunk and limbs to a particular position in space. Tendon compliance acts like a spring in series with the muscle fibers so that movement of the joint, for example, the fingertip, is not faithfully transmitted back to the muscle itself. Since some of the information about movement comes to the nervous system via muscle spindles, it could be argued that tendon compliance confounds the nervous system's ability to control joint position. Of course, this would be most severe for muscles in series with long tendons.

A most extreme case of muscle-tendon units that must maintain joint position and that are vulnerable to tendon compliance are the digital flexors. These muscles maintain the position of fingertips but the muscles themselves are located remotely from the fingertips in the proximal forearm, presumably to decrease the inertia and bulk of the hand (Hildebrand, 1974). How can these muscle-tendon units be "designed" to provide adequate control of joint position while still maintaining their remote position? The strategy appears to be the use of much stiffer tendons to compensate for the inability to further reduce the intrinsic compliance of the system. This conclusion was made after making mechanical measurements at physiological loads of each digit of the flexor digitorum superficialis (FDS) and flexor digitorum profundus (FDP) muscles. Loading each tendon to the appropriate force resulted in no significant difference in tendon strain between any of the tendons or between muscle types

---

Therapist's Comments

Another fascinating example of the dramatic influence of tendon compliance during jumping is the recent demonstration that, during a jump that begins from a squat position, the medial gastrocnemius fascicles shorten before joint movement, stretching the Achilles tendon. Then, during the jump the fascicle length remains relatively constant (isometric) and the tendon actually recoils at a high velocity producing the movement. If the fibers were to shorten at the high velocity to produce the movement, the fiber force would be quite low based on the force-velocity relationship of the muscle. The Achilles tendon is probably the perfect candidate for energy storage and release as shown in this chapter, based on the very long tendon that is in series with muscles containing short fibers (gastrocnemius and soleus).

(FDP versus FDS). Average absolute strain observed for the FDP and FDS tendons at the maximum tetanic tension (1.20±0.38%, n=39 measurements from 40 tendons from 5 specimens) was less than half of that predicted to occur in upper extremity muscles of this architectural design (Lundberg et al., 1997).

The issue of tendon compliance will be returned to during the discussion of the gait cycle (page 153). Tendons can also play a significant role in the energetics of locomotion (Alexander & Bennet, 1977). At this point, let us state that the relative amount of tendon compared with muscle fibers will determine the magnitude of the increase in operating range of the muscle-tendon unit so that, in some ways, tendon length : fiber length ratio is a parameter that reveals design of a muscle-tendon unit in the same way as PCSA and fiber length represent design parameters of muscle.

Joint Moments

Definition of Torque

In the musculoskeletal system, muscles generate and transmit force, via tendons, to bones. If muscles generate sufficient force, bones move. Bones are not free to move in space but are usually constrained to rotate about a joint axis. Therefore a mechanical system must be quantitatively described using the concept of torque. The equation used to calculate torque is as follows:

$$\tau = \vec{r} \times \vec{F} \qquad \text{(Eq. 3-4)}$$

in which τ is torque, r is the moment arm, F is the applied force, and $\times$ represents the vector cross-product of the two quantities (Fig. 3-9A). Thus, a force F, is applied a distance r away from an axis (open circle, Fig. 3-9A) that is free to rotate. The arrows above the moment arm and force variables signify that they are vector quantities. That is, both have magnitude as well as direction. This is another way of saying that the orientation between r and F is important. If

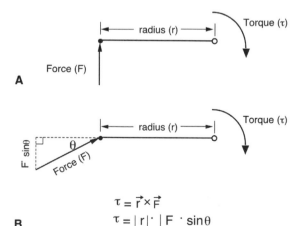

FIGURE 3-9. (A) Schematic diagram illustrating the definition of torque (τ) which is composed of a force (F), a moment arm or radius (r). **(B)** Change in torque as the force is applied to the axis at an angle θ. The component of force tending to rotate the axis is F·sinθ, which is equal to the moment arm (r).

this equation is expanded, the torque can be expressed as follows:

$$\tau = |\,r\,|\cdot|\,F\,|\cdot\sin\theta \qquad\text{(Eq. 3-5)}$$

in which the vertical bars around r and F represent the vector magnitudes, and θ is the angle between the direction of force application and the axis of rotation. The basis for this expression can be seen in Figure 3-9B in which the force, F, is applied at an angle θ relative to the axis of force generation. The component of force that causes rotation is $F\cdot\sin\theta$, the short side of the triangle shown as a dotted line. $F\cdot\sin\theta$ is the perpendicular distance between the point of force application and the axis of rotation, and this term is referred to as the moment arm.

Moment arm is measured in distance units such as meters. Because the $\sin\theta$ term is dimensionless, torque has units of Newton-meters (force-distance units). Another common unit of torque is foot-pounds (such as are used in the automobile industry, and, interestingly, on isokinetic dynamometer machines used in rehabilitation). Proper representation of torque always requires use of the correct units that includes both force units and distance units.

Applying this idea to the musculoskeletal system, "strength" actually represents torque. All real-world performance (sprinting, lifting weights, getting out of bed, writing, squeezing a grip device) represents manifestations of torque generation by the musculoskeletal system. If the implications of this statement are grasped, it is clearly incorrect to conclude that a person is "strong" simply because their muscles generate large forces. This may sound sacrilegious and it may even be the case, but it is not necessarily required. It would be just as ridiculous to conclude that a person is strong simply because they have large moment arms. Based on the above discussion, it is clear that at least three strategies exist for changing torque: changing force, changing moment arm, or changing the angle between the two (all strategies are illustrated in Fig. 3-10).

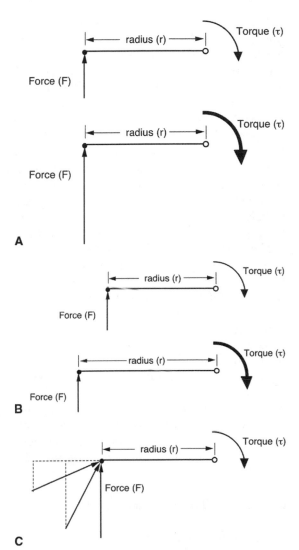

FIGURE 3-10. Three different strategies for changing torque. **(A)** Torque increases as force increases (bold curved line signifies increased torque). **(B)** Torque increases as moment arm increases. **(C)** Torque increases as the angle between force application and axis of rotation increases toward 90°.

Torque Examples

A common experience of torque generation is seen when a large force is required to remove the lid from a can of paint. Using a screwdriver is the most common method, because of its long handle (moment arm), it generates a large torque and thus a large upward force on the lid

(Fig. 3-11A). The downward imposed force is transferred via a fulcrum (the lip of the can) to produce an upward output force. Similarly, the human triceps muscle (Table 1-1) can generate a contractile force that is transmitted via the elbow joint to produce elbow extension (Fig. 3-11B). With this in mind, it is interesting to compare elbow extensor strength of various animals. In the animal kingdom, it is well known that baboons have elbow extension strength three to six times that of humans. However, analysis of baboon triceps muscles reveals that the muscles are approximately the same size as those of humans. Observation of the baboon's ulna reveals the basis for the great extension strength: The long olecranon process (moment arm) extends 3–4 cm posteriorly from the elbow joint (axis of rotation) (Hildebrand, 1974). Similarly, animals that are excellent diggers may have an olecranon process equally as long as the proximal portion of the ulna. Therefore when real-world strength or performance is mentioned, it must be in terms of a torque or joint moment. When trying to understand the generation of a particular joint moment in the musculoskeletal system, both the force producing the moment and moment arm about which that force is acting must be considered.

Muscle Force Producing the Moment

Determination of the muscle force that produces a joint moment is simple in principle but extremely difficult in practice. As discussed in Chapter 2, muscle force varies with muscle length (length-tension relationship), muscle velocity (force-velocity relationship), and activation level (fiber recruitment). If the muscle length, velocity, and recruitment level are known, then muscle force can be predicted. In practice, this is easier said than done because of the technical problems of defining these parameters noninvasively. Muscle length and velocity can be estimated based on external bony movement, but muscle fiber movement is not the same as muscle-tendon unit movement. Higher resolution methods such as magnetic resonance imaging (MRI), ultrasound, or direct measurement are required to obtain these values. Activation level is typically estimated using the electromyogram (EMG) of the muscle. To determine the relative level of activation, the measured EMG may be expressed relative to the EMG measured when the muscle is fully activated by the individual. Of course, this approach assumes that the muscle can be sampled adequately and still necessitates the determination of the maximum force of contraction which is almost never available. (However, see below for some clever approaches to human muscle force measurement and estimate.)

Moment Arm Producing the Moment

Determination of joint moment arm requires an understanding of the anatomy and movement (kinematics) of the joint of interest. For example, some joints can be considered to rotate about a fixed point. A good example of such a joint is the elbow. At the elbow joint, where the humerus and ulna articulate, forearm rotation occurs primarily about a fixed point, referred to as the joint "center of rotation." In the case of the elbow joint, the position of the center of rotation remains relatively constant throughout the joint range of motion. However, in other joints (for example, the knee), because the articulating surfaces of the tibia and femur are not perfect circles, the center of rotation moves in space as the knee joint rotates. In the case of the knee, it is not appropriate to discuss a single center of rotation, but rather a center of rotation corresponding to a particular joint angle, or, using the terminology of joint kinematics, the instant center of rotation (ICR), that is, the center of rotation at any "instant" in time or space. The change in ICR as a function of joint angle traces a curve which, for the case of the knee, is known as the "screw axis," since it is not a fixed point in space (Crowninshield, Pope, & Johnson, 1976; Smidt, 1973).

Identification of the joint ICR is difficult in practice. The most common method for ICR determination implements the technique of rigid body kinematics (Panjabi, 1979). Using

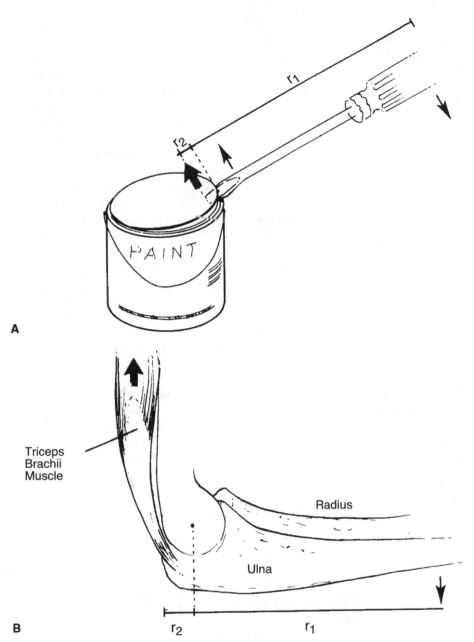

FIGURE 3-11. Common examples of torque generation. **(A)** Torque on a screwdriver provides a large upward force to remove the lid of a paint can. Input moment arm is r_1 while output moment arm is r_2 and the fulcrum is the edge of the paint can. **(B)** Triceps muscle force is applied via moment arm r_2 to the olecranon process to generate an elbow extension torque via moment arm r_1.

rigid body kinematics, two points are identified on two rigid bodies before and after rotation, and the axis about which the bodies rotate is identified using simple algebraic methods. (See Lieber & Boakes [1988] for an example of application of this method.) Often such measurements are taken from radiographs. Such methods have been used a great deal in orthopedic surgery, for example, to define the normal kinematics of joints that are surgically replaced. The intention is to design artificial joints that mimic the kinematics of normal joints.

Having defined a joint ICR, the moment arm is defined as the perpendicular distance from point of force application to the axis of rotation. This is illustrated in Figure 3-12 for a simulated elbow joint. In Figure 3-12A, the elbow joint is almost fully extended. Let the angle, θ, between the brachialis muscle and the ulna be relatively small, e.g., $\theta=20°$. Let the distance between the brachialis insertion site and the elbow instant center be 5 cm. In this case, the perpendicular distance between the point of force application and the elbow ICR is shown by the dotted line in Figure 3-12A and is equiv-

alent to 5 cm $\times$ sin(20°) = 1.7 cm. Thus, because the joint is nearly fully extended, this presents an unfavorable mechanical advantage to the muscle—the moment arm is relatively small. Much of the force generated by the muscle will simply compress the joint, not rotate it. Contrast this situation with the conditions shown in Figure 3-12B, in which the joint has now been flexed to $\theta=50°$. Now, the moment arm equals 5 cm $\times$ sin(50°) = 4.3 cm. For a simple hinge joint (a joint with a fixed ICR), the maximum moment arm is attained at $\theta=90°$. If moment arm versus joint angle was plotted for this simple hinge joint, a simple sine function that has a maximum of 5 cm occurring at $\theta=90°$ of flexion could be obtained. Such a relationship can be generated for any joint. In general, the curves for human joints are not as simple as the one previously illustrated.

Methods for Human Muscle Force Determination

Hopefully, it is clear that almost all clinical measurements are actually joint moment measurements rather than direct muscle force mea-

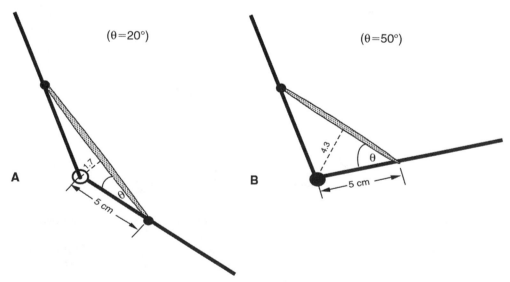

FIGURE 3-12. Schematic example of altered moment arm with change in joint angle. **(A)** At an acute joint angle ($\theta=20°$) moment arm is relatively small (1.7 cm). **(B)** At larger joint angles ($\theta=50°$) moment arm increases considerably to 4.3 cm. This is because the angle between the muscle force and point of force application changes.

surements. Many people discuss these values in terms of muscle "force" but it is actually a misnomer. However, there are valid reports in the literature of muscle force obtained under a variety of conditions. How can this be? The earliest estimates of muscle force based on torque measurements simply measured the torque using some type isokinetic dynamometer and then estimating moment arm using plane X-rays (Schantz, Randall, Hutchinson, Tyden, & Astrand, 1983). Later, the method of moment arm measurement was refined to represent more physiological conditions using, for example, magnetic resonance images (Rugg, Gregor, Mandelbaum, & Chiu, 1990). Finally, in the most recent implementation, ultrasound probes in the region of the joint have been used to make precise moment arm measurements during muscle contraction enabling muscle force calculations (Ito, Akima, & Fukunaga, 2000; Magnusson, Aagaard, Rosager, Dyre-Poulsen, & Kjaer, 2001).

However, accurate muscle force measurements have also been made by applying ingenious measuring devices directly to human tendons. In an early example, a transducer was surgically placed around a human Achilles tendon and individuals walked, ran, or jumped as instructed, providing muscle force values directly without the need for moment arm calculation (see Color Plate Section, Fig. C-5A). This method was based on work that had been performed at UCLA by the biomechanist Dr. Bob Gregor (who studied cat locomotion) and was applied to human locomotion studies by the Finnish biomechanist, Professor Paavo Komi. Komi et al. (1996) later refined the method by making it less invasive using a small fiber optic probe that was inserted into the tendon via a 19-gauge needle (Color Plate Section, Fig. C-5B). This method has the advantage of being less invasive and smaller so that it is applicable to a wider variety of human tendons. However, it suffers from the disadvantage that the fiber optic probe only measures relative force change and must be calibrated using the indirect methods described above in which moments are

converted to forces after measuring moment arms. Finally, muscle force has been measured directly using intraoperative muscle stimulation of a muscle-tendon unit in which the insertion tendon has been removed before surgical transfer. This is extremely invasive, is only applicable to situations in which the muscle will be released from its insertion due to planned surgery, and thus is not widely applicable (Color Plate Section, Fig. C-5C) (Freehafer, Peckham, & Keith, 1979). However, it has the tremendous advantage of providing an actual direct muscle force value.

Presentation of the various strengths and weaknesses of the myriad methods used for studying human muscle function should impress the student with the creativity, ingenuity, and tenacity that scientists have demonstrated in their quest to understand human muscle function. No single method is best for every application. The serious investigator must carefully consider their experimental needs and the quality and quantity of data needed. Then, the most appropriate method should be used that satisfies those requirements.

Muscle-Joint Interaction During Isometric Torque Production

For a given muscle-joint system, muscle force-generating properties and joint kinematics can be defined. Unfortunately, the detailed relationship between the many human muscles and joints has not been thoroughly studied. To clearly understand the stated problem, refer to Figure 3-13. A hypothetical length-tension relationship, which is expressed as a force-joint angle relationship is placed in Figure 3-13A. In Chapter 2, the length-tension curve for single frog muscle fibers (Fig. 2-4) was shown. The muscle force-joint angle relationship will be some portion of this curve. For the purpose of discussion, assume that muscle force increases and then decreases as a trigonometric sine function as the joint rotates (Fig. 3-13A). (The detailed forms of both muscle and moment arm

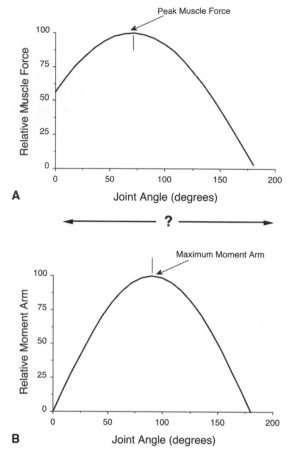

FIGURE 3-13. Conceptual question posed by the relative angular location of the angle at which maximum muscle force occurs and the angle corresponding to maximum moment arm. **(A)** Muscle force as a function of joint angle with peak force at about 70°. **(B)** Moment arm as a function of joint angle with peak moment arm at about 90°. Small vertical lines represent peaks of each curve. Horizontal arrows emphasize the fact that relative angular relationship between these two relationships is generally unknown.

curves are relatively arbitrary and only intended to illustrate muscle-joint interaction.) A typical moment arm curve is shown in Figure 3-13B. Since the moment is simply the product of muscle force and moment arm, the joint moment results from the product of these two curves. However, the key questions that must

be addressed are, "What is the relative angular relationship between the muscle and joint properties (arrows in Figure 3-13)? That is, is muscle force maximum at the same angle where moment arm is maximum? If not, at what joint angle is muscle force maximum?" If the two curves are offset relative to one another (vertical dotted lines), their product can be dramatically altered (see page 137). Understanding the relationship between muscle and joint properties is important from the point of view of understanding the normal design of the musculoskeletal system. It is also important in providing a scientific basis for surgical procedures that involve movement or transfer of muscles from one position to another (Lieber & Fridén, 1997; Lieber, Pontén, & Fridén, 1996). The relationship between muscles and joints must be understood to mimic the natural function of the musculoskeletal system and to recreate this relationship using surgical intervention. Specifically, the relative angular relationship between the two curves in Figure 3-13 must be defined.

Joint Angle Corresponding to Maximum Muscle Force

Examination of current physiology texts reveals a good deal of wishy-washiness regarding the definition of the joint angle that corresponds to maximum muscle force. Typically, it is stated that muscle force is maximum when the joint is in a neutral position, or when the muscle is at resting length. What is the basis for such statements? Unfortunately, there is little scientific basis for such a statement. Recent studies of torque generation in animals and humans have produced conflicting results. Some studies have concluded that the joint angle at which muscle force was at its maximum was either outside the normal range of motion, or at one extreme end of the range of motion.

Torque Generation in the Frog Hindlimb

The relationship between sarcomere length and joint angle in the frog has been discussed (Lieber & Boakes, 1988). Recall that frog muscle is the only skeletal muscle for which the sarcomere length-tension relationship is available (Fig. 2-4). Therefore, definitive determination of the relationship between sarcomere length and joint angle can be determined only for the frog musculoskeletal system so it is first used to understand basic principles. First, the results from this detailed experiment will be presented followed by a more complex example from the human upper extremity.

In the frog study, the semitendinosus muscle was examined during knee rotation. In the frog, the semitendinosus is a biarticular hamstring muscle that crosses both the knee and hip. The frog pelvis, femur, tibia, and semitendinosus muscles were isolated and placed in a specially designed jig, surrounded by physiological saline solution (Fig. 3-14). With the hip at 90° of flexion, the knee joint was flexed throughout its range of motion, from 0° to 180° of flexion. During joint flexion, sarcomere length was measured by laser diffraction. Laser diffraction is a method based on the fact that the A-I band periodicity acts a diffraction grating to incident laser light. Because of destructive and constructive interference, a diffraction pattern is produced that is proportional to sarcomere length (for details, see Lieber, Yeh, & Baskin, 1984). The relationship between sarco-

mere length and joint angle, shown in Figure 3-15A, presents a striking illustration of the manner in which muscle force can change during joint flexion. Note that with the joint fully extended (180°), the muscle was highly lengthened to a sarcomere length of 3.6 μm, the sarcomere length corresponding to zero active tension on the sarcomere length-tension curve (Fig. 2-4). When the knee was flexed, the muscle shortened and sarcomere length decreased to approximately 2.0 μm, the sarcomere length corresponding to maximum tetanic tension. It is interesting to note that, in this muscle-joint system, the muscle would produce no force with the joint fully extended (sarcomere length 3.6 μm) and maximum force (sarcomere length 2.0 μm) with the joint fully flexed. In the same experimental system, the knee joint kinematics were also studied, and the knee was shown to behave essentially as a simple hinge joint, as illustrated in Figure 3-15B. Finally, in the same system, the muscle was stimulated, the joint was rotated throughout the same range of motion, and the torque was directly measured. The torque-joint angle relationship shown in Figure 3-15C was obtained. The combined results of this study are illustrated schematically in Figure 3-16A and graphically in Figure 3-16B. Note that maximum torque (the optimal joint angle) was obtained at 120° of flexion, which was neither the angle at which muscle force was maximum (160°) nor the angle at which moment arm was maximum (90°). Thus torque production in this system (and probably other musculoskeletal systems, Lieber & Shoemaker, 1992) resulted from the interaction between muscle and joint properties and not either property alone.

Generalized Design of Musculoskeletal Torque Generators

Unfortunately, the details of this section cannot be fully written as yet. However, several main points can be made, which provide a basis for understanding any musculoskeletal torque generating system. Recall that in the frog system above, as the knee flexed, sarcomere length

---

Box 3-3. Is a Person Strongest at the Joint Angle Where Their Muscle Generates the Highest Force?

No, not necessarily. Muscle force and moment arm both change throughout the range of motion. Torque (which is what "strength" represents), is the product of muscle force and moment arm. The joint angle where torque is maximum is not necessarily the joint angle where either muscle force or moment arm is maximum. Unfortunately, most of the detailed torque generating properties of human joints are unknown. However, using animal models, it has been clearly demonstrated that muscles need not generate their highest forces in any particular place within the normal range of motion.

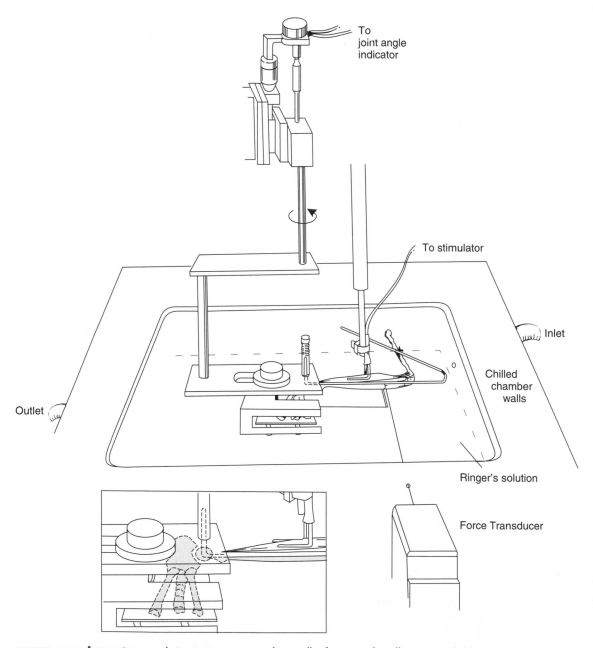

FIGURE 3-14. Apparatus used to measure experimentally frog semitendinosus sarcomere length, hip and knee joint angle, and joint torque. The frog bone-muscle complex is secured to the rotating arm of the jig. Stimulating electrodes flank the semitendinosus muscle. Joint angle is changed by rotating the arm, and joint angle is read directly from a goniometer. The femur and tibia are stabilized throughout the experiment. (From: Mai, M.T., Lieber, R.L. (1990). A model of semitendinosus muscle sarcomere length, knee and hip joint interaction in the frog hindlimb. *Journal of Biomechanics, 23*, 271–279.)

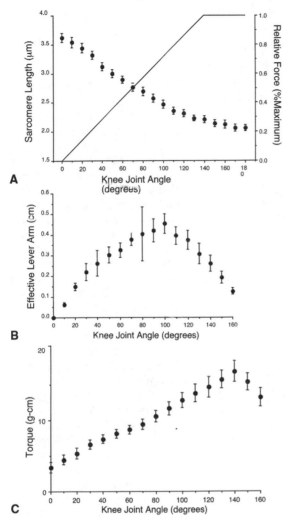

FIGURE 3-15. (A) Sarcomere length (left axis in μm) versus knee joint angle. All sarcomere lengths are on the descending limb of the length-tension curve. Solid line and right axis represent the approximate muscle force corresponding to the measured sarcomere length. **(B)** Moment arm versus knee joint angle. Symbols and solid line represent mean values ± standard error from 10 muscles. Note that muscle force and moment arm vary significantly throughout the joint range of motion. **(C)** Knee joint torque versus joint angle for the frog semitendinosus muscle during knee joint rotation. Data shown are ± mean standard error for all frogs. Note that torque increases relatively linearly from 0° to 140° and drops off sharply from 140° to 160°. (Data from: Lieber, R.L., Boakes, J.L. (1988). Sarcomere length and joint kinematics during torque production in the frog hindlimb. *American Journal of Physiology, 254*, C759–C768.)

decreased from 3.6 μm to 2.0 μm. Why? Did this have to be the case? The answer is no. The mechanical reason for the relatively large sarcomere length change (1.6 μm) during joint rotation was that the number of sarcomeres arranged in series along the fibers was such that when muscle-tendon length decreased from full extension to full flexion, to take up that length change, each sarcomere was required to shorten 1.6 μm. Clearly, if there had been twice as many sarcomeres arranged in series, each sarcomere would have only shortened half as much, or 0.8 μm. For example, suppose a muscle-joint system were configured such that, by extending from 40° to 80°, the muscle went from its minimum to its maximum length (Fig. 3-17A). Now, suppose the muscle fiber length were significantly increased. What happens to joint range of motion? Clearly, because more sarcomeres are in series to take up the length change, joint range of motion increases. Now the muscle can extend from 70° to 145°—a total of 75° (compared to the previous 40°; Fig. 3-17B). Therefore, by increasing fiber length, active range of motion has increased from 40° to 75° (Fig. 3-18). This demonstrates the intimate interaction between the muscle and the joint about which it rotates.

Based on this example, the ratio between muscle fiber length (number of sarcomeres in series) and moment arm influences the amount of sarcomere shortening that will occur during joint rotation (Equation 3-6). This ratio can be calculated for any muscle joint system as

$$\text{Ratio} = \frac{\text{Fiber Length}}{\text{Moment Arm}} \qquad \text{(Eq. 3-6)}$$

and will determine the relative influence of the muscle on the muscle-joint torque generator (Table 3-1, page 140). If fiber length is long compared with moment arm, relatively little sarcomere length change will occur during joint rotation, and muscle force change will contribute little to the joint moment. If, however, fiber length is short and moment arm is long, the sarcomeres will change length a great deal during joint rotation, and so will muscle

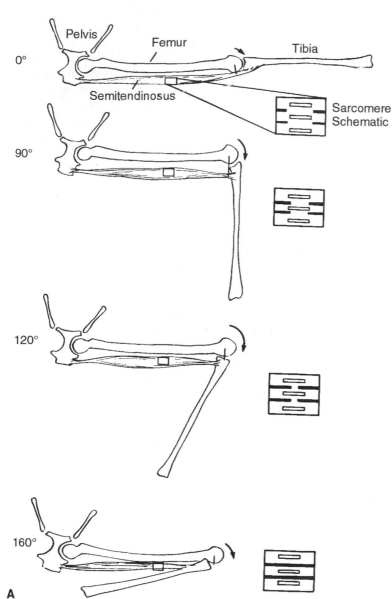

FIGURE 3-16. (A) Schematic relationship between relative muscle force, relative effective lever arm, and relative joint torque as a function of knee joint angle. Length of curved arrow at knee represents torque magnitude. Thin vertical line at knee represents magnitude of the moment arm. **(B)** Graphical representation of relationship diagrammed in **(A)**. Note that throughout the range of motion, muscle force and effective lever arm interact to produce torque. Note that maximum muscle force and maximum effective lever arm (filled circles) do not coincide with the optimal joint angle. (Data from: Lieber, R.L., Boakes, J.L. (1988). Muscle force and moment arm contributions to torque production in frog hindlimb. *American Journal of Physiology, 254*, C769–C772 and Lieber, R.L., Boakes, J.L. (1988). Sarcomere length and joint kinematics during torque production in the frog hindlimb. *American Journal of Physiology, 254*, C759–C768.)

(continued)

force. This dramatically affects the muscle contribution to the joint moment (Zajac, 1992).

Human Musculoskeletal Torque Generators
LOWER EXTREMITY
In the frog muscle-joint system presented above, a specific case was presented in which muscle, bone, and joint properties could be measured directly to determine their relative influence in torque generation. Obviously, such invasive experiments cannot be performed on humans. However, using ingenious assumptions and collecting the available experimental torque data from the literature for the hip, knee, and ankle joint, Drs. Melissa Hoy and Felix Zajac (Hoy, Zajac, & Gordon, 1990; Zajac & Gordon, 1989) developed a model of torque production in the human lower limb. They predicted muscle force based on architectural measurements from cadaver specimens (Fig.

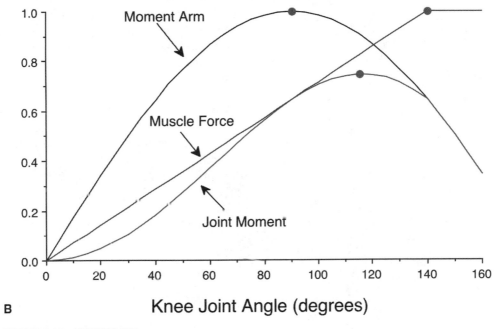

B

Knee Joint Angle (degrees)

FIGURE 3-16. *(CONTINUED)*

3-19A), moment arm from skeletal studies (Fig. 3-19B), and predicted the torque produced by each muscle group (Fig. 3-19C). By making small adjustments in the various model assumptions, they fit their data to actually measured torque data obtained during human voluntary contraction. Comparison of the three components of Figure 3-19 immediately yields the conclusion that muscle force, moment arm, and torque are not simply scaled versions of one another. Inspect Figure 3-19C (torque), and determine which of its components most strongly influences it. Doesn't Figure 3-19A look more like 3-19C than 3-19B? This leads to the conclusion that generally muscle force is probably the major determinant of peak joint torque. However, note the many exceptions: Soleus torque and gastrocnemius torque are similar despite the fact that the soleus produces almost twice the contractile force that the gastrocnemius does. Why? The gastrocnemius must have a larger moment arm (Fig. 3-19B). As another example, the gluteus medius and maximus generate approximately the same force. Yet the hip extension torque of the gluteus medius is over four times that of the glu-

teus maximus due to its large moment arm. Look for other relationships in the figure itself.

In their analysis of the lower limb, Hoy et al. (1990) also showed that the ratio between fiber length and moment arm varied considerably between muscle-joint systems. For example, in the lower extremity, fiber length : moment arm ratios varied from 80 (for the gluteus maximus) to about 1.0 (for the soleus). Other values are shown in Table 3-1. In the upper extremity, combining the architectural data of Lieber et al. (1990) with the joint kinematic data of Horii et al. (Horii, An, Cooney, & Linscheid, 1991), these ratios vary from 11 (for the extensor carpi radialis brevis) to about 2.0 (for the flexor carpi ulnaris). Again, other intermediate values are given in Table 3-1.

What has been demonstrated here is yet another design parameter of the musculoskeletal system. In addition to the previously described muscle architectural properties (fiber length, physiological cross-sectional area, tendon length), there is also the fiber length/moment arm ratio (Equation 3-6), which determines the relative influence of muscle on the muscle-joint torque generator. In fact, if either

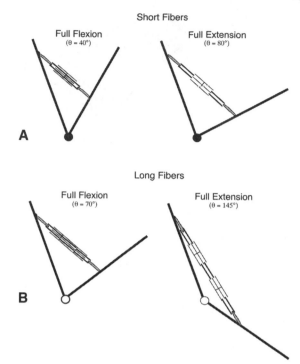

FIGURE 3-17. Schematic illustration of muscle active range of motion changing due to altered muscle fiber length. **(A)** Short muscle fibers result in only 40° range of motion from 40° to 80° of flexion. **(B)** Long muscle fibers result in a range of motion of about 75° from 70° to 145° of flexion.

fiber length or moment arm is altered (*e.g.*, due to surgery or trauma), the joint strength and range of motion can be dramatically altered.

TORQUE GENERATION IN THE HUMAN WRIST

As discussed above, it is not yet routinely possible to measure either muscle force or moment arm directly in human systems. However, a number of indirect methods have been used to obtain the necessary information to create a model to describe torque generation in the human wrist. To predict the muscle forces and wrist extension moments generated by the prime movers of the wrist, a biomechanical model previously described was implemented (Loren et al., 1996). This model was based on experimental measurement of prime wrist mover muscle architecture (Lieber, Fazeli, & Botte, 1990) and the mechanical properties of

each wrist tendon (Loren & Lieber, 1995). Moment arms were then measured on cadaveric extremities (Loren et al., 1996) using a stepwise regression procedure (Burkholder & Lieber, 1996) in which data were fit and differentiated with respect to joint angle to yield moment arms. The details of the methods are not critical, just that muscle forces and moment arms were used to predict joint torque values. Equations that described the moment arms of the prime wrist movers were as follows:

$$r_{FCU}(\theta) = -14 + 0.028 \cdot \theta \qquad \text{(Eq. 3-7)}$$

$$r_{ECU}(\theta) = 7.2 + .0022 \cdot \theta^2 - 4.1 \cdot 10^{-9} \cdot \theta^5 \qquad \text{(Eq. 3-8)}$$

$$r_{FCR}(\theta) = -15 + 0.082 \cdot \theta \qquad \text{(Eq. 3-9)}$$

$$r_{ECRB}(\theta) = 16 + 0.16 \cdot \theta + .00087 \cdot \theta^2 - .000058 \cdot \theta^3 \qquad \text{(Eq. 3-10)}$$

$$r_{ECRL}(\theta) = 10 + 0.17 \cdot \theta \qquad \text{(Eq. 3-11)}$$

Therapist's Comments

One question that always comes up when I talk about the relationship between sarcomere length-tension relationship and joint moment arms is "Can this information be applied to exercise?" I think so. Although this is not a definitive answer, as shown in this text, muscles are strengthened when subjected to high forces (Chapters 4 and 6). Thus, strictly speaking, if one were to perform exercise at the joint angle in which the *muscle* produced the maximum force, it may not be the same joint angle at which the patient is strongest (See, for example, Fig. 3-16B). Thus, if the frog, described in Figure 3-15, was to "hop" into my clinic, I would be tempted to exercise the semitendinosus muscle with the knee in full flexion and the hip at 90° even though the torque (strength) at this angle is low. This is a provocative concept that requires explicit testing once more of these relationships are known for human muscle (such as the wrist example given below).

in which $r_i(\theta)$ represents the moment arm for the selected muscle (in mm), wrist joint angle (θ) is in degrees, negative angles refer to wrist flexion, and the subscript refers to the specific muscle (Fig. 3-20).

Based on the relatively complete data set regarding wrist muscle and joint properties, a few general trends emerged. Wrist extensors were predicted to operate primarily on the plateau and descending limb of their sarcomere length-tension curve (Fig. 3-21) with all muscles generating maximal force in full extension. Only the ECRB was predicted to operate at sarcomere lengths corresponding to less than 80% P_o in the normal range of motion. Wrist flexors were predicted to operate predominantly on the shallow and steep ascending limbs of their length-tension curve with both flexors generating maximal force in full wrist extension (Fig. 3-21). Note that in full flexion, it is possible for wrist flexors to generate forces that are less than 50% P_o.

Such a design presents interesting implications for the design of the wrist as a torque motor. Both flexor and extensor muscle groups generate maximum force with the wrist fully extended. As the wrist extends, maximum isometric extensor force increases due to extensor shortening up the descending limb of the length-tension curve and maximum isometric flexor force increases due to flexor lengthening up the ascending limb of the length-tension curve. This effect is superimposed upon an increasing extensor moment arm as the extensor muscles elevate off of the wrist under the extensor retinaculum and a decreasing flexor moment arm as the flexors juxtapose the wrist beneath the flexor retinaculum. Combining the muscle and joint effects, extensor muscle force is amplified by an increasing extensor moment arm and flexor muscle force is attenuated by a decreasing flexor moment arm (Fig. 3-20). Interestingly, because the flexors as a group develop significantly greater force than the extensors (due to their larger physiological cross-sectional area), the net result is a nearly constant ratio of flexor to extensor torque over the wrist range of motion (Fig. 3-22). In fact, while at the muscle level, the flexors are considerably stronger than the extensors (Brand,

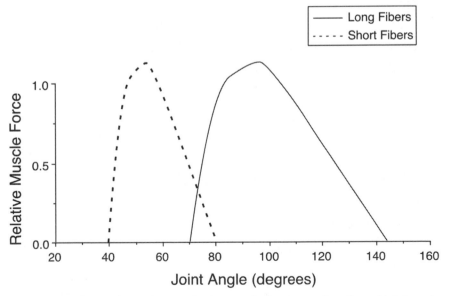

FIGURE 3-18. Comparison of approximate muscle force as a function of joint angle for the two "muscles" in Figure 3-17. Note that the muscle with the long fibers (solid line) has a range of motion of 75° while the muscle with the short fibers (dotted line) has a range of only 40°.

Beach, & Thompson, 1981; Lieber, Fazeli, & Botte, 1990), when including the wrist kinematics, extensor moment slightly exceeds flexor moment. Additionally, wrist resistance to angular perturbation increases as the wrist is

TABLE 3-1	Fiber Lengths and Moment Arms of Limb Muscles[a]

Muscle	Fiber Length (m)	Fiber Length/ Moment Arm Ratio
Leg muscles		
Adductor longus	.132	2.80
Adductor magnus	.144	2.71
Rectus femoris	.082	1.70
Iliopsoas	.127	6.54
Gluteus maximus	.180	79.5
Gluteus medius	.081	5.79
Gluteus minimus	.064	13.9
Pectineus	.130	5.27
Tensor fascia latae	.118	2.80
Gracilis	.345	6.26
Sartorius	.566	10.8
Hamstrings	.107	1.76
Biceps femoris (short head)	.173	4.38
Vasti	.084	1.78
Gastrocnemius	.048	1.47
Soleus	.024	.926
Other plantarflexors	.038	5.77
Dorsiflexors	.101	3.08
Wrist muscles		
Extensor carpi radialis longus	76	11
Extensor carpi radialis brevis	48	4
Extensor carpi ulnaris	50	8.3
Flexor carpi radialis	51	3.4
Flexor carpi ulnaris	41	2.6

[a]Data compiled from: Hoy, M.G., Zajac, F.E., Gordon, M.E. (1990). A musculoskeletal model of the human lower extremity: The effect of muscle, tendon, and moment arm on the moment-angle relationship of musculotendon actuators at the hip, knee, and ankle. *Journal of Biomechanics, 23,* 157–169; Lieber, R.L., Fazeli, B.M., Botte, M.J. (1990). Architecture of selected wrist flexor and extensor muscles. *Journal of Hand Surgery, 15A,* 244–250; Horii, K.N., An, W.P., Cooney, Linscheid, R.L. (1991). Kinematics and tendon excursion of wrist movers. *Journal of Hand Surgery, 18A,* 83–90; and Loren, G.J., Shoemaker, S.D., Burkholder, T.J., Jacobson, M.D., Fridén, J., Lieber, R.L. (1996). Influences of human wrist motor design on joint torque. *Journal of Biomechanics, 29,* 331–342.

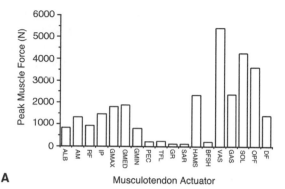

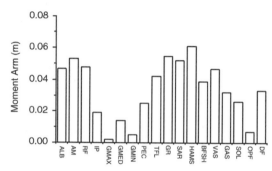

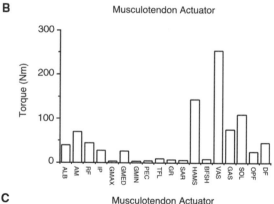

FIGURE 3-19. Bar graphs of muscle force **(A)**, moment arm **(B)**, and torque **(C)** for various muscles of the lower limb. Note that torque is not an exactly scaled representation of either moment arm or muscle force. (Data from: Hoy, M.G., Zajac, F.E., Gordon, M.E. (1990). A musculoskeletal model of the human lower extremity: The effect of muscle, tendon, and moment arm on the moment-angle relationship of musculotendon actuators at the hip, knee, and ankle. *Journal of Biomechanics, 23,* 157–169.)

moved to full extension because both flexor and extensor moments increase in a similar fashion (Fig. 3-22). To summarize the results from these studies, coordination between muscle and joint properties results in a torque system that is balanced throughout the range of motion in spite of varying muscle force and joint moment arms. This balance is achieved at the expense of

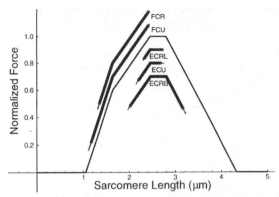

FIGURE 3-21. Predicted operating range of the prime movers of the wrist superimposed upon a human sarcomere length-tension curve. Abbreviations are the same as Figure 3-20. (Data From: Lieber, R.L., Fridén, J. (1998). Musculoskeletal balance of the human wrist elucidated using intraoperative laser diffraction. *Journal of Electromyography and Kinesiology, 8,* 93–100.)

maximum moment generation at the wrist and therefore, we conclude that this system is not simply designed to operate near maximum force as is often assumed in musculoskeletal models. Importantly, experimental support for this theoretical model was recently published providing support for both the concept and the experimental approach (Gillard, Yakovenko, Cameron, & Prochazka, 2000).

Performance in the Musculoskeletal System

At this point it is useful to review that, in our discussions of muscles, tendons, and joints, a number of intrinsic and extrinsic design parameters in the musculoskeletal system that are related to different aspects of performance have been discovered. Some are related only to the isolated muscle, joint, or tendon properties (*e.g.,* fiber length, moment arm, tendon compliance) and others are related to the interaction between these systems (*e.g.,* fiber length : moment arm ratio, fiber length : tendon ratio). All of these parameters are listed in Table 3-2. Note that it is possible to alter muscle, muscle-joint, muscle-tendon, and torque motor properties in numerous ways and in numerous combinations. It is not surprising to see such

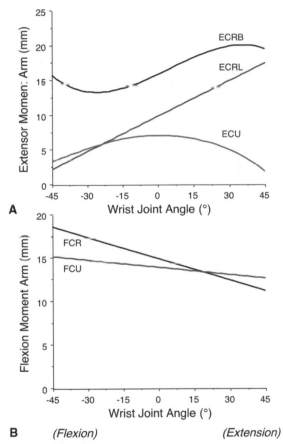

FIGURE 3-20. Graph of wrist muscle moment arms as a function of wrist joint angle from equations 3-7 to 3-11. **(A)** Wrist extensors, **(B)** Wrist flexors. Abbreviations: FCU, flexor carpi ulnaris; FCR, flexor carpi radialis; ECU, extensor carpi ulnaris; ECRB, extensor carpi radialis brevis; ECRL, extensor carpi radialis longus. (Data from: Loren, G.J., Shoemaker, S.D., Burkholder, T.J., Jacobson, M.D., Fridén, J., Lieber, R.L. (1996). Influences of human wrist motor design on joint torque. *Journal of Biomechanics, 29,* 331–342.)

> ### Therapist's Comments
>
> To reinforce the idea that the relationship between muscle and joint, as described above, for the wrist is not unique in the human body, we have performed a similar study in the lower extremity in which we measured the change in biceps femoris long head fascicle length with movement of the hip and knee (Chleboun et al., 2001). We estimated the sarcomere length change based on sarcomere length in a cadaver biceps femoris to relate the length-tension relationship to joint position change as shown above for the wrist. We found that this biarticular muscle was predicted to operate over a small portion of the ascending limb, and primarily over the plateau and the descending limb of the length-tension relationship. It is interesting that two very different anatomical positions (*i.e.,* hip and knee both flexed to 90° and hip and knee both at 0°) occupied the plateau of the length-tension relationship.

variation in design from muscle-to-muscle and joint-to-joint. It would be naïve and closed-minded to think that all joint systems must be designed identically. However, these parameters provide some understanding of the underlying design of a particular system of interest (*e.g.,* design for high force production, speed, etc.).

Physiological Range of Motion

The normal voluntary active range of motion (ROM) has been defined clinically for a number of joints and is commonly used during physical examination to diagnose deficiency or disease. However, before proceeding directly to the ROM discussion, the way in which muscle contractile properties vary as a function of architecture must be covered, because different architectural arrangements will have a profound impact on voluntary ROM.

Force-Generating Properties of Muscles with Different Architectures

In Chapter 2 we showed that muscle architecture had a profound influence on muscle force-

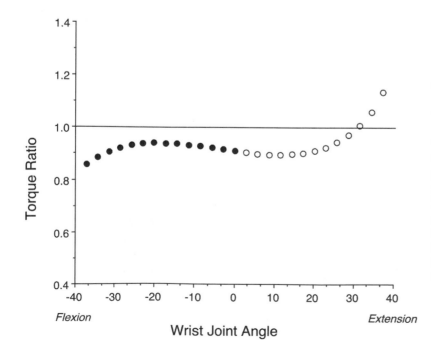

FIGURE 3-22. Ratio of wrist flexion torque-to-wrist extension torque throughout the wrist range of motion. Note that the torque ratio is nearly one throughout the entire range of motion despite changing muscle forces and moment arms. Filled circles represent flexed angles while open circles represent extended angles. Note that wrist extensor moment slightly exceeds wrist flexor moment.

TABLE 3-2	Design Parameters of the Musculoskeletal System
Parameter	**Property Affected**
Fiber length	Velocity or excursion
Fiber area	Fiber force
Physiologic cross-sectional area	Maximum muscle force and torque
Tendon length	Increased range, damping, and energy storage
Moment arm	Maximum torque
Tendon length/fiber length ratio	Relative stiffness of a muscle-tendon unit
Fiber length/moment arm ratio	Relative muscle-joint influence
Fiber type distribution	Muscle speed and endurance
Motor unit distribution	Relative muscle control

generating properties. Recall that muscle force is proportional to physiological cross-sectional area (PCSA), whereas muscle speed (or excursion) is proportional to fiber length. For example, suppose there were two muscles with dramatically different designs but identical muscle fiber types, as illustrated in Figure 3-23. Both muscles have approximately the same amount of contractile material (mass), but the arrangement of this material is quite different. The muscle in Figure 3-23A, shown as the biceps brachii, has relatively long fibers that extend almost the entire length of the muscle and are parallel to the muscle's force-generating axis. In architectural lingo this is the classic parallel-fibered muscle. Contrast this with the muscle shown in Figure 3-23B shown as a vastus lateralis, which has relatively short fibers that extend a short length relative to the muscle length and are tilted by about 30° to the muscle's force-generating axis. This is the classic pennated muscle. It must be emphasized that the intrinsic length-tension and force-velocity properties of these two muscles are identical; i.e., the properties of the composite sarcomeres are identical. It is the arrangement of the sarcomeres that imparts the functional differences

upon the two muscles. In Figure 3-24A, the schematic length-tension curves of the two muscles is plotted. Note that muscle A, with its longer fibers, has a greater absolute working range compared with muscle B. This is because, for a given muscle length change, the sarcomeres in muscle A lengthen less because the length change is distributed over a greater number of sarcomeres. However, note also that muscle A generates a lower tension than muscle B, because muscle B contains a much greater PCSA. Muscle B is perhaps designed for force production whereas muscle A is designed for excursion. This concept is well illustrated by the force-velocity curves plotted in Figure 3-24B. Note that muscle A has a maximum contraction velocity (V_{max}) that is much greater than muscle B, again because of its long fibers. Each sarcomere within the fiber contracts at the same velocity, whether in muscle A or muscle B. However, by placing more sarcomeres in series in muscle A, the overall muscle velocity is greater. Again, note that the maximum tetanic tension (P_o), for muscle B is much greater than that observed for muscle A, because of its greater PCSA.

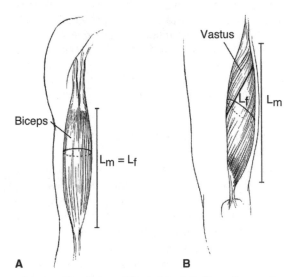

FIGURE 3-23. Schematic representation of muscles with different architectures. **(A)** Muscle with long fibers and small PCSA. **(B)** Muscle with short fibers and large PCSA.

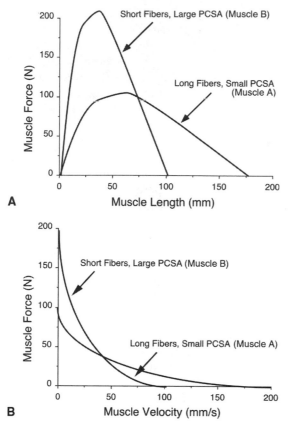

FIGURE 3-24. (A) Schematic length-tension relationships of muscles A and B shown in Figure 3-23. Note that the muscle in 3-23A has a longer working range and lower maximum tetanic tension due to long fibers and small PCSA. **(B)** Force-velocity relationships of muscles shown in Figure 3-23. Note that the muscle in 3-23A with longer fibers has a higher contractile velocity but a lower maximum tetanic tension.

Range of Motion as a Function of Architecture

Therefore, muscles with longer fibers have a longer functional range than muscles with shorter fibers. As discussed previously, does this imply that muscles with longer fibers are associated with joints that have larger ROMs? The answer is no. It is true that a muscle with longer fibers does have a longer working range. However, the amount of muscle length change that occurs as a joint rotates strongly depends on the muscle moment arm as previously de-

fined. This idea is illustrated in Figure 3-25, in which a simulated "muscle" is attached using two different moment arms. In Figure 3-25A, the moment arm is much less than in Figure 3-25B. This means that in Figure 3-25A, the muscle will change length much less for a given

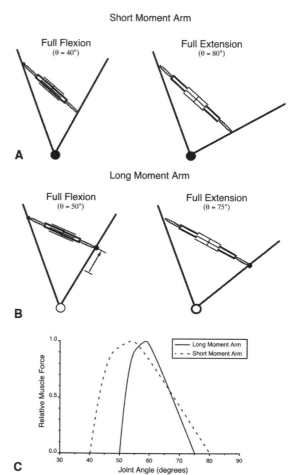

FIGURE 3-25. Effect of changing moment arm on active range of motion (ROM). In this example, the muscle in Figure 3-17A was attached with two different moment arms. **(A)** 40° range of motion for "normal" muscle. **(B)** Moment arm increase results in a decrease in range of motion to 25°. In **(B)**, the active ROM is smaller since the moment arm is greater, and therefore, more sarcomere length change occurs for a given angular rotation. **(C)** Comparison of force versus joint angle (range of motion) for muscles with short (dotted line) or long (solid line) moment arms.

change in joint angle compared to the same change in joint angle in Figure 3-25B. As a result, the active ROM for the muscle-joint system shown in Figure 3-25A will be much greater than that which is shown in Figure 3-25B in spite of the fact that their muscular properties are identical. In fact, in the current example, increasing moment arm decreased range of motion from 40° to only 25° (Fig. 3-25C).

Muscles that are, for instance, designed for speed because of their long fibers may not actually produce large velocities if they are placed in position with a large moment arm. The increased moment arm causes a greater joint moment, and the muscle is best suited for torque production. Similarly, a muscle that appears to be designed for force production due to the large PCSA, if placed in position with a small moment arm, may actually produce high-joint excursions or angular velocities.

TORQUE GENERATION IN THE HUMAN WRIST EXTENSORS

The interplay between muscle and joint properties and the concept of musculoskeletal design is well illustrated by examination of muscles and joints of the human wrist. First, consider the muscles themselves. Inspection of the architecture graph (Fig. 1-18) reveals that the ECRB is a muscle with shorter fibers and larger PCSA compared with the ECRL. The simplest functional comparison between these two muscles would be to state that the ECRB has a design that favors force production whereas the ECRL has a design that favors excursion. However, these muscles are synergistic at the wrist and both appear to be activated synchronously (Bäckdahl & Carlsöö, 1961; McFarland, Krusen, & Weathersby, 1962; Riek & Bawa, 1992). Seeing this difference and beginning to understand the interplay between muscle and joint properties, we might speculate that the design of the wrist muscle-joint system taken together might compensate for differences between the muscles. In other words, even though the muscles had different architectural designs,

perhaps the torque motors were similar. If the ECRB had a wrist moment arm that was muscle smaller than the ECRL, the fiber length change per joint angle rotation could actually be the same in the two muscle groups and their torque generating properties much more similar. Was this the case? It turned out not to be. First, the moment arms of the two muscles acting in wrist extension were measured using traditional biomechanical methods (Loren et al., 1996). It was discovered that the ECRB moment arm was actually much greater than the ECRL moment arm (Fig. 3-20). This meant that, not only did the joint moment arm not compensate for the differences between muscles, it actually accentuated the differences (Fig. 3-26). Why is this a good design? From a design point of view, high moment arm : fiber length ratio results in a torque motor in which large fiber length changes produce large force changes during joint rotation and, thus, this motor would vary torque output greatly as the joint rotated. This is more or less the design of the ECRB torque motor for wrist extension motions, based on its relatively short fibers and large moment arm. In

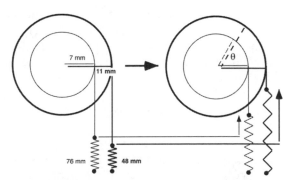

FIGURE 3-26. Schematic diagram of the interrelationship between fiber length and moment arm for the ECRB and ECRL torque motors. The ECRB (bold print, thick lines) with its shorter fibers and longer moment arm changes sarcomere length about 2.5 times as much as the ECRL with its longer fibers and smaller moment arm. (Data from: Lieber, R.L., Ljung, B-O., Fridén, J. (1997). Intraoperative sarcomere measurements reveal differential musculoskeletal design of long and short wrist extensors. *Journal of Experimental Biology, 200*, 19–25.)

contrast, the significantly longer fibers and smaller moment arm of the ECRL results in a torque motor with different functional properties. The ECRL-based motor retains a more constant torque output with joint rotation because, for a given amount of joint rotation, force changes less. This differential muscle-joint interaction may provide insight into the diversity of design between muscles. The ECRB and ECRL muscles as a synergistic group have a maximum tetanic tension of 25.6 kg and a V_{max} (converted to joint angle velocity) of approximately 2,800 °/s. For a single muscle to generate that much force while maintaining such a high V_{max}, the fiber length would have to be 76 mm (as for the ECRL to maintain the same V_{max}) and the cross-sectional area would have to be about 4.2 cm² (the sum of the two muscles' physiological cross-sectional areas to maintain the same maximum force). Using the simple equation for muscle physiological cross-sectional area (Sacks & Roy, 1982), this single muscle would weigh 33.7 g, which is over 30% greater than the sum of the two muscle masses (Lieber, Fazeli, & Botte, 1990). Having two muscles as synergists thus accomplishes the same task at the velocity extremes with a much lower overall mass. This not only saves "energy" because less tissue must be maintained, it also provides less inertial resistance to movement, which may be beneficial at high velocities.

"OPTIMAL" ARCHITECTURE FOR A PARTICULAR FUNCTION

In theory, it is possible to arrange a given quantity of sarcomeres (i.e., a fixed muscle mass) to produce almost any combination of cross-sectional area and maximum shortening velocity simply by adjusting the fiber length. This can be illustrated by a thought exercise in which muscle fiber length is changed mathematically while maintaining constant muscle mass and the effect on performance is calculated. Based on the relationship between muscle mass, PCSA, and fiber length (Equation 1-1), increasing fiber length requires a decrease in PCSA, and thus, a decrease in muscle force

(Fig. 3-27A). In contrast, as fiber length increases, sarcomere velocity decreases for a given angular velocity, resulting in increased "dynamic" muscle force (i.e., muscle force at a fixed velocity, Fig. 3-27B). These two opposing effects illustrate the interaction between isometric force production (resulting from PCSA) and dynamic force production (resulting from sarcomere number and velocity). Since the PCSA effect is an exponential decrease with increasing fiber length and the sarcomere velocity effect is a modest linear increase with increasing fiber length, their product demonstrates an "optimal" design—a design in which force is maximum for a muscle of a given mass operating at a specified velocity (Fig. 3-27C). Interestingly, when theoretical optimal fiber lengths were calculated for a variety of mouse muscles and then experimentally measured, the measured values were close to their theoretical optima (Lieber, 1997).

To summarize, muscle design may or may not be a reflection of its actual use in the physiological muscle-joint torque-generating system. It does seem, in general, that muscle fiber length and muscle moment arm are positively correlated (McClearn, 1985). Thus, muscles with long fibers tend to have long moment arms, but this is not necessarily the case. Muscle architectural features may represent muscle adaptation to kinematic criteria. However, definitive support for this suggestion awaits further study.

Isokinetic Dynamometers Used in Physical Assessment

It is important to be able to characterize human performance objectively in sports and rehabilitation, not only to evaluate patient progress but also to ascertain the efficacy of clinical treatment. Using objective criteria such as maximum joint moment and ROM, it is possible to evaluate the efficacy of many surgical and rehabilitative procedures. One of the most commonly used tools for musculoskeletal assess-

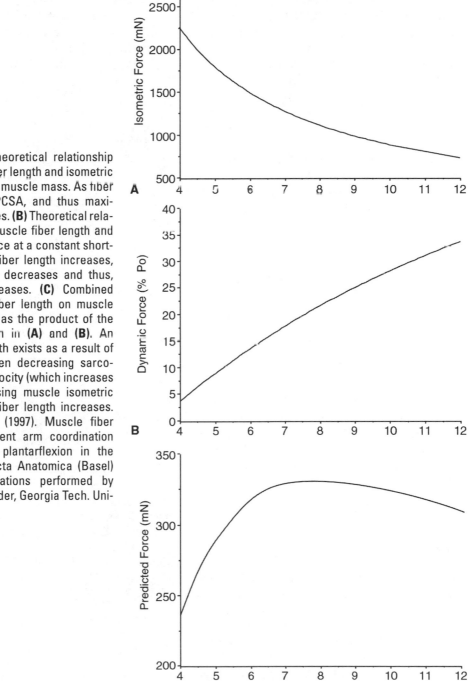

FIGURE 3-27. **(A)** Theoretical relationship between muscle fiber length and isometric force for a constant muscle mass. As fiber length increases, PCSA, and thus maximum force decreases. **(B)** Theoretical relationship between muscle fiber length and dynamic muscle force at a constant shortening velocity. As fiber length increases, sarcomere velocity decreases and thus, muscle force increases. **(C)** Combined effect of varying fiber length on muscle tension, calculated as the product of the relationships shown in **(A)** and **(B)**. An "optimal" fiber length exists as a result of the tradeoff between decreasing sarcomere shortening velocity (which increases force) and decreasing muscle isometric force capacity as fiber length increases. (From: Lieber, R.L. (1997). Muscle fiber length and movement arm coordination during dorsi- and plantarflexion in the mouse hindlimb. Acta Anatomica (Basel) 159, 84–89; Calculations performed by Dr. Thomas Burkholder, Georgia Tech. University.)

ment is the isokinetic dynamometer. This is a device that measures joint moment while maintaining a constant joint velocity (isokinetic = "same motion"). If joint velocity is set to zero, an isometric joint moment versus joint angle relationship is generated, which, as described above, represents the interaction between muscle and joint properties. It is clearly not appropriate to ascribe any portion of a moment versus joint angle curve to either muscle or joint properties alone.

Physiological Cross-Sectional Area and Fiber Length Influence on Isokinetic Torque

Consider the underlying physiological processes that make up the isokinetic joint moment. At this point, only the ideal case will be considered, i.e. instantaneous and complete activation of the entire muscle throughout the joint range of motion. As the joint begins to move, dynamic muscle contractile properties determine the muscle force developed based on their force-velocity relationships. It can be assumed that joint kinematics are velocity independent and, thus, variations in the moment-angle curves as a function of velocity represent variations in muscle force. How should such isokinetic data be interpreted? What should be expected? First, the moment achieved during isokinetic contraction (concentric muscle contraction) must necessarily be less than that achieved during isometric contraction because the muscle has a typical force-velocity relationship (Fig. 2-7). Second, the muscle force generated during isokinetic contraction will be a function of the muscle's PCSA and its fiber length. The reason that isokinetic muscle force varies with PCSA is obvious because isometric force is directly proportional to PCSA. The reason that muscle force varies with fiber length is less obvious although straightforward. Recall that isokinetic moment measurements are obtained while the joint is limited to a specific isokinetic movement. This means that the muscle is also forced to maintain a certain (although not necessarily constant) shortening velocity. Since shortening velocity is fixed, the longer the muscle fibers, the higher the relative muscle

force that can be sustained during shortening. This is because longer muscle fibers have more sarcomeres in series and, with longer fibers, each sarcomere will have a slower absolute contraction velocity, allowing it to stay higher on its force-velocity curve (i.e., closer to P_o). This idea is illustrated in Figure 3-28A, in

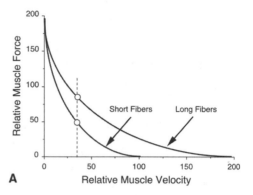

A

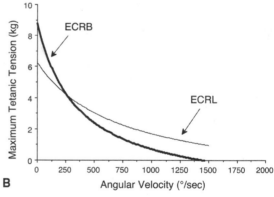

B

FIGURE 3-28. (A) Force-velocity relationships of two muscles with different fiber lengths but identical strengths. Note that the muscle with longer fibers maintains a higher force at a given velocity (dashed vertical line) due to a smaller sarcomere shortening velocity. Difference between muscles becomes smaller as shortening velocity decreases. **(B)** Torque-angular velocity relationship for the radial wrist extensors, ECRB and ECRL. Note that, at an angular velocity of 240 °/sec, the ECRL becomes the "stronger" muscle even though the ECRB is "stronger" under isometric conditions. These data demonstrate that, while muscle architecture may predict the isometric properties of a muscle, joint kinematics and joint velocity may strongly influence an understanding of in vivo design.

which force is measured from two hypothetical muscles that are shortening at the same velocity. Note that, for a given shortening velocity (vertical dotted line), the muscle with longer fibers maintains a higher force compared to the muscle with shorter fibers. This means that the muscle with longer fibers generates the greater force.

Such an influence of fiber length on force production is seen in the example of the long and short radial wrist extensor design presented earlier (Fig. 3-26). As described previously (Fig. 1-18) the ECRB has a higher physiological cross-sectional area and thus a higher predicted maximum tetanic tension than the ECRL because of its greater number of shorter muscle fibers (Lieber, Fazeli, & Botte, 1990). Yet, because these fibers are shorter, for a given angular velocity (assuming similar fiber-type proportions), force relative to maximum isometric tension decreases to a greater extent in the ECRB (Fig. 3-28B). Using the architectural properties of the two muscles, along with nominal values for the maximum contraction velocity (V_{max}) of mammalian muscle (Close, 1972), the force-velocity relationship for each muscle can be determined. The exact values for V_{max} and the force-velocity curvature are not important in making this comparison as long as the ECRB and ECRL fiber-type distributions are not dramatically different from one another. The contraction velocity at which the ECRL becomes stronger is approximately 80 mm/s which, on the basis of the two muscle moment arms, corresponds to an angular velocity of approximately 240°/sec (Fig. 3-28B). This results in a design in which the ECRB is stronger isometrically but, as angular velocity increases, the ECRL becomes the stronger muscle.

Fiber Length and Physiological Cross-Sectional Area in Force Production

Recall that a muscle with long fibers was designed for speed or excursion, whereas a muscle with a high PCSA was designed for force production. It is clear that, in the intact muscle-joint system, this is not necessarily the case. For example, in Figure 3-28, the muscle with

---

Box 3-4. When Are Two Muscles Better Than One?

When they are synergistic with very different architectural designs. By placing muscles together with very different architectural properties (for example, the wrist extensors, ankle dorsiflexors, and ankle plantarflexors) a much wider range of contractile properties is made possible with a much smaller muscle mass. To perform the same task with a single "supermuscle" would typically require muscles masses that are 30–50% greater than observed in nature.

---

longer fibers was actually designed for high excursion from the muscle point-of-view alone, but, when considering the muscle and joint together, it was designed for force production—it generated a greater force during movement compared to the muscle with shorter fibers. This "equivalence" of fiber length or PCSA as design strategies to increase force was explicitly proposed by Gans and DeVries (1987). The take-home lesson in these types of discussions is that it is better to understand the underlying physiology than to try to memorize a few facts about muscle design. In this way, you can simply reason out a particular situation in terms of force or speed production.

The joint moment-isokinetic velocity relationship has been studied in a number of circumstances for variously aged populations of both genders. These data serve as normative values in evaluating limb and/or health status. Early in the development of the isokinetic dynamometer, Perrine and Edgerton (1978) measured the torque-isokinetic relationship on healthy individuals and attempted to interpret the data in terms of muscle force-velocity properties (Fig. 3-29). The torque-isokinetic velocity relationship looked (dangerously) similar to the isolated muscle force-velocity relationship. The main deviation between the two was that the torque observed at very low velocities was much lower than was expected based on extrapolation of the torque-velocity relationship to zero velocity (dotted lines in Fig. 3-29). Perrin

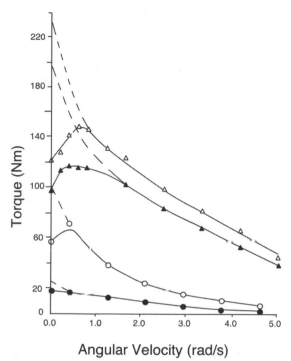

FIGURE 3-29. Isokinetic torque-angular velocity relationship elucidated by Wickiewicz et al. (1983) on quadriceps (open triangles), hamstrings (filled triangles), plantarflexors (open circles), and dorsiflexors (filled circles). Dotted lines extending to slow velocities represent the theoretical force-velocity curve of Hill (1938). Note that forces at low angular velocities are much lower than predicted. This may represent an "override" of the nervous system to prevent very high muscle forces.

and Edgerton interpreted this deviation as representing a safety factor in the neural system that prevented overactivation of the muscle to dangerously high force levels. Since that time, others have repeated the experiments and obtained similar results; however, the underlying explanation for the deviation is not completely known. It is difficult to rigorously interpret torque-velocity data because a number of factors are typically unknown. These include the following:

1. Muscle physiological cross-sectional area (PCSA).

2. The fraction of the muscle's PCSA that is activated.
3. Absolute moment arm as a function of joint angle and velocity.
4. Muscle fiber length as a function of joint angle and velocity.
5. Tendon length as a function of joint angle and velocity.
6. Inertial properties of the joint.

These factors may be only roughly estimated or even ignored in experimental studies of isokinetic torque and the extent to which they affect the conclusions of the study depend on the particular study. These factors will be considered independently as the limitations of isokinetic dynamometers are presented.

Limitations of Isokinetic Dynamometers

The first issue considered is the lack of information regarding muscle PCSA. As discussed in Chapter 2, muscle PCSA is almost never the same value as any anatomical PCSA measured in one of the traditional anatomical planes. Thus, to date, the best estimates of intact human PCSAs are derived from combination studies in which muscle volume is first determined using an imaging method such as CT scanning, MRI, or even ultrasound (Fukunaga et al., 1992). Then, PCSA is calculated using a modified form of Equation 1-1 in which measured muscle volume is substituted for calculated muscle volume and PCSA is calculated as:

$$PCSA = \frac{Muscle\ Volume \cdot \cos\theta}{Fiber\ Length} \qquad (Eq.\ 3\text{-}12)$$

Simply determining this value for PCSA is a study in itself and thus, in almost all reports, this value is ignored or assumed based on published data in the literature. If the purpose of the study is to simply measure changes in performance, this is probably not a problem. However, if the purpose of the study is to establish values for force per unit area or test for absolute muscle size differences between genders or age groups, this may pose a serious limitation. A second unknown in most studies is the activa-

tion of the muscle itself during isokinetic testing. This is important for at least two reasons. First, if the muscle is not maximally activated, the torque measured cannot be interpreted in terms of the muscle's maximum tetanic force, but must be interpreted relative to the force generated at the same activation level. Many estimate the relative muscle activation level based on EMG data, which are scaled to the EMG values obtained during maximum isometric activation by the same individual. Of course, this approach assumes that the amount of muscle activated scales with EMG and that, during isometric activation, muscle activation is maximal. Of these two, the latter is questionable (Enoka & Fuglevand, 1993) and the extent to which the former is true probably depends on the muscle group studied. The third factor, absolute moment arm of the muscle is typically estimated by imaging the joint during the same type of rotation that occurs during isokinetic testing. Most of these types of measurements have been performed on the knee and ankle joints, the major target of isokinetic tests (Smidt, 1973). The problem with these estimates is that they usually measure the joint at rest and, when a muscle is activated causing the tendon to become taut, its moment arm can increase. This has been clearly demonstrated for the dorsiflexors (Ito, Akima, and Fukunaga, 2000). Since torque is directly proportional to

moment arm, errors in moment arm-estimate directly affect the accuracy of torque measurements. Again, if the investigation deals with change in torque, it is usually safe to assume that moment arm has remained constant over the short period of study. If however, absolute torques are interpreted in terms of absolute muscle forces, precise measures of moment arm are required.

The two unknowns that are most important and also most difficult to obtain are muscle fiber and tendon length/velocity during isokinetic motion. The reason these are important factors is obvious: muscle force is highly dependent on length and velocity as previously discussed (Chapter 2, pages 51 to 66). To "account" for variations in muscle or tendon length during isokinetic movements, some individuals report an "angle specific" joint torque, i.e., torque generated at a specified joint angle. The idea is to report torques at the same fiber length, regardless of speed. However, this is not correct for the following reason: because muscle force varies with velocity (due to the force-velocity relationship) and tendon elongation varies with muscle force (due to its stress-strain relationship), tendon elongation varies with muscle velocity. Or stated in another way, muscle fiber length varies with isokinetic velocity so that, even if a torque is measured at a specified angle, this does not represent identical fiber lengths.

This phenomenon was recently explicitly studied using ultrasound measurements by Fukunaga and colleagues (Ichinose, Kawakami, Ito, Kanehisa, & Fukunaga, 2000). These authors measured muscle fiber length of the vastus lateralis (VL) muscle during isokinetic testing protocols to try to understand the physiological basis for isokinetic torque generation itself and to explicitly test the assumption regarding "angle specific" torque measurements. They measured VL fiber length at two different angular velocities across a large knee joint range of motion. Importantly, they found that, in spite of the fact that angular velocity was maintained at a constant level (Fig. 3-30A), and

---

Box 3-5. What Is "Iso" About Isokinetic Testing?

Most isokinetic testing machines are good enough to keep the angular velocity constant during testing. However, detailed real-time studies of quadriceps muscles have shown that muscle fiber velocity and moment arm are basically never constant during the test. This means that it is extremely problematic to interpret isokinetic data in terms of the muscles generating the torque. The results from these types of studies are often vastly overstated and overinterpreted.

thus, the movement really was "isokinetic," nothing else was constant during the movement. Most importantly, muscle fiber velocity was never constant throughout the joint range of motion, especially at the higher velocity of 150°/sec (Fig. 3-30B). This was due to all of the factors that have been discussed: variable knee extensor moment arm, variable tendon compliance, and variable muscle activation. Thus, although isokinetic torque values may be expressed as norms for a given population (*e.g.,* Caucasian females older than 80 years), the underlying basis for the actual values obtained is elusive. As a result, isokinetic dynamometry

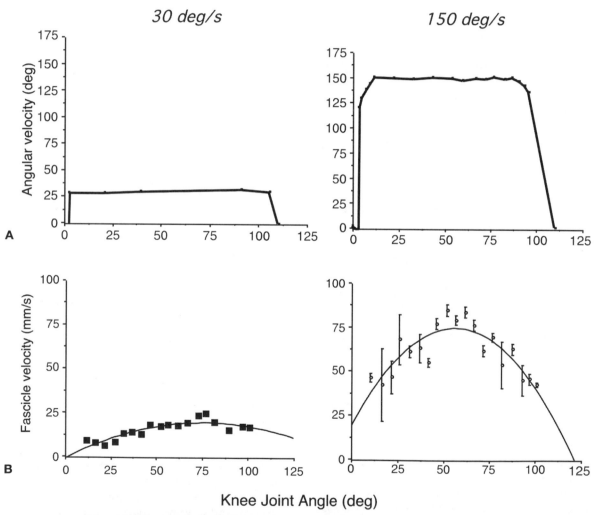

FIGURE 3-30. Muscle fiber velocity measured using ultrasound during isokinetic dynamometry. Note that, in spite of the fact that joint angular velocity is "constant," muscle fiber velocity is not at all constant. **(A)** Angular velocity of joint during isokinetic testing at 30°/sec (left) and 150 °/sec (right). **(B)** Muscle fiber velocity during isokinetic testing at 30°/sec (left) and 150 °/sec (right). Note greater variations in fiber velocity at higher angular velocities. (Data from: Ichinose, Y., Kawakami, Y., Ito, M., Kanehisa, H., Fukunaga, T. (2000). In vivo estimation of contraction velocity of human vastus lateralis muscle during "isokinetic" action. *Journal of Applied Physiology, 88,* 851–856.)

Therapist's Comment

Another example of problems in isokinetic dynamometry is the fact that the angular velocity of many "normal" activities is far beyond the maximal angular velocity of the isokinetic devices. For example, glenohumeral rotation during throwing is about 6000°/sec whereas most machines are limited to ~300°/sec. Another example is the angular velocity of the knee and ankle just before lift off during jumping is about 720°/sec. Finally, as Dr. Lieber points out in this chapter, the joint angular velocity is maximum at a time when fascicle length is constant thus shortening velocity of the fascicles is near zero. These facts render this "tool" a less-than-reliable indicator of muscle performance.

should be used and interpreted with extreme caution. The numbers themselves may be repeatable, but the underlying basis for the values themselves for changes in the values is elusive.

A practical note regarding this testing method is that the time required to recruit muscle fibers typically ranges from 50–200 msec. Thus, it is not wise to use any torque data obtained during this startup portion of the dynamic torque curve. At high angular velocities, this may represent most of the torque record itself. During recruitment and acceleration, the limb is accelerating from stationary to the selected speed of motion, and, unfortunately, at the end of the limb acceleration phase, the limb strikes the testing bar (even if it was already in contact) and generates a force spike simply due to the impact. As a result, torques measured in this deceleration region can be artificially high and not represent torque generated by the muscle, rather, representing instead the impact torque of a decelerating limb onto a measuring tool. There are some who think this impact force is even dangerous to the subject. As a result of limitations such as these, several manu-

facturers have installed electronic damping circuits to minimize the observation of these mechanical artifacts. One must be sure that the damping itself does not mask the intended measurement.

The Gait Cycle

Muscle-joint interaction has been discussed under very specific conditions: isometric, isokinetic, and isotonic conditions. However, what muscle forces and lengths are observed during normal movement? This activation of muscles and joints during normal movement has been studied both in animals and in humans (Basmajian & DeLuca, 1985). Goslow et al. presented a description of feline muscle-tendon unit length, joint angles, and gait speeds (Goslow, Reinking, & Stuart, 1973). In several cats, they measured isolated bone dimensions and bone movement (using real-time radiography at the prestigious Harvard Museum of Comparative Zoology) during walking at various speeds. They then related the various muscle lengths and dimensions to the cats' movement and to the known pattern of muscle electrical activation (Engberg & Lundberg, 1969).

This new knowledge of muscle and joint properties will now be applied to a discussion of the typical action of muscles and joints during walking and running. You will see that the gait cycle is a wonderfully orchestrated sequence of electrical and mechanical events that culminate in the coordinated propulsion of a body through space (Fig. 3-31). First, the different phases of the gait cycle will be defined, and then skeletal, electrical, and muscular changes that occur during the various phases will be discussed. Finally, these data will be interpreted in terms of what has been learned about muscle's static and dynamic properties.

Phases of the Gait Cycle

In its most general form, the gait cycle is divided into two phases: stance and swing (Table 3-3, Figure 3-31). These phases refer to the ac-

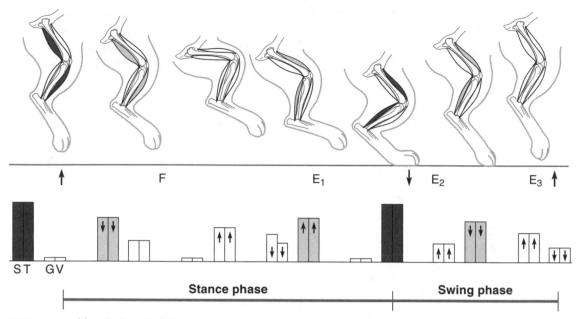

FIGURE 3-31. Muscle length, joint angle, and activation patterns during the cat gait cycle. (Muscle length and joint angles from Goslow, G.J., Reinking, R., Stuart, D. (1973). The cat step cycle: Hind limb joint angles and muscle lengths during unrestrained locomotion. *Journal of Morphology, 141*, 1–42.; EMG data from: Engberg, I., Lundberg, A. (1969). An electromyographic analysis of muscular activity in the hindlimb of the cat during unrestrained locomotion. *Acta Physiologica Scandinavica, 75*, 614–630.) Activation of each muscle group is shown as a different shading pattern. Darker shading represents higher activation. Lower bar graphs represent activation patterns for muscles during that gait phase. Step cycle phase and toe off and toe strike are shown immediately beneath the line. S: semitendinosis, T: tibialis anterior, G: gastrocnemius, V: vasti.

TABLE 3-3	Components of the Phillippson Gait Cycle		
Swing Phase		**Stance Phase**	
F	*E₁*	*E₂*	*E₃*
Flexion phase as foot is lifted from ground	Extension of limb until foot contacts ground	"Yield" phase as foot contacts ground and supports body	Propulsive phase as limb extends and propels body into space

tion of a limb that is either in contact with the ground and, therefore, providing some body support (stance) or a limb that is airborne, preparing for the next step (swing). Both stance and swing phases are subdivided into portions that refer to the action of the various muscular groups causing the movement. During swing

phase, the limb flexors are sequentially activated at the knee, hip, and ankle to lift the limb off of the ground. The limb extensors are then activated to extend the knee and place the foot onto the ground. These two phases are referred to as F and E₁-, respectively, referring to "flexion" and the first portion of "extension." Together, they comprise the swing phase (Table 3-3). Next, the extensor muscles are activated to higher levels, and as the foot strikes the ground, muscles and skeleton absorb the shock of ground impact, yielding somewhat under the weight of the body. These events comprise the E_2 or "yield" phase of gait. Finally, in a synchronized movement, all extensors propel the body until the foot finally leaves the ground to begin another swing phase. This final propulsive phase is known as E_3. It is obvious that these phases, referred to as the Phillippson step cycle (Philippson, 1905), are named for the kinematics of functional muscle groups that are active during the various phases (Table 3-4). As will be shown there is much more to be considered during gait than simply which muscle is "on" and which is "off."

Muscle Group Activities During the Gait Cycle

As stated above, the accomplishment of a step should be viewed as a coordinated effort between the neural control system (brain and spinal cord), the muscular system, and the skeletal system. A more detailed view of the muscle

TABLE 3-4	Muscle Actions During Different Phases of the Cat Gait Cycle[a,b]			
	Swing		**Stance**	
Muscle Group	**F**	**E_1**	**E_2**	**E_3**
Extensors				
Hip	PL	AL	ISO	AS
Knee	PL	AS	AL	AS
Ankle	PL	AS	AL	AS
Flexors				
Hip	AS	ISO	AL	AL
Knee	AS/AL	AL	PS	AS/AL
Ankle	AS	AL	PL	AL

[a]Adapted from: Goslow, G.J., Reinking, R., Stuart, D. (1973). The cat step cycle: Hind limb joint angles and muscle lengths during unrestrained locomotion. *Journal of Morphology, 141*, 1–42.

[b]PL, passive lengthening; AL, active lengthening; AS, active shortening; PS, passive shortening; ISO, isometric.

groups involved in gait is summarized in Figure 3-31 for one cycle. In this example, certain specific muscles will be discussed as typical for the function of that muscle group. The iliopsoas (IP) will be considered a typical hip flexor, the semitendinosis (ST) a knee flexor, and the tibialis anterior (TA) an ankle dorsiflexor. The semimembranosus (SM) will be considered a typical hip extensor, the vastus lateralis (VL) a knee extensor, and the medial gastrocnemius (MG) and soleus (S), ankle plantarflexors. Muscle actions are much more complex than might be anticipated. In fact, the notion that muscles simply contract and cause joint rotation is incorrect and oversimplified.

During the flexion phase (F), the limb flexors (IP, ST, and TA) are activated, resulting in active flexor muscle shortening, to elevate the foot off of the ground (Fig. 3-31; Table 3-4). As a result, the hip, knee, and ankle flex. During this same period, because of active shortening of the flexors, the extensors (SM, VL, MG, S) are passively stretched. As the body mass moves forward, the limb extensors are activated, and the flexors shut off to permit initiation of limb extension (E_1). During E_1, the extensors are activated, causing limb extension, and now the extensors actively shorten. Due to (low) electrical activity in the flexors, flexors actively lengthen. As the foot strikes the ground (E_2, the yield phase of stance), the extensors are highly active. However, the mass and momentum of the body are so great that in spite of this high extensor activity, the knee and ankle joints are forced to flex or yield. Obviously, forced flexion of the hip, knee, and ankle during active extensor activity will result in active lengthening of the VL, MG, and S, respectively. Recall from the force-velocity relationship that active lengthening (eccentric contraction) results in high muscle forces. Thus, during this E_2 phase, the extensor muscles are well suited for absorbing a great deal of external kinetic energy and acting as "brakes" to make sure the joints do not collapse under the load of the body. Because this portion of the gait cycle includes eccentric muscle contraction, it is not surprising that muscle injury and soreness are sometimes associated with muscle activity seen during this phase of the gait cycle (Chapter 6). It is also not surprising that during E_2 the flexors are completely silent, since gravity and momentum are doing what the flexors would do anyway. In the last portion of stance, the lengthening extensors have generated enough force to reverse the transient joint flexion back into extension, and the flexors dramatically change from active lengthening to active shortening. This transition from lengthening to shortening (the so-called stretch-shorten cycle) has significant energetic consequences, which will be discussed later. Active shortening of the extensors during late E_3 results in pronounced joint extension and propels the body forward into space. The flexors, that were electrically silent during E_2, begin to be activated during the late stages of E_3 (in preparation for F) and are, therefore, actively lengthened.

Muscle Force Modulation During the Gait Cycle

During gait most muscle groups experience periods of active shortening, active lengthening, and passive lengthening (Table 3-4). It is exciting to understand the underlying events of this complex sequence of events, which is routinely referred to as simply "walking" or "running." Some of the fine points of gait, which relate these gross muscle and joint changes to the muscle's physiological properties and to the joint's kinematic properties should be considered before moving on. Several questions come to mind upon gross inspection of the gait cycle. First, how much does muscle force modulation really matter in accomplishing the gait cycle? Muscle force changes in response to length (length-tension relationship) and velocity (force-velocity relationship), but how do these relationships figure into physiological action of muscles during gait? Several elegant studies of gait and mathematical modeling of gait suggest that muscle length changes, during the time when muscles are active, are relatively small. In other words, when muscle force is increasing in flexors during the E_3 phase of gait, it

is not simply because sarcomere length is changing, resulting in greater overlap of thick and thin filaments and an increase in potential force. In this case, it is primarily due to increased muscle fiber recruitment.

Muscle Length Changes During the Gait Cycle

Most investigators agree that the total length muscle change that occurs during the gait cycle is typically less than 20% of the total physiological range of the muscle (the physiological muscle range is that observed when the joint is forced to go from full flexion to full extension; see pages 157–159). For example, in the study of four ankle extensors previously mentioned, Goslow et al. (1973) measured skeletal joint angles and muscle physiological properties and calculated muscle-tendon lengths during locomotion in the cat. They showed that the four ankle extensor muscles (medial gastrocnemius, lateral gastrocnemius, soleus, and plantaris) only changed length by about 20% and they generated their maximum forces at different ankle angles, ranging from 40° to 100°, and that the angle corresponding to maximum muscle moment arm was 120°. Again, here is a situation in which muscle force and moment arm are not optimized at the same angle. It can be concluded then that the musculoskeletal system is not solely designed to produce a high force at a particular angle. As a second example, Gregor et al. (1988) showed that during the stance phase of gait when the soleus (SOL) first actively lengthens and then actively shortens, the total length excursion is only about 10% of its maximum length (and is probably even less when one considers the fact that the Achilles tendon can actually absorb some of the length change). A final example comes from a study in frogs in which semimembranosus muscle length was studied in detail and it was shown that, during a maximal hop, sarcomere length changed from about 2.4 μm to 1.9 μm, a total excursion of only 20% and at sarcomere lengths corresponding to about 90% maximum force generation (Lutz & Rome, 1996). These types of studies show that muscle length changes during active locomotion tend to be relatively small.

Sarcomere Length Operating Range During Gait

You have seen that absolute length changes during locomotion tend to be small, but can more be learned about muscle design by investigating the absolute ranges on the length-tension curve over which muscles operate? It is difficult to hypothesize, a priori, the "best" sarcomere length operating range of muscle. From a purely mechanical point of view, operation at or near the plateau of the active force-length relation is appealing and is often tacitly presented as fact in physiology textbooks because this is the sarcomere length range that results in maximal force production. Indeed, as shown in Chapter 2, the basic shape of the force-length relationship has a profound influence on the nature of force generation in skeletal muscle (Fig. 2-4). From a control point of view, sarcomere operation on the ascending limb might be considered appealing as this range is inherently mechanically stable—any length perturbation creates an opposing force that restores sarcomere length to a stable value (Julian & Morgan, 1979). Sarcomere operation on the descending limb may be less appealing since it has been stated that this portion of the length-tension curve is inherently unstable with increasing length resulting in decreasing force, etc. (Hill, 1953).

One approach to addressing this issue is to evaluate all of the published data of sarcomere length operating ranges to elucidate some general trends or principles (Burkholder & Lieber, 2001). This survey included muscles reported in 83 separate studies covering a total of 51 different muscles from 8 different species yielding a total of 91 data sets. Specifically, the data were obtained from studies of 6 bird, 10 cat, 3 fish, 8 frog, 1 horse, 23 human, 13 mouse, 17 rabbit, and 10 rat muscles. Minimum and maximum sarcomere length of these muscles are displayed as a histogram in Figure 3-32 and

superimposed on a normalized force-length curve in Figure 3-33. The summarized report yielded an average minimum sarcomere length of $81\pm17\%$ of optimal length (L_o) and an average maximum length of $117\pm21\%$ L_o. The average sarcomere length operating range was $100\pm14\%$ L_o suggesting that $L_o\pm14\%$ L_o would make a reasonable first approximation for a "generic" muscle in the absence of other data.

These data support the idea that, for most of the muscles and species studied, muscle force generation tends to be close to optimal and length range is relatively small.

As a final means of emphasizing the relative importance of muscle length and velocity in producing force, consider the unique changes that are predicted to occur in the frog semitendinosus muscle (ST) during hopping. The frog semitendinosus muscle is biarticular, as it is in the human. During the hop, both the hip and knee are extending at a relatively high velocity (Calow & Alexander, 1973). Since the ST is anatomically placed to produce a knee flexion and hip extension moment, extension of the hip will shorten the muscle and extension of the knee will lengthen the muscle. Again, here you can see the general phenomenon that, during normal motions, muscle lengths do not change dramatically. To reiterate, this is mechanically favorable because to replace the biarticular ST with a monoarticular hip extensor and knee flexor, both monoarticular muscles would have to shorten at relatively high velocities, placing them lower on their force-velocity relationship and requiring their PCSAs to be huge in order to create the necessary torque. Accomplishing the same task with the biarticular ST is extremely mechanically efficient. How can we determine the detailed action of the ST during a frog hop? Obviously, it is technically impossible to measure sarcomeres directly during hopping. However, it is possible to measure sarcomere length-joint angle relationships, measure joint angle changes during frog hopping, and to infer the sarcomere behavior (Lieber & Boakes, 1988; Mai & Lieber, 1990). This is what is illustrated in Figure 3-34. Note that, as the frog hop progresses, sarcomere length begins at about 2.0 μm and ends at about 2.6 μm (Fig. 3-34A). Based on the understanding of the frog sarcomere length-tension relationship (Fig. 2-4) you know that such a sarcomere length increase down the descending limb of the length-tension relationship, would, under isometric conditions, decrease muscle force about 25% due to decreased filament overlap. Such a force decrease is not seen. Note in the force record (Fig. 3-34B) corresponding to this length change that force dramatically increases during the hop. Why? The answer lies in the change in muscle velocity (Fig. 3-34C). In the

first portion of the hop, the muscle is shortening slightly, but shortening velocity is decreasing. Due to the force-velocity relationship, decreased muscle velocity results in increased force (See Fig. 2-7). For a brief moment, the muscle is actually isometric! Next, presumably due to the action of other muscles, the ST is forced to lengthen. This forced lengthening results in high muscle forces due to the discontinuity in the force-velocity relationship which occurs when proceeding from shortening to lengthening (See Fig. 2-7). Therefore, the muscle force record (Fig. 3-34B) is not influenced as much by the muscle length as it is by the

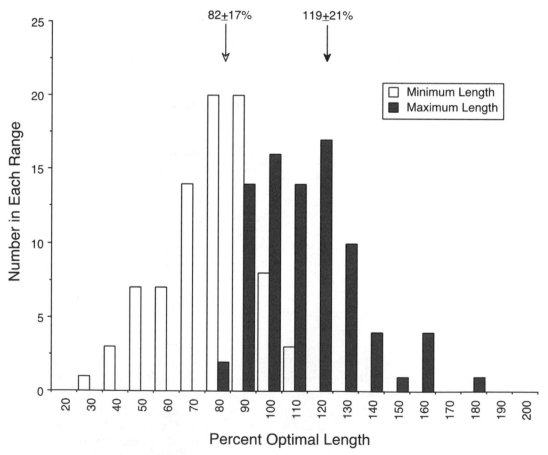

FIGURE 3-32. Histogram of minimum and maximum sarcomere lengths summarized from 91 separate data sets assembled from 51 different muscles in 8 different species. Average minimum sarcomere length was 81±17% of optimal length (L_o) and average maximum length was 117±21% L_o. (Data from: Burkholder, T.J., Lieber, R.L. (2001). Sarcomere length operating range of muscles during movement. *Journal of Experimental Biology, 204*, 1529–1536.)

FIGURE 3-33. Range of sarcomere length operating ranges reported, graphically superimposed upon a normalized sarcomere length-tension curve. The ranges are ordered from minimum length to maximum length within a study and are color coded according to the species from which the data were obtained. (Data from: Burkholder, T.J., Lieber, R.L. (2001). Sarcomere length operating range of muscles during movement. *Journal Experimental Biology, 204*, 1529–1536.)

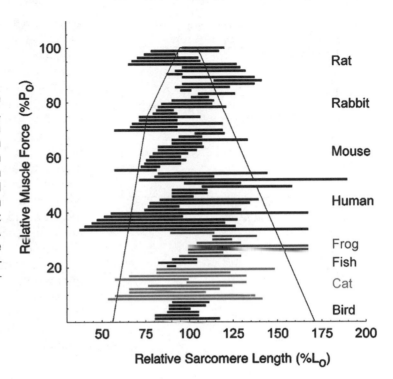

muscle velocity. Incidentally, a recent "reversal" from shortening to lengthening was implicated in causing the repetitive strain injury known as "tennis elbow" (Lieber, Ljung, & Fridén, 1997). Although the data are highly speculative in nature, they do point out the way in which knowledge of sarcomere length changes can be used to infer normal function and even pathophysiology.

Biomechanics of Biarticular Muscles

The sarcomere length record of Figure 3-34A also raises interesting points regarding the physiological function of a biarticular muscle such as the ST. Note first that the ST undergoes shortening and then lengthening during the single coordinated hopping movement. This results directly from the relative hip and knee moment arm magnitudes, hip and knee joint angular velocities, and the relative timing of the actions at the two joints. Therefore, the view that a skeletal muscle simply contracts to cause

joint rotation is not well founded. In this case the velocity of the muscle itself reverses direction due to the sophisticated balance between muscle and joint properties.

The second observation is that the ST is obviously not shortening during the entire movement. In fact, it must be concluded that the ST is not "hopping" the frog, it is actually being "hopped!" The ST is being actively stretched by other muscles that are extending the knee. Therefore, although it could be concluded that, based on anatomical considerations, the ST is a hip extensor and a knee flexor, it is not flexing the knee at all in this motion! Physiological function may not, therefore, be obvious based only on anatomical configuration.

How is the ST caused to lengthen? The best guess to date is that other muscles are stretching the ST, resulting in its active lengthening. The most likely candidates for the other muscles are the knee extensors. Thus, it has been hypothesized that the ST acts as an "activatable sling" at the knee joint, providing a route of force transmission from the mono-

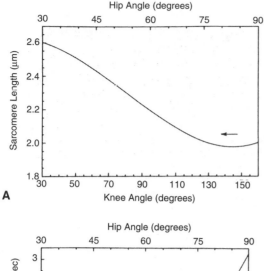

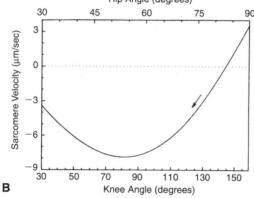

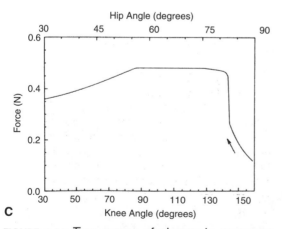

FIGURE 3-34. Time course of change in sarcomere length **(A)**, sarcomere velocity **(B)**, and muscle force **(C)** during a model frog hop, assuming full muscle activation. (From: Mai, M.T., Lieber, R.L. (1990). A model of semitendinosus muscle sarcomere length, knee and hip joint interaction in the frog hindlimb. *Journal of Biomechanics, 23*, 271–279.)

articular knee extensors to the hip joint (Fig. 3-35A). Through the ST muscle, the mono-articular knee extensors (equivalent to humans' vasti muscles) are able to extend the hip joint during jumping (Lieber, 1990). Such a mechanism may operate in the mammalian ST as well as other biarticular muscles (Van Ingen Schenau, 1989). For example, a similar relationship could occur between the gastrocnemius muscle (which crosses the knee and ankle) and the TA (which crosses only the ankle) whereby the dorsiflexion moment generated by the TA could be transferred, via the gastrocnemius into knee flexion (Fig. 3-35B; Table 3-5). Should such a mechanism operate physiologically, it would have a profound impact on the interpretation of studies that ascribe externally measured or calculated moments to specific muscle groups. This is because the force generators for motion that occur at a particular joint need not even cross that joint. (For example, the TA could affect knee flexion.) It would also dramatically affect the interpretation of joint weakness that is observed at a particular site. For example, suppose that the ST muscle discussed above was used during standing to extend the hip, but also to transmit vasti moments to the hip. Difficulty in standing might be an observation and, incorrectly might conclude that the hip extensors were weak. In fact, it may be that the vasti are actually the weak muscles, unable to provide the extra moment needed to stand. This idea that muscles at re-

---

Box 3-6. Can Knee Extension Strength Help Hip Extension?

Yes. And not only that, dorsiflexion can provide power for knee flexion. This is because numerous muscles are biarticular—they cross two joints. As a result they can mechanically couple an action at one joint to another joint. In fact, by activating "sets" of muscles, mechanical power can be coupled all the way from the ankle to the hip. This effect may require that we reconsider our association of movement dysfunction with strength at a single joint.

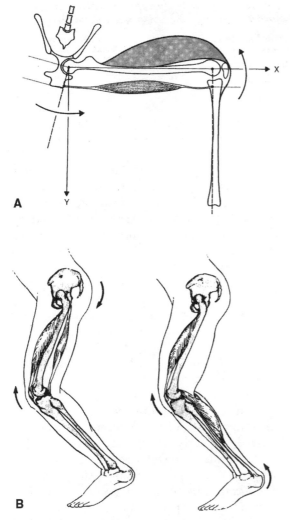

FIGURE 3-35. (A) Schematic representation of transfer of frog knee extension into hip extension by the biarticular semitendinosus muscle. In this scenario, knee extension is converted into hip extension by the biarticular semitendinosus. (From: Mai, M.T., Lieber, R.L. (1990). A model of semitendinosus muscle sarcomere length, knee and hip joint interaction in the frog hindlimb. *Journal of Biomechanics, 23*, 271–279.) **(B)** Joint moment transfer by biarticular human muscles. Transfer of knee extension into hip extension by the biarticular semitendinosus (left panel) and transfer of knee extension into plantarflexion by the biarticular gastrocnemius (right panel). Other examples are proposed in Table 3-5.

mote sites could affect joints that they do not cross (*e.g.,* the vasti affecting the hip joint) might require new thinking regarding the basis of joint weakness or movement abnormalities.

Gait Cycle Timing at Increased Velocities

Given this relatively standardized description of the gait cycle, the modifications of gait that occur as speed is changed should be addressed. As gait speed increases, what happens to the relative time of each gait cycle portion? Clearly, the time in each phase must decrease, but does it decrease to the same extent? The answer is no. Goslow et al. (1973) showed that as gait speed increases, the proportion of the gait cycle devoted to stance decreases and is mirrored by a dramatic increase in the proportion of the gait cycle devoted to swing. During low-speed walking, stance phase occupied about 60% of the cycle whereas swing occupied about 40%. However, at high speed locomotion, in spite of the decreased absolute time of each phase, the swing phase occupied over 75% of the total cycle time. Within the swing phase, both F and E_1 increased their relative proportion, although F increases to a greater extent. In stance, the relative proportion of E_2 and E_3 both decreased in proportion, but the greatest decrease was seen in E_3, which occupied nearly 60% of the gait cycle at slow speeds and only 15% of the cycle at high speeds. It is obvious that the relative amount of time spent in contact with the ground decreases as gait speed increases.

Energy Expenditure During Gait

One theme that emerges from the discussion of movement is that the musculoskeletal system appears to be designed so that energy is not wasted, which makes sense. The design of a machine that performs useful work is based in part on the energetic requirements and availability to that machine. Muscle is an extremely

TABLE 3-5	Examples of Interaction Between Monoarticular and Biarticular Muscles		
Muscle Group	**Action**	**Biarticular Muscle Link**	**Resultant Action**
Quadriceps	Knee extension	Hamstrings	Hip extension
Dorsiflexors	Dorsiflexion	Gastrocnemius	Knee flexion
Gluteals	Hip extension	Rectus femoris	Knee extension
Gluteals	Hip extension	Iliopsoas	Spine flexion
Gluteals	Hip extension	Rectus femoris and Gastrocnemius	Plantarflexion

efficient machine. Current estimates of the energetics of muscle contraction are that approximately 30% of the energy within the ATP molecule can, under optimal conditions, be converted to mechanical work (He, Bottinelli, Pellegrino, Ferenczi, & Reggiani, 2000). Compare this to a typical internal combustion engine such as is found in an automobile which may have an energetic efficiency of only a fraction of a percent and you can appreciate why engineers are eagerly involved in the study of the molecular motors that make up muscle (Spudich, 1994). What are the strategies used in the musculoskeletal system to conserve energy?

Muscles as Springs

One simple yet powerful concept that was proposed by the eminent comparative physiologist Dr. Dick Taylor at Harvard University, was that muscles, during locomotion, can act as springs to absorb energy and then release the stored energy to create mechanical work during cyclic motion. The mass of the body interacts with the "springs" of the muscles and tendons to produce a movement that is reminiscent of a spring oscillating up and down. Recall from basic physics that, as a spring oscillates, kinetic energy is transferred to potential energy as the spring is compressed and then back to kinetic energy as the spring recoils. In the human body, the situation, albeit much more complex structurally and physiologically can be considered a mass-spring system. One major difference is that the "springs" are actually muscles and tendons (Alexander, 1988; Alexander & Bennet,

1977) and there is a metabolic "cost" associated with activating the muscle and thus, making the spring "stiff." In a classic study, Taylor and colleagues (Hoyt & Taylor, 1981) measured the relationship between running speed and metabolic cost in horses. They found that, during running, the energetic cost of locomotion was not constant across speeds but rather showed a clear minimum at a particular speed (Fig. 3-36). Interestingly, this speed of minimum energy expenditure was also the speed at which the animal would choose to run if it were allowed to choose the speed. When the "cost" of locomotion at that speed became too high, the animal would change its running style (e.g., from a trot to a gallop in horses) to re-establish a new, lower cost of locomotion. Humans also behaved similarly in this regard—the self-selected walking speed was shown to be approximately the most metabolically inexpensive speed. The most economical gait was observed at low speeds. As walking speed increased, there became a point when the cost of walking became high and running was more energetically favorable, causing a walk-run transition. These data indicate that the individual will generally attempt to move in a manner that minimizes energy expenditure. More recent studies from the same laboratory demonstrated that this transition might actually occur at a point in which muscle force reached a critical level (Farley & Taylor, 1991). Thus, rather than minimizing energetic cost, these authors hypothesized that the trot-gallop transition occurred to decrease maximum muscle force and thus prevent the possibility of injury.

The mechanical model used to describe this type of locomotion is the so-called "inverted

FIGURE 3-36. Energy expenditure in a horse during different types of locomotion at different velocities. Oxygen consumption was measured in a horse that walked at different speeds (triangles) and trotted at different speeds (circles). For each type of gait, a most efficient speed was observed. Walk-to-trot gait transition occurred near the speed at which the cost for walking at a particular speed exceeded the cost for trotting at that same speed. (Data from: Hoyt, D.F., Taylor, C.R. (1981). Gait and energetics of locomotion in horses. *Nature, 292*, 239–240.)

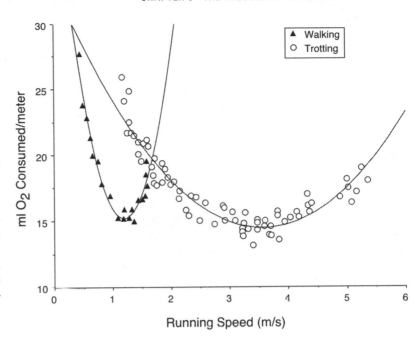

pendulum" model (Fig. 3-37), in which a "mass" (the torso of an animal or human) is placed on top of a "spring" (the legs or locomotory apparatus). As is well known in physics, the natural frequency of oscillation of a pendulum increases if the spring stiffness increases or if the mass decreases. Changes in either mass or stiffness are referred to as "tuning" a pendulum to operate at a desired frequency. Does such

"tuning" occur in humans during locomotion? Yes, there is evidence that it does.

Several interesting experiments in human locomotion were performed by Dr. Clare Farley and colleagues (Ferris & Farley, 1998), who treated the leg muscles as "springs" whose stiffness could be altered simply by changing the level of recruitment of the muscle group. These ideas were tested by allowing humans to

Box 3-7. Why Is Walking Like Hopping on a Pogo Stick?

During walking, cyclic muscle activation and movement causes the body center of mass to move in a smooth up-and-down arc relative to the ground. This can be considered as a mass "bouncing" on a spring, where the spring is the entire leg. Within the leg, contracting muscles "energize" the tendons by stretching them and the tendons then "rebound" by giving some of the energy back to the walking individual later in the gait cycle. As a result, cyclic activation of muscle is like repetitive stretching and release of a "springing" tendon.

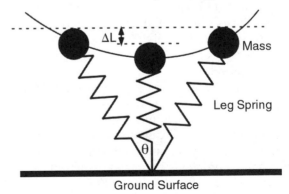

FIGURE 3-37. Schematic drawing of the "inverted pendulum" model of locomotion. In this model, a mass oscillates on top of a spring. (Modified from: Farley, C.T., Glasheen, J., McMahon, T.A. (1993). Running springs: Speed and animal size. *Journal of Experimental Biology, 185*, 71–86.)

hop over surfaces of different stiffnesses and measuring the level of activation by electromyography of the appropriate muscle groups as well as the movement of the body. If the goal of the locomotion activity was to maintain a "tuned" inverted pendulum, then the level of activation should have been changed to compensate for a particular surface stiffness. In other words, if the surface was stiff (*e.g.*, walking on concrete) the muscle activation level could be relatively low to achieve a certain stiffness. If, however, the surface was compliant (*e.g.*, walking on a 6-inch thick piece of foam rubber) the muscle activation level must be increased to achieve the same stiffness level. This is exactly what was observed (Fig. 3-38). As the stiffness of the surface was increased, the calculated stiffness of the leg was decreased (Kleg in Fig. 3-38A). As a result of this "real-time" stiffness adjustment, the total contact time with the ground (Fig. 3-38B) as well as the leg+ground stiffness (Kleg in Fig. 3-38C) remained constant. Subsequently, these authors have shown that leg stiffness was primarily adjusted by modifying ankle stiffness (Farley et al., 1998; Farley & Morgenroth, 1999), and that this adjustment happened within the first step onto a new surface (Ferris, Liang, & Farley, 1999). These data demonstrate tremendously rapid and sophisticated adjustments by the nervous system. Therapists who are aiding individuals in gait or observing individuals walking over various surfaces must be aware of this capability of the nervous system.

It appears, to a first approximation, that the inverted pendulum model is useful in describing cyclic activity of limbs during locomotion. Such information is important in the interpretation of gait information from individuals suffering from problems that impair their ability to move at a certain velocity or who lack the ability to activate certain muscle groups across a range of useful levels. It even seems to explain differences in muscle activation under conditions of hypogravity such as those observed in space flight in which the quantitative but not the

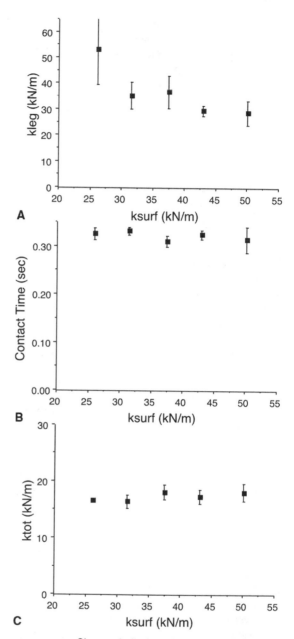

FIGURE 3-38. Change in limb stiffness as an individual walks from a "stiff" to a "compliant" surface. Limb stiffness is estimated from the surface electromyogram. Kleg represents leg stiffness, while Ktot represents total leg plus ground stiffness. (Data from: Farley, C.T., Houdijk, H.H., Van Strien, C., Louie, M. (1998). Mechanism of leg stiffness adjustment for hopping on surfaces of different stiffnesses. *Journal of Applied Physiology, 85*, 1044–1055.)

Box 3-8. Which Requires More Calories, Walking a Mile or Running a Mile?

Interestingly, they require about the same amount of energy. Individuals select the gait style (*e.g.,* walking or running) in part, to minimize energy consumption. At a certain speed, it takes less energy to run than to walk and the transition from walking to running occurs. It also takes more muscle force and the transition to running decreases muscle force, perhaps preventing injury. Overall, running requires more energy per unit time, but this increase is componsated for by the fact that you cover a certain distance more rapidly. The net result is an almost constant amount of energy consumed per unit distance!

---

qualitative effect of gravity is altered (Farley & McMahon, 1992). Future studies are required to exploit the concept of muscle energy storage in locomotion to the benefit of patients with movement disorders.

Direct Force and Length Measurements During Locomotion

Several animal studies reported either muscle force or muscle length values that were obtained during normal gait. These are extremely technically difficult experiments to perform, but they provide the most direct evidence for the complex interaction between muscles and the other connective tissues that occur during locomotion. The most widely studied muscles are the cat ankle extensors, which have been studied during the stance phase at locomotion of various speeds. This information has been used to try to understand how different muscles are used during activities of different intensities. Because the mechanical arrangement of the muscles is somewhat redundant (*i.e.*, both muscles produce plantarflexion when activated), it is not clear what strategy will be used by the nervous system to activate

the different muscles under different conditions. Typically, comparisons are made between the SOL and the MG muscles to provide insights into fiber type specific activity during locomotion, because the SOL is composed only of slow fibers (in cats) and the MG is composed primarily of fast fibers (Chapter 2, pages 79–90).

The experimental approach used to investigate this problem involves measurement of muscle electrical activity via electromyograms (EMGs), muscle length (usually using analysis of film of walking cats), and muscle force (which recently has been measured by implanting force transducers on the individual tendons of the various muscles) (Hoffer et al., 1989; Hoffer & Narahara, 1967; Walmsley, Hodgson, & Burke, 1978; Whiting, Gregor, Roy, Edgerton, 1984). These investigators generally agree that, at low speeds, the first muscle to be activated is the SOL, whereas only at higher speeds (requiring higher joint moments) the faster contracting and stronger MG is recruited. At still higher speeds, the SOL is nearly maximally activated, and any increases in extension moment that produce the higher locomotion speeds are produced by recruiting the MG to higher and higher levels. This "order" of activation is consistent with the "size principle" previously discussed (Chapter 2, pages 98–102) and leads to the general concept that muscles with a preponderance of slow fibers are activated at very low levels of exertion, even for postural stabilization, and muscles with a greater fraction of fast fibers are recruited for tasks requiring higher forces (such as faster locomotion or walking up a hill). The basic assumption used in this logic is that the slow fibers of the soleus muscle behave in a manner similar to the slow fibers within the predominantly fast MG muscle. It is difficult to rigorously test this assumption.

One might also be interested in determining the actual muscle forces achieved relative to the maximum tetanic tension of the muscle. In other words, how much "extra" force is available during normal movement that is not normally used? This question was addressed by performing in vivo force measurements of cat triceps surae muscle force during walking and then measuring maximum tetanic tension in the same muscles in a terminal in situ physiologic experiment (Fowler et al., 1989). One of the most surprising results was that the muscle tension measured in the soleus muscle during walking often exceed its maximum force (P_o). This could obviously be accomplished for the ankle extensors simply by the eccentric contractions that normally occur during E_2. However, the explanation was not quite this simple. As mentioned, these investigators measured muscle velocity and muscle force in vivo during gait and compared those force and velocity values to those achieved during termi-nal in situ force-velocity experiments (Gregor et al., 1988). A schematic of the results for the soleus is shown in Figure 3-39. The classic force-velocity curve for the soleus (shown by the dotted line in Figure 3-39) was shown to often lie below the in vivo force-velocity relationship measured during locomotion. In other words, during normal gait, at a given velocity, the muscle generated more force than would be expected based on its known force-velocity relationship. How is this possible?

Muscle-Tendon Interaction During Gait

The apparent answer to the dilemma lies in the method of measuring muscle velocity in vivo. Usually, such measurements are made from external movies taken of the animal during gait.

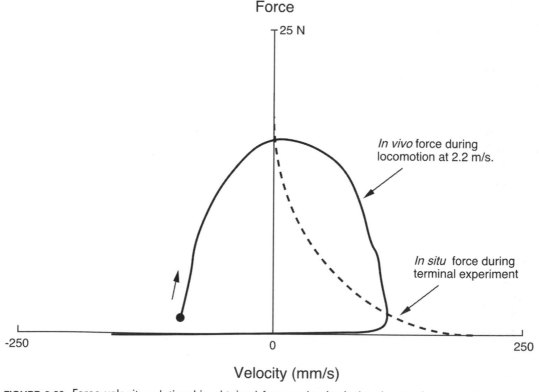

FIGURE 3-39. Force-velocity relationship obtained from an in situ isolated cat soleus muscle compared to actual in vivo force-velocity relationship measured during locomotion. Note that forces of the muscle-tendon unit lie above the in situ force-velocity curve. (From: Gregor, R.J., Roy, R.R., Whiting, W.C., Lovely, R.G., Hodgson, J.A., Edgerton, V.R. (1988). Mechanical output of the cat soleus during treadmill locomotion: In vivo vs. in situ characteristics. *Journal of Biomechanics, 21,* 721–732.)

Then, based on external bony landmarks, muscle origin-to-insertion distances are calculated, from which in vivo "muscle" velocity is obtained. However, in reality, this length represents the in vivo muscle-tendon length and the calculated value is the muscle-tendon velocity. It is now thought that the tendon length change that accompanies muscle activation during gait (at least in the ankle extensors) has a dramatic impact on this relationship. The current explanation goes something like this: During E_2, as the toe of the cat strikes the ground and the ankle is forced to plantarflex, the MG is actively lengthened at a very high tension, which also lengthens the Achilles tendon. Then, as the muscle-tendon unit progresses from E_2 to E_3, the tendon begins to recoil so that it is shortening faster than the muscle. Stated another way, the energy that was stored in the tendon "spring" during E_2 is now released as the tendon shortens, and the muscle is not required to shorten as fast to achieve the overall muscle-tendon unit velocity. This would explain why the estimated in vivo force-velocity relationship was above the in situ curve—the muscle fiber velocity was underestimated in the in vivo situation since tendon compliance was not considered. Complete resolution of this dilemma will await separate measurement of muscle length and tendon length during gait. However, measurements by Griffiths (1991) and Hoffer et al. (1989) have tended to confirm this explanation, but the jury is still out (Fig. 3-4). Here a new function for the tendon is presented—that of elastic energy storage. Energy storage by tendinous structures has already been demonstrated for a number of animals, especially those with long tendons in series with large muscles (Alexander, 1988). If elastic energy storage were to be used during gait, it would be expected that the perfect time would be during the E_2-E_3 transition as the muscle goes from lengthening to shortening at very high tensions. Several authors have pointed out that this stretch-shorten cycle can dramatically increase locomotion efficiency (Alexander, 1988).

In the same way that energy storage by muscles acting as "springs" can make locomotion more efficient, energy storage by tendons in series with muscles can also increase the efficiency of locomotion. Such an effect would be most pronounced in animals that demonstrate long tendons in series with muscle fibers. One obvious example is the Achilles tendon of the hopping kangaroo. Morgan and colleagues (Morgan et al., 1976; Morgan, Proske, & Warren, 1978) measured the mechanical properties of the triceps surae musculature along with the properties of the Achilles tendon. They also measured the joint motions and muscle activation associated with kangaroo hopping at a variety of speeds. These authors estimated that, by cyclic energy storage and release in the kangaroo, the animal saved about 30% of the energy that would be required if all of the shortening and force generation were to be done by muscle tissue alone. One of the main reasons for this energy savings is that the muscles were able to shorten at lower velocities, thus generating higher relative forces on their force-velocity curves. The second reason for the energy savings is the fact that energy "stored" during the E_2 phase of locomotion is then "used" or "released" during the E_3 phase. Such cyclic storage and release of energy is analogous to a child hopping on a pogo stick. The kangaroo is effectively hopping on the "pogo stick" of its Achilles tendon. Probably, such extreme energy storage is not as important for humans. In fact, it has been shown that in the kangaroo rat (a smaller version of the kangaroo, with scaled proportions), energy storage and locomotion efficiency does not seem to be occurring (Biewener & Blickhan, 1988). The explanation is that the kangaroo rat is more concerned with escaping predators (requiring stiff tendons for high acceleration) than efficient locomotion. Alexander and colleagues (1988) have used the energy storage argument to predict fairly accurately, the "optimal" stiffness for tendons relative to the muscles to which they are attached (Ker, Alexander, & Bennett, 1988).

Physiological Functions of Tendons
A variety of the mechanical and physiological properties of tendons have been described. To

summarize several of their roles, the four major functions are reiterated as follows:

1. The most obvious function of tendons is that they connect muscles to bones.
2. By virtue of their compliance, tendons can absorb length changes during high-impact motions (shock absorption), which allows muscles to lengthen at lower eccentric velocities. This in turn lowers the muscle tension achieved, which might prevent muscular injury (Chapter 6). Tendons probably function physiologically in the high compliance region of their stress-strain curves.
3. Due to their significant but limited compliance, tendons also increase the functional range of the muscle-tendon unit. This is because they allow sarcomeres to shorten during contraction, and they lengthen to absorb some of the passive tension.
4. During stretch-shorten cycles, high forces elongate tendons. The subsequent muscle shortening is accompanied by release of stored tendon elastic strain energy. This increases locomotion efficiency. In addition, since tendons recoil and take up some of the length of the muscle-tendon unit, this keeps muscle fiber velocity low, which keeps potential muscle tension higher.

Implications for Physical Therapy

What are some of the implications of these concepts on current physical therapy practice? The most obvious implication is that, to fully understand the nature of strength, one must understand torque. When measuring strength you are measuring the interaction between muscle and joint properties. At the joint angle where torque is maximum, muscle force and joint moment arm are involved to varying degrees and neither muscle nor joint properties need be maximized. Therefore, the first thing you must choose in strength testing is the appropriate joint angle. At what angle is the most "muscle" information obtained? At what angle is the most "joint" information obtained? This ques-

tion must be answered on a case-by-case basis, and unfortunately, there is not enough data on human muscles and joints to answer it completely. However, on theoretical grounds a number of statements can still be made. Always assume that you are neither at the angle at which muscle force is maximum nor the angle at which joint moment arm is maximum (refer to Figure 3-16B).

To determine the basis for strength changes, consider all of the facts that you have learned so far. Strength (torque) can be altered due to changes in muscle force or muscle moment arm. In situations such as simple immobilization, when muscles can become weak due to fiber atrophy (Chapter 5) and muscle force decreases, you might suspect that muscle force is the main reason that strength has decreased. Since torque is simply the product of muscle force and joint moment arm, a decrease in muscle force due to atrophy will simply be represented as a decrease in the joint torque. However, it is not necessary to have muscle atrophy to have weakness. Recall that muscle force can also dramatically change in response to the level of excitation, which recruits a varying number of muscle fibers. Changes in muscle force can, therefore, simply be a result of decreased electrical drive to the muscle. This could be detected as a change in EMG. Therefore, the various pieces of the puzzle—EMG, muscle force, and moment arm—must be on hand to make an unambiguous diagnosis of the physiological basis for a strength change.

Finally, a surgical procedure that moves a muscle from one position to another can cause weakness. What is the basis for the weakness? Again, due to the surgical procedure itself, the muscle may have atrophied (note the statement "may have atrophied," since surgical procedures can result in muscle hypertrophy, as outlined in Chapter 4). Muscle atrophy might be the reason for the weakness. However, suppose that the muscle moment arm was altered by the surgical procedure itself. Could this not also produce weakness? Yes, increased moment arm (and, therefore, decreased fiber length/moment arm ratio) causes the muscle to change force faster as the joint rotates. Now, if the muscle passes through its entire length-tension range, joint torque will be extremely low despite the fact that muscle force is exactly the same. In addition to a change in moment arm, a surgical procedure can change the muscle fiber length (Chapter 4, pages 189–191). The functional effect would be similar: Sarcomere length would change at a different rate as the joint rotates.

If the muscle's ability to adapt is considered, the situation becomes even more interesting. In spite of the relatively predictable structure and function of muscle tissue, it is one of the most plastic tissues in the body. The nature of muscle adaptation not only provides insights in a muscle's history but can also be exploited in rehabilitation to return a muscle's properties to normal. Muscle adaptation will be discussed in the next chapter and will provide the substance for the remainder of the book.

■ Chapter Summary

In this chapter, you were shown the way in which muscles, tendons, and bones interact to produce movement. A major conclusion was that torque production results from interaction between muscles and joints and not from either muscles or joints alone. Also, muscle architecture has a profound effect on muscle force, excursion, and range of motion and may be considered one design parameter of the musculoskeletal system. Finally, the beautifully orchestrated sequence of events known as the gait cycle was investigated. The biomechanical interaction between muscles and tendons that can produce dramatic energy savings during locomotion was detailed as well. As mentioned, these concepts are just now being applied to sports medicine and therapy. Further advances in treatment will undoubtedly follow as more practitioners become aware of these concepts.

REFERENCES

Alexander, R., Bennet, C.H. (1977). Storage of elastic strain energy in muscle and other tissues. *Nature, 265*, 114–117.

Alexander, R.M. (1988). *Elastic mechanisms in animal movement.* Cambridge, MA: Cambridge University Press.

Amiel, D., Frank, C., Harwood, F., Fronek, J., Akeson, W. (1984). Tendons and ligaments: a morphological and biochemical comparison. *Journal of Orthopaedic Research, 1*, 257–265.

Bäckdahl, M., Carlsöö, S. (1961). Distribution of activity in muscles acting on the wrist (an electromyographic study). *Acta Morph Neerl-Scand, 4*, 136–144.

Basmajian, J.V., DeLuca, C.J. (1985). *Muscles alive. their functions revealed by electromyography.* Baltimore, MD: Williams & Wilkins.

Biewener, A., Blickhan, R. (1988). Kangaroo rat locomotion: design for elastic energy storage or acceleration? *Journal of Experimental Biology, 140*, 243–255.

Brand, P.W., Beach, R.B., Thompson, DE. (1981). Relative tension and potential excursion of muscles in the forearm and hand. *Journal of Hand Surgery, 3A*, 209–219.

Burkholder, T.J., Lieber, R.L. (1996). Stepwise regression is an alternative to splines for analyzing noisy data. *Journal of Biomechanics, 29*, 235–238.

Burkholder, T.J., Lieber, R.L. (2001). Sarcomere length operating range of muscles during movement. *Journal of Experimental Biology, 204*, 1529–1536.

Butler, D.L., Grood, E.S., Noyes, F.R., Zernicke, R.F. (1978). Biomechanics of ligaments and tendons. In *Exercise and Sport Sciences Review. Volume 25* (pp.125–182). Baltimore, MD: The Franklin Institute Press.

Calow, L.J., Alexander, R.M. (1973). A mechanical analysis of a hindlimb of a frog. *Journal of Zoology, 171*, 293–321.

Chleboun, G.S., France, A.R., Crill, M.T., Braddock, H.K., Howell, J.N. (2001). In vivo measurement of fascicle length and pennation angle of the human biceps femoris muscle. *Cells Tissues Organs, 169*, 401–409.

Close, R.I. (1972). Dynamic properties of mammalian skeletal muscles. *Physiology Review, 52*, 129–197.

Crowninshield, R., Pope, M.H., Johnson, R.J. (1976). An analytical model of the knee. *Journal of Biomechanics, 9*, 397–405.

Engberg, I., Lundberg, A. (1969). An electromyographic analysis of muscular activity in the hindlimb of the cat during unrestrained locomotion. *Acta Physiologica Scandinavica, 75*, 614–630.

Enoka, R.M., Fuglevand, A.J. (1993). Neuromuscular basis of the maximum voluntary force capacity of muscle. In M.D. Grabiner (Ed.) *Current Issues in Biomechanics* (pp. 215–235). Champaign, IL: Human Kinetics.

Farley, C.T., Houdijk, H.H., Van Strien, C., Louic, M. (1998). Mechanism of leg stiffness adjustment for hopping on surfaces of different stiffnesses. *Journal of Applied Physiology, 85*, 1044–1055.

Farley, C.T., McMahon, T.A. (1992). Energetics of walking and running: Insights from simulated reduced-gravity experiments. *Journal of Applied Physiology, 73*, 2709–2712.

Farley, C.T., Morgenroth, D.C. (1999). Leg stiffness primarily depends on ankle stiffness during human hopping. *Journal of Biomechanics, 32*, 267–273.

Farley, C.T., Taylor, C.R. (1991). A mechanical trigger for the trot-gallop transition in horses. *Science, 253*, 306–308.

Ferris, D.P., Farley, C.T. (1998). Interaction of leg stiffness and surfaces stiffness during human hopping. *Journal of Applied Physiology, 82*, 15–22.

Ferris, D.P., Liang, K., Farley, C.T. (1999). Runners adjust leg stiffness for their first step on a new running surface. *Journal of Biomechanics, 32*, 787–794.

Fowler, E.G., Gregor, R.J., Hodgson, J.A., Roy, R.R. (1989). The contribution of individual muscles to the ankle moment produced in the cat hindlimb. *Journal of Biomechanics, 22*, 1101–1110.

Freehafer, A.A., Peckham, P.H., Keith, M.W. (1979). Determination of muscle-tendon unit properties during tendon transfer. *Journal of Hand Surgery, 4A*, 331–339.

Fukunaga, T., Ichinose, Y., Ito, M., Kawakami, Y., Fukashiro, S. (1997). Determination of fascicle length and pennation in a contracting human muscle in vivo. *Journal of Applied Physiology, 82*, 354–358.

Fukunaga, T., Ito, M., Ichinose, Y., Kuno, S., Kawakami, Y., Fukashiro, S. (1996). Tendinous movement of a human muscle during voluntary contractions determined by real-time ultrasonography. *Journal of Applied Physiology, 81*, 1430–1433.

Fukunaga, T., Roy, R.R., Shellock, F.G., Hodgson, J.A., Day, M.K., Lee, P.L., Kwong, F.H., Edgerton, V.R. (1992). Physiological cross-sectional area of human leg muscles based on magnetic resonance imaging. *Journal of Orthopaedic Research, 10*, 928–934.

Gans, C., De Vries, F. (1987). Functional bases of fi-ber length and angulation in muscle. *Journal of Morphology, 192*, 63–85.

Gillard, D.M., Yakovenko, S., Cameron, T., Prochazka, A. (2000). Isometric muscle length-tension curves do not predict angle-torque curves of human wrist in continuous active movements. *Journal of Biomechanics, 33*, 1341–1348.

Goslow, G.J., Reinking, R., Stuart, D. (1973). The cat step cycle: Hind limb joint angles and muscle lengths during unrestrained locomotion. *Journal of Morphology, 141*, 1–42.

Gregor, R.J., Roy, R.R., Whiting, W.C., Lovely, R.G., Hodgson, J.A., Edgerton, V.R. (1988). Mechanical output of the cat soleus during treadmill locomotion: in vivo vs. in situ characteristics. *Journal of Biomechanics, 21*, 721–732.

Griffiths, R.I. (1991). Shortening of muscle fibres during stretch of the active cat medial gastrocnemius muscle: The role of tendon compliance. *Journal of Physiology (London), 436*, 219–236.

He, Z.H., Bottinelli, R., Pellegrino, M.A., Ferenczi, M.A., Reggiani, C. (2000). ATP consumption and efficiency of human single muscle fibers with different myosin isoform composition. *Biophysical Journal, 79*, 945–961.

Hildebrand, M. (1974). *Analysis of vertebrate structure*. New York, NY: John Wiley and Sons.

Hill, A.V. (1938). The heat of shortening and the dynamic constants of muscle. *Proceedings of the Royal Society of London Series B: Biological Sciences, 126*, 136–195.

Hill, A.V. (1953). The mechanics of active muscle. *Proceedings of the Royal Society of London Series B, 141*, 104–117.

Hoffer, J.A., Caputi, A.A., Pose, I.E., Griffiths, R.I. (1989). Roles of muscle activity and load on the relationship between muscle spindle length and whole muscle length in the freely walking cat. *Progress in Brain Research, 80*, 75–85.

Hoffer, J.O., Narahara, H.T. (1967). Enhanced permeability to sugar associated with muscle contraction. *Journal of General Physiology, 50*, 551–561.

Horii, K.N., An, W.P., Cooney, Linscheid, R.L. (1991). Kinematics and tendon excursion of wrist movers. *Journal of Hand Surgery, 18A*, 83–90.

Hoy, M.G., Zajac, F.E., Gordon, M.E. (1990). A musculoskeletal model of the human lower extremity: the effect of muscle, tendon, and moment arm on the moment-angle relationship of musculotendon actuators at the hip, knee, and ankle. *Journal of Biomechanics, 23*, 157–169.

Hoyt, D.F., Taylor, C.R. (1981). Gait and energetics of locomotion in horses. *Nature, 292*, 239–240.

Ichinose, Y., Kawakami, Y., Ito, M., Kanehisa, H., Fukunaga, T. (2000). In vivo estimation of contraction velocity of human vastus lateralis muscle during "isokinetic" action. *Journal of Applied Physiology, 88,* 851–856.

Ikai, M., Fukunaga, T. (1968). Calculation of muscle strength per unit cross-sectional area of human muscle by means of ultrasonic measurement. *Internationale Zeitschrift fur Angewante Physiologie Einschliesslich Arbeitsphysiologie,* 26, 26–32.

Ito, M., Kawakami, Y., Ichinose, Y., Fukashiro, S., Fukunaga, T. (1998). Nonisometric behavior of fascicles during isometric contractions of a human muscle. *Journal of Applied Physiology, 85,* 1230–1235.

Ito, M., Akima, H., Fukunaga, T. (2000). In vivo moment arm determination using B-mode ultrasonography. *Journal of Biomechanics, 33,* 215–218.

Julian, F.J., Morgan, D.L. (1979). Intersarcomere dynamics during fixed end tetanic contractions of frog muscle fibers. *Journal of Physiology (London), 293,* 365–378.

Kannus, P. (2000). Structure of the tendon connective tissue. *Scandinavian Journal of Medicine and Science in Sports, 10,* 312–320.

Kawakami, Y., Ichinose, Y., Fukunaga, T. (1998). Architectural and functional features of human triceps surae muscles during contraction. *Journal of Applied Physiology, 85,* 398–404.

Kawakami, Y., Lieber, R.L. (2000). Interaction between series compliance and sarcomere kinetics determines internal sarcomere shortening during fixed-end contraction. *Journal of Biomechanics, 33,* 1249–1255.

Ker, R.F., Alexander, R.M., Bennett, M.B. (1988). Why are mammalian tendons so thick? *Journal of Zoology, 216,* 309–324.

Komi, P.V., Belli, A., Huttunen, V., Bonnefoy, R., Geyssant, A., Lacour, J.R. (1996). Optic fibre as a transducer of tendomuscular forces. *European Journal of Applied Physiology and Occupational Physiology, 72,* 278–280.

Kuno, S., Fukunaga, T. (1995). Measurement of muscle fibre displacement during contraction by real-time ultrasonography in humans. *European Journal of Applied Physiology, 70,* 45–48.

Lieber, R.L. (1990). Hypothesis: Biarticular muscles transfer moments between joints. *Developmental Medicine and Child Neurology, 32,* 456–458.

Lieber, R.L. (1997). Muscle fiber length and moment arm coordination during dorsi- and plantarflexion in the mouse hindlimb. *Acta Anatomica, (Basel), 159,* 84–89.

Lieber, R.L., Boakes, J.L. (1988). Sarcomere length and joint kinematics during torque production in the frog hindlimb. *American Journal of Physiology, 254,* C759–C768.

Lieber, R.L., Brown, C.G., Trestik, C.L. (1992). Model of muscle-tendon interaction during frog semitendinosus fixed-end contractions. *Journal of Biomechanics, 25,* 421–428.

Lieber, R.L., Fazeli, B.M., Botte, M.J. (1990). Architecture of selected wrist flexor and extensor muscles. *Journal of Hand Surgery, 15A,* 244–250.

Lieber, R.L., Fridén, J. (1997). Intraoperative measurement and biomechanical modeling of the flexor carpi ulnaris-to-extensor carpi radialis longus tendon transfer. *Journal of Biomechanical Engineering, 119,* 386–391.

Lieber, R.L., Leonard, M., Brown-Maupin, C. (2000). Muscle contraction effects on aponeurosis and tendon load-strain properties. *Cells Tissues Organs, 166,* 48–54.

Lieber, R.L., Leonard, M.E., Brown, C.G., Trestik, C.L. (1991). Frog semitendinosus tendon load-strain and stress-strain properties during passive loading. *American Journal of Physiology, 261,* C86–C92.

Lieber, R.L., Ljung B-O, Fridén, J. (1997). Sarcomere length in wrist extensor muscles. Changes may provide insights into the etiology of chronic lateral epicondylitis. *Acta Orthopaedica Scandinavica, 68,* 249–254.

Lieber, R.L., Pontén, E., Fridén, J. (1996). Sarcomere length changes after flexor carpi ulnaris-to-extensor digitorum communis tendon transfer. *Journal of Hand Surgery, 21A,* 612–618.

Lieber, R.L., Shoemaker, S.D. (1992). Muscle, joint, and tendon contributions to the torque profile of frog hip joint. *American Journal of Physiology, 263,* R586–R590.

Lieber, R.L., Yeh, Y., Baskin, R.J. (1984). Sarcomere length determination using laser diffraction. Effect of beam and fiber diameter. *Biophysical Journal, 45,* 1007–1016.

Loren, G.J., Lieber, R.L. (1995). Tendon biomechanical properties enhance human wrist muscle specialization. *Journal of Biomechanics, 28,* 791–799.

Loren, G.J., Shoemaker, S.D., Burkholder, T.J., Jacobson, M.D., Fridén, J., Lieber, R.L. (1996). Influences of human wrist motor design on joint torque. *Journal of Biomechanics, 29,* 331–342.

Lundberg, S.R., Enguidanos, S.T., Kramer, S.K., Abrams, R.A., Loren, G.J., Lieber, R.L. (1997). Tendon biomechanical properties correlate with human digital flexor muscle function. *Transactions of the Orthopaedic Research Society, 22,* 6.

Lutz, G.J., Rome, L.C. (1996). Muscle function during jumping in frogs. I. Sarcomere length change, EMG pattern, and jumping performance. *American Journal of Physiology, 271,* C563–C570.

Magnusson, S.P., Aagaard, P., Rosager, S., Dyre-Poulsen, P., Kjaer, M. (2001). Load-displacement properties of human triceps surae aponeurosis in vivo. *Journal of Physiology (London)* (in press).

Mai, M.T., Lieber, R.L. (1990). A model of semitendinosus muscle sarcomere length, knee and hip joint interaction in the frog hindlimb. *Journal of Biomechanics, 23,* 271–279.

McClearn, D. (1985). Anatomy of raccoon (Procyon lotor) and caoti (Nasua narica and N. nasua) forearm and leg muscles: Relations between fiber length, moment-arm length, and joint excursion. *Journal of Morphology, 183,* 87–115.

McFarland, G.B., Krusen, U.L., Weathersby, H.T. (1962). Kinesiology of selected muscles acting on the wrist: Electromyographic study. *Archives of Physical Medicine and Rehabilitation, 43,* 165–171.

Morgan, D.L. (1976). Separation of active and passive components of short-range stiffness of muscle. *American Journal of Physiology, 232,* C45–C49.

Morgan, D.L., Proske, U., Warren, D. (1978). Measurements of muscle stiffness and the mechanism of elastic storage of energy in hopping kangaroos. *Journal of Physiology, 282,* 253–261.

Myllyharju, J., Kivirikko, K.I. (2001). Collagens and collagen-related diseases. *Annals of Medicine, 33,* 7–21.

Panjabi, M.M. (1979). Centers and angles of rotation of body joints: A study of errors and optimization. *Journal of Biomechanics, 12,* 911–920.

Perrine, J.J., Edgerton, V.R. (1978). Muscle force-velocity and power-velocity relationships under isokinetic loading. *Medicine and Science in Sports and Exercise, 10,* 159–166.

Philippson, M. (1905). L'autonomie et la central sation dans le systeme nerveux des animaux. *Trav Lab Physiol Inst Solvay (Bruxelles), 7,* 1–208.

Riek, S., Bawa, P. (1992). Recruitment of motor units in human forearm extensors. *Journal of Neurophysiology, 68,* 100–108.

Rugg, S.G., Gregor, R.J., Mandelbaum, B.R., Chiu, L. (1990). In vivo moment arm calculations at the ankle using magnetic resonance imaging (MRI). *Journal of Biomechanics, 23,* 495–501.

Sacks, R.D., Roy, R.R. (1982). Architecture of the hindlimb muscles of cats: Functional significance. *Journal of Morphology, 173,* 185–195.

Schantz, P., Randall, F.E., Hutchinson, W., Tyden, A., Astrand, P.O. (1983). Muscle fibre type distribution, muscle cross-sectional area and maximal voluntary strength in humans. *Acta Physiologica Scandinavica, 117,* 219–226.

Smidt, G.L. (1973). Biochemical analysis of knee flexion and extension. *Journal of Biomechanics, 6,* 79–92.

Spudich, J.A. (1994). How molecular motors work. *Nature, 372,* 515–518.

Van Ingen Schenau, G. (1989). From rotation to translation. Constraints on multijoint movement and the unique role of biarticular muscles. *Journal of Human Movement and Science 8,* 301–337.

Walmsley, B., Hodgson, J.A., Burke, R.E. (1978). Forces produced by medial gastrocnemius and soleus muscles during locomotion in freely moving cats. *Journal of Neurophysiology, 41,* 1203–1216.

Whiting, W.C., Gregor, R.J., Roy, R.R., Edgerton, V.R. (1984). A technique for estimating mechanical work of individual muscles in the cat during treadmill locomotion. *Journal of Biomechanics, 17,* 685–694.

Wickiewicz, T.L., Roy, R.R., Powell, P.L., Edgerton, V.R. Muscle architecture of the human lower limb. *Clinical Orthopaedics and Related Research, 179,* 275–283.

Woo, S.L.-Y., Gomez, M.A., Amiel, D., Ritter, M.A., Gelberman, R.H., Akeson, W.H. (1981). The effects of exercise on the biomechanical and biochemical properties of swine digital flexor tendons. *Journal of Biomechanical Engineering, 103,* 51–56.

Zajac, F.E. (1989). Muscle and tendon: properties, models, scaling, and application to biomechanics and motor control. *Critical Reviews in Biomedical Engineering, 17,* 359–411.

Zajac, F.E. (1992). How musculotendon architecture and joint geometry affect the capacity of muscle to move and exert force on objects: A review with application to arm and forearm tendon transfer design. *Journal of Hand Surgery, 17A,* 799–804.

Zajac, F.E., Gordon, M.E. (1989). Determining muscle's force and action in multi-articular movement. In J. Holloszy (Ed.) *Exercise and Sport Sciences Review.* (pp. 187–230). Baltimore, MD: Williams & Wilkins.

CHAPTER 4

Skeletal Muscle Adaptation to Increased Use

Chapter Overview

This chapter changes gears. The first three chapters focused on a presentation and understanding of the design and function of the neuromusculoskeletal system. From this point and through the remainder of the book its ability to adapt—its plasticity, will be discussed. An understanding of neuromuscular plasticity forms the physiological basis of physical therapy. The goal of therapy is to improve function. Developing modalities that improve function relies on an understanding of the factors that cause such functional changes. In this chapter, specific cases in which the level of muscle use is increased will be given close attention. Each case represents a "model" in which use is increased either in an animal or human subject. To provide a broad understanding of neuromuscular adaptation to increased use, we discuss five diverse experimental models. You will see that, in spite of the fact that various models are used to increase levels of use, the adaptations are fairly consistent. The "cleanest" model of adaptation—chronic electrical stimulation—will be discussed first and the chapter will end with the most physiological—voluntary exercise. Each model will build upon the information gleaned from the previous model and consistent themes will emerge. The goal is to provide a broad understanding of how a muscle adapts when the level of use is increased to be able to exploit this plasticity to the benefit of the patient.

Educational Objectives

● To be able to describe the basic experimental "models" of adaptation to increased use.
● To be able to explain the strengths and weaknesses of each model in its ability to provide an understanding of adaptation to increased use.
● To be able to define the factors that cause adaptation to increased usage.
● To provide clinical examples that parallel the experimental models of increased use.
● To be able to predict changes in muscles which occur after experimental and clinical examples of increased usage.

Introduction

Despite the relatively dogmatic presentation of skeletal muscle structure and function in Chapters 1 through 3, for didactic purposes, the chapters did not include the fact that skeletal muscle is one of the most adaptable (plastic) tissues in the body. Thus, virtually every structural aspect of muscle that has been discussed so far can change given the proper stimulus. This includes architecture, fiber type distribution, tendon length, fiber diameter, myosin heavy chain profile, mitochondrial distribution, capillary density, fiber length, etc. This fact alone underscores the dynamic ability of a muscle to respond to altered use and provides the therapist with the "good news" that therapeutic modalities can actually change musculoskeletal tissues. What are the factors that control each skeletal muscle property? This is difficult to answer without a more specific question, but it is clear that the main reason a skeletal muscle changes any of its properties is a change in the level of muscle activity relative to "normal." Interestingly, "normal" is different for different muscles and even for different fibers within the same muscle. It is difficult to make sweeping generalizations regarding adaptation; however, the unifying concepts presented in the following models will allow you to "think" the way a muscle does. Hopefully, an understanding of muscle adaptation will enable you, the therapists, to exploit muscle's amazing plasticity to the benefit of your patients. Do not be intimidated about treading into these very basic science models for this understanding. This is powerful science and you have complete access to it. What is missing currently are individuals armed with this information who will try to apply it therapeutically.

Adaptation to Chronic Electrical Stimulation

Chronic electrical stimulation provides one of the "cleanest" views of muscle adaptation to increased use. This model has long been used by basic scientists to study skeletal muscle adaptation since it induces a repeatable, quantifiable amount of "exercise." Unlike complex models of human exercise, which may produce conflicting results even when different laboratories are performing identical exercise protocols, results from chronic electrical stimulation studies are highly consistent among laboratories. Thus, a collection of such studies has been synthesized in a manner that provides a fairly global view of muscle structural and physiological changes that occur in response to the stimulation.

In this model, a well-defined progression of muscular changes is observed that enables investigation of the mechanism and time-course of muscle adaptation. In addition, observations of muscular changes following electrical stimulation provide insights into other forms of muscle adaptation such as those that occur following immobilization, disease, surgery, or exercise.

Experimental Method for Chronic Muscle Stimulation

Normally, skeletal muscles that play a postural role (such as the multifidus muscles, soleus and vastus intermedius muscles), and thus have a high proportion of slow fibers, are physiologically frequently activated at low frequencies. Conversely, muscles with a very high proportion of fast fibers may be activated only intermittently with high frequency bursts of electrical activity. The fact that electrical activity and muscle properties seem to be intimately interrelated, provides an experimental basis for understanding muscle plasticity. The best documented effects of electrical stimulation on skeletal muscle are those that occur after chronic, low-frequency stimulation (similar to the activity of a "slow" muscle) is imposed upon a predominantly "fast" muscle. Experimentally, a cuff electrode is wrapped around a peripheral nerve and the wire leads from the electrode are routed to a neuromuscular stimulator. The stimulator may even be small enough to implant within animal or the leads may exit and externally connect to a stimulator (Fig. 4-1). Such experiments have been performed over the past 40 years in mammalian models such as the cat, the rat, and the rabbit with the results indicating that adaptations are not species specific.

If the stimulator is activated at a nominal frequency of about 10 Hz and allowed to operate 8–24 hours per day, a well-defined progression of changes is observed whereby the fast muscle first changes its metabolic and then its contractile properties to completely "transform" into a "slow" muscle. Below is a description of the details of the transformation process, which is based on experimental data from a number of laboratories. For didactic purposes, the results have been com-

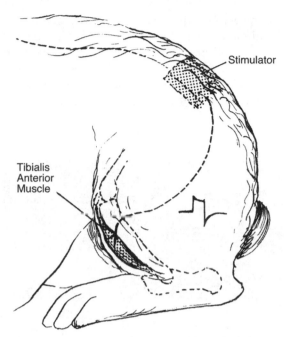

FIGURE 4-1. Experimental model used for chronic activation of rabbit skeletal muscle. This model is one of the most consistent methods used to study muscle plasticity. Stimulating electrodes are implanted directly into a muscle (shown) or placed around a motor nerve and routed to either a subcutaneous stimulator or leads, which exit and connect to an external stimulator (not shown). The stimulator activation pattern is then chronically imposed upon the muscle as a substitute for or in addition to normal neural activity.

bined, primarily representing the work of Drs. Brenda Eisenberg (Chicago, USA), Dirk Pette (Konstanz, Germany), and Stanley Salmons (Liverpool, England). Before describing the details of the transformation process, a few general statements should be made. Transformation has been documented in a number of different muscles and species so that the effects observed are probably not species or muscle specific. The fast-to-slow transformation that occurs is detectable using all of our modern techniques such as measurement of muscle contractile, ultrastructural, histochemical, biochemical, molecular, and morphological properties. In all cases, following transformation,

the new slow fibers are almost completely indistinguishable from normal slow skeletal muscle fibers (Eisenberg, Brown, & Salmons, 1984; Eisenberg & Salmons, 1981; Pette, 1990; Salmons & Henriksson, 1981; Salmons & Vrbova, 1969). It is also generally accepted, based on time-series studies and single fiber biochemistry, that the changes that occur result from a true transformation of a single fast fiber into a slow fiber and not from selective loss of fast fibers with subsequent slow fiber regeneration or proliferation. The fast fibers actually *become* slow fibers.

How does the transformation occur? Remember that this muscle is being completely rearranged while it is still physiologically active. This is analogous to rebuilding the engine of a car while it is driving down the freeway. Next, the details of the various muscle cellular components as the adaptation occurs will be discussed.

Time Course of Muscle Fiber Transformation

If low frequency stimulation is applied 8–24 hours per day, the total transformation process requires about 8 weeks. If the stimulator is active for a shorter period of time, the transformation takes longer or may not fully occur. The earliest observed changes occur within a few hours after the onset of stimulation where the

Box 4-1. Electrical Stimulation Can Make Muscles Weaker?

Absolutely. Chronic electrical stimulation is the best model used by physiologists to cause repeatable and consistent changes in skeletal muscle—the most obvious being muscle fiber atrophy and muscle weakness. This should be viewed as a deliberate response by the muscle to become a "metabolic machine" in response to chronic use and not some sort of degeneration. The small muscle fiber size that results from chronic stimulation may facilitate transport of oxygen into the cell and metabolites out of the cell.

sarcoplasmic reticulum (SR) membrane network begins to swell (Fig. 4-2A). The significance of this morphological change is not clear but it is routinely observed. Within the next 2–12 days, increases are measured in the volume percent of mitochondria, oxidative enzyme activity, number of capillaries per square millimeter, total blood flow, and total oxygen consumption, reflecting a profoundly increased muscle metabolic activity (Figs. 4-2B, 4-2C). Histochemically, these metabolic alterations are reflected as an increased percentage of FOG fi-

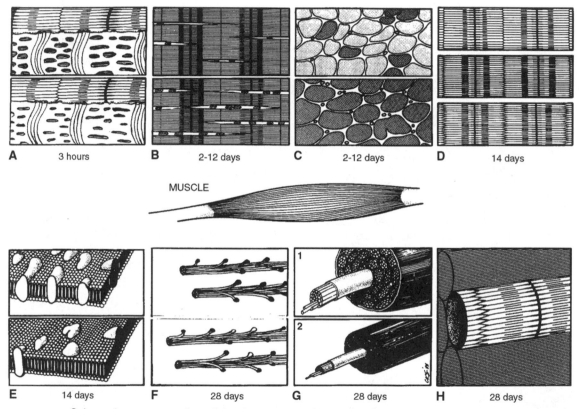

FIGURE 4-2. Schematic representation of the time course of muscular adaptation to chronic stimulation transforming from a fast to a slow fiber. In each panel the normal fiber is shown in the upper panel and the stimulated fiber in the lower panel. (A) SR begins to swell after three hours of stimulation. (B) After 2–12 days of chronic stimulation, an increase in the volume percent of mitochondria is observed. (C) After 2–12 days of chronic stimulation, an increase in capillary density and increase in type FOG (represented as "darkly" staining in this simulated SDH stain) fibers is observed. (D) After 14 days, the Z-band begins to increase in width. (E) After 14 days, a decrease in the amount and activity of calcium ATPase is observed. (F) After 28 days, the myosin profile is altered with different myosin monomers incorporating into single filaments (this figure is schematic and actual structural changes associated with myosin incorporation are not known). (G) After 28 days, muscle mass and fiber area are decreased. (H) After 28 days, the Z-band is the full width of a normal slow-contracting muscle and the density of T-system has decreased. At this point, the transformed fast contracting muscle is indistinguishable from a normal slow contracting muscle. (Modified from: Lieber, R.L. (1988). Time course and cellular control of muscle fiber type transformation following chronic stimulation. *ISI Atlas of Science, 1*, 189–194.)

bers at the expense of FG fibers (Fig. 4-2C). The increase in oxidative enzymes and capillary density are manifested functionally as a decrease in muscle fatigability. At this point, the width of the Z-band begins to increase toward the wider value observed for normal slow muscle (Fig. 4-2D). (Again, the significance of Z-disk width change is not known). The amount and activity of the calcium transport ATPase decreases and changes its particle distribution within the SR bilayer (Fig. 4-2E). Here is an important point: just because activity increases, does not mean that all muscle proteins must also increase. Some proteins increase in amount (i.e., are upregulated) and others decrease in amount (i.e., are downregulated). The "choice" which the muscle makes depends on the goal of the adaptation. As the muscle is receiving information consistent with being chronically active at fairly low levels, it alters its genetic expression pattern to create a structure consistent with this functional requirement. In the case of decreased expression of amount and activity of SR calcium transport proteins, this can be detected physiologically as a prolonged time-to-peak twitch tension and a prolonged relaxation time of a muscle twitch or as a decrease in the fusion frequency (Fig. 4-3). Here is a case in which a structural change in the muscle has a clear physiological correlate. However, as noted above (for the SR and Z-disk), it is not always possible to correlate a precise functional effect of a structural change. Note that, for every stimulation frequency shown in Figure 4-3, the stimulated muscle demonstrates partial tetanic fusion while the control muscle completely relaxes between stimuli. This is due to the lower ability of stimulated muscle to release and uptake calcium during activation and relaxation. The net result is that the stimulated muscle tension record completely fuses at a lower frequency than the control leg. Effectively, the muscle generates more tension per unit activation energy, which would appear to be a good strategy if the goal is posture-type control. In fact, even the physical appearance of the stimulated muscle approaches that of the more pos-

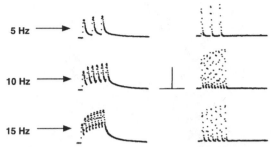

FIGURE 4-3. Comparison of the form of unfused tetani between a stimulated leg (left panel) and control leg (right panel) of the rabbit tibialis anterior. Note that at every frequency, the stimulated leg demonstrates partial tetanic fusion while the control leg completely relaxes between stimuli due to the decrease in activity and/or amount of calcium transport proteins within the SR. As a result, the stimulated leg tension record completely fuses at a lower frequency than the control leg. Calibration bar in center of figure. Vertical bar = 500 g, horizontal bar = 500 ms. Muscle temperature = 37.2°C. This muscle was transcutaneously stimulated at 10 Hz × 1 hour/day × 5 days/week × 4 weeks. (From: Lieber, R.L. (1986). Skeletal muscle adaptability iii: Muscle properties following chronic electrical stimulation. *Developmental Medicine and Child Neurology, 28,* 662–670.)

tural muscles by taking on a "deep red" appearance (Fig. 4-4). Finally after about 4 weeks of continuous stimulation, an alteration in the myosin light chain profile is observed whereby the normally fast muscle, containing only light chains LC1f, LC2f, and LC3f, now contains light chains characteristic of slow fibers, i.e., LC1s and LC2s (Fig. 4-2F). Recall from Chapter 2 that the precise role of the light chains is not fully understood. However, the fact that the light chains associated with slow fibers are expressed is consistent with the fast muscle fiber becoming more like a slow muscle fiber. The heavy chain profile may also be altered at this time. Finally, after such a prolonged "dose" of increased activity, muscle fiber cross-sectional area, maximum tetanic tension, and muscle mass have decreased significantly (Fig. 4-2G). The Z-band is now the full width of that normally observed in a slow fiber and the density of

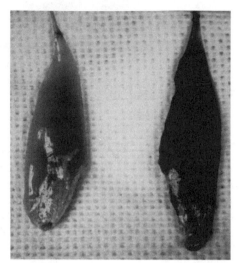

Control   **Experimental**

FIGURE 4-4. Photograph of control (left) and experimentally stimulated (right) rabbit tibialis anterior muscles whose contractile properties are shown in Figure 4-3. Note the dark (actually deep red) appearance of the stimulated muscle, which reflects the dramatic capillary proliferation and myoglobin content.

the T-system greatly decreased (Fig. 4-2H). The muscle is now indistinguishable from a normal slow skeletal muscle in every respect. Two things can be concluded from this typical time-course of transformation:

1. Muscle metabolic enzymes, capillaries, SR and T-system, are much more easily changed than contractile proteins.
2. Although chronic stimulation does increase muscle endurance capacity, it is not an effective means for increasing fiber size in normal muscle.

The decrease in skeletal muscle mass and fiber area should not be viewed as an atrophic or degenerative response, *i.e.*, an undesirable "overuse" type of injury. Rather, it appears that fiber atrophy represents a deliberate adaptive response of the muscle fiber to chronic stimulation—perhaps to decrease diffusion distances from the muscle fiber to the interstitial spaces, which contain the capillaries. As an

aside, it is interesting that chronic low frequency electrical stimulation is the best way to make a muscle weaker. This should certainly raise some eyebrows in the therapeutic community because electrical stimulation is commonly used to treat muscle atrophy. More will be said about this later in this chapter (page 202).

Cellular Regulation of Transformation

Chronic stimulation experiments have also provided insights into the cellular control of factors that determine muscle fiber types. The elegantly coordinated transformation sequence suggests that chronic stimulation induces a shift in the protein synthesis and degradation machinery within the muscle cell. Transformation occurs at slightly different rates along the length of individual fibers, suggesting that the nuclei of transforming fibers do not act in a completely uniform manner (remember that, during development, muscle fiber nuclei retained some independence, with nuclei under the neuromuscular junction preferentially expressing the gene for the acetyl choline receptor and nuclei near the muscle-tendon junction preferentially expressing the gene for adhesion proteins). Such nonuniformity is seen, for example, if a single fast fiber is stained histochemically for fiber type during the transformation process—some regions will contain slow myosin and others will contain fast myosin. In fact, during transformation, many regions show both fast and slow myosins. In other words, individual muscle fibers may be composed of dif-

---

Box 4-2. Which is Easier to Change, Muscle Endurance or Speed?

Endurance, and other metabolic changes are much more readily changed compared to changes involving speed. Changes in speed reflect a difference in the contractile motor myosin and thus change in fiber types. Muscles can adapt to altered metabolic demands within days of initiation of the change, whereas changes in contractile proteins such as myosin, may require weeks of continued activity.

ferent myosin types. This presents some interesting contractile possibilities, which are only currently being investigated. Although it is generally agreed that many and perhaps even most muscle fibers may express multiple myosin isoforms, the functional significance of multiple myosins is not known (Bottinelli, Betto, Schiaffino, & Reggiani, 1994a; Bottinelli, Betto, Schiaffino, & Reggiani, 1994b; Lutz, Cuizon, Ryan, & Lieber, 1998; Schiaffino & Reggiani, 1996).

It is known that alterations in the amount and type of proteins present in the cell can result from numerous different mechanisms including alterations in DNA replication (duplication of the DNA template coding for a protein), change in transcription rates (the rate at which mRNA copies are made from the DNA template), alteration in translation rates (the rate at which protein is translated on the ribosomal machinery based on mRNA codes), and changes in protein degradation rates. Which of these several mechanisms operates within the transforming muscle cell? Do changes in different proteins occur by the same mechanism?

In an effort to address this question, Williams and colleagues (Williams, Salmons, Newsholme, Kaufman, & Mellor, 1986) measured the concentration of mRNA coding for a glycolytic enzyme (aldolase) and mRNA coding for an enzyme involved in oxidative phosphorylation (cytochrome b) in muscles that were chronically stimulated at 10 Hz for 5 or 21 days. They documented an asynchronous change in mRNA levels coding for the two proteins. This should not be surprising since different muscle functions may have a different time-course of adaptation. After 21 days, aldolase mRNA fell to one-fourth of normal levels during which cytochrome b mRNA increased 5-fold, paralleling the observed decrease and increase of glycolytic and oxidative enzymes, respectively. However, after only 5 days of stimulation, aldolase mRNA concentration had decreased significantly but cytochrome b mRNA concentration remained unchanged. These data suggested that chronic stimulation resulted in reciprocal changes in the expression of the aldolase and cytochrome b

genes at the level of transcription since changes in the amount of mRNA coding for the different enzymes was found to parallel changes in protein level. However, because of the different time courses, the transcriptional changes might have occurred by different regulatory mechanisms. This raises the likely scenario that different proteins might be controlled by different factors. Additionally, other nontranscriptional mechanisms have been demonstrated in other models. As more data are presented more general statements will be made about this.

Adaptation to Chronic Stretch

The next model of increased use is one that is still causing great interest in the scientific community. This is the model whereby the length of a muscle is chronically increased by immobilizing a joint in a fixed position or by surgical intervention. In spite of the fact that only muscle length is changed, without concomitant muscle stimulation, this type of treatment represents an extremely intense increased use model since the imposed treatment is "experienced" by the muscle 24 hours per day for the duration of the experiment.

Experimental Method for Fiber Length Alteration

To chronically stretch a muscle requires joint fixation in an extreme position. For example, to stretch the soleus muscle chronically, the ankle is immobilized in a fully dorsiflexed position. Conversely, to stretch the tibialis anterior, the ankle is immobilized in full plantarflexion.

The seminal experiments on chronic stretch were performed in England by the muscle cell biologists Drs. Pamela Williams and Geoffrey Goldspink (1971, 1973). They immobilized mouse ankles fully dorsiflexed to stretch the soleus muscles (Fig. 4-5) and measured the resulting changes in the number of serial sarcomeres along the length of the muscle. The results were impressive. After only 4 weeks of immobilization in dorsiflexion, the number of sarcomeres in soleus muscle fibers had in-

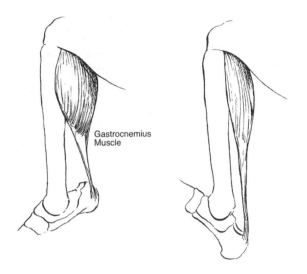

Plantarflexion   Dorsiflexion

FIGURE 4-5. Experimental method for chronic length change of the gastrocnemius muscle. Ankles are immobilized either in full dorsiflexion (right) to stretch the gastrocnemius or in full plantarflexion (left) to shorten the gastrocnemius muscle. After the immobilization period, muscle morphological and contractile properties may be determined.

creased dramatically by approximately 20% such that the "resting" sarcomere length of the stretched soleus was nearly that of an unstretched, normal soleus. Consider the sequence of events that must have occurred: the soleus muscle-tendon unit was stretched secondary to ankle dorsiflexion, thereby creating an increased sarcomere length. Next, the muscle, "sensing" this increase, synthesized new sarcomeres to return sarcomere length to "normal." In a similar experiment, these investigators immobilized the muscles with the ankle fully plantarflexed, thus shortening the soleus and, after 4 weeks, the number of sarcomeres decreased by about 40%. They measured the length-tension properties of the immobilized muscles and found that the muscles generated their maximum tetanic tension at a length very close to the length at which they were immobilized. Their interpretation of the data was that the muscle adjusted sarcomere number to reset L_o to the immobilization length. Extending this conclusion, others often state dogmatically that

muscles will change serial sarcomere number after a chronic length change (due to immobilization, transplantation or transposition) such that optimal sarcomere length is achieved at the most common joint position. This may be an overstatement (see below) but does have support in the basic science literature. A better way to make this statement is that muscles *may* change serial sarcomere number secondary to the chronic length change.

The muscles immobilized in the shortened position were shown to be much stiffer, much more resistant to passive stretch. Williams and Goldspink interpreted this latter result as the muscle "protecting" itself from overstretch of the sarcomere. With so few sarcomeres, they felt that the increased stiffness would prevent sarcomere length from increasing to the length beyond which force could be generated. They also demonstrated that the entire process occurred even in the absence of the nerve since nearly identical results were obtained when the nerve was severed before the experiment. The control center for the adaptive process was within the muscle itself.

Age-Specific Adaptation to Chronic Length Change

Another factor influencing the extent of sarcomere number adaptation was the age of the animal at the time of immobilization. Tardieu and her colleagues immobilized in full dorsiflexion

---

Box 4-3. When Does Immobilization Not Cause Muscle Atrophy?

Immobilization will not result in muscle atrophy if it involves significant muscle stretch. Chronic muscle stretch provides a powerful hypertrophic influence on skeletal muscle. Thus, immobilization of an ankle fully plantar flexed results in tremendous atrophy of the plantar flexors while immobilization in full dorsiflexion results in much less atrophy or even hypertrophy in some cases. It is therefore not correct to think of "immobilization" and "atrophy" as necessarily going hand in hand.

the ankles of young and old rabbits and examined soleus muscle fiber and tendon lengths after 18 days in this lengthened position (Tabary, Tabary, Tardieu, Tardieu, & Goldspink, 1972). They found, as expected that the length of the muscle-tendon unit increased dramatically in both old and young animals. However, young animals increased muscle-tendon length by shortening muscle fiber length and lengthening tendon length whereas older animals increased muscle-tendon length only by lengthening their muscle fibers. This suggests that the tissue type that is most amenable to adaptation is age-dependent. You might speculate that these findings are significant when it comes to understanding muscle adaptation in pediatric patients.

Location of Sarcomere Adaptation

A second surprising result was demonstrated in follow-up experiments in which Williams and Goldspink (1971) determined the location of the new sarcomeres added during stretch. The investigators fed animals radioactive adenosine so that any new sarcomeres synthesized would be radioactive (adenosine is incorporated into the structural ADP of the actin monomers) and thus, visible using modern autoradiographic methods (a procedure whereby a film emulsion is placed over the tissue and the radioactive areas "expose" the film grains causing dark spots on the tissue). Where do you suppose the newly synthesized sarcomeres were located? Throughout the tissue? At specific locations? The answer was that most of the newly synthesized sarcomeres were located at the fiber ends, near the muscle-tendon junction (Fig. 4-6). Control experiments demonstrated that this change only occurred if the muscle was stretched, since immobilization with the ankle in the neutral position produced no such change. The location of highest adaptive capacity was thus seen to be the muscle-tendon junction. Interestingly, this is one location within the muscle of extremely high mitochondrial and protein synthetic activity (Eisenberg & Milton, 1984).

Labelling Density in Different Muscle Regions:

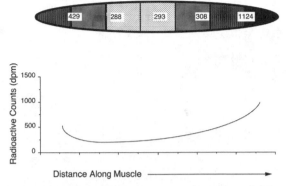

FIGURE 4-6. Sohomatic representation of spatial location of radioactive adenosine label following chronic stretch of mouse soleus muscle. Darker shading represents higher labeling (numbers superimposed on shading patterns). Most of the radioactive label was located at the fiber ends suggesting that sarcomere addition occurred mainly at the ends of the fibers and not throughout the muscle length. Lower panel represents graphical form of the labeling density along the muscle length in counts per minute (cpm). (Based on data in: Goldspink, G. (1983). Alterations in myofibril size and structure during growth, exercise, and changes in environmental temperature. In L. D. Peachey, (Ed.), *Handbook of Physiology* (pp. 539–554). Baltimore, MD: American Physiological Society.)

In a similar immobilization experiment, Edgerton and his colleagues at UCLA investigated the differential sensitivity of various muscles to immobilization-induced sarcomere number alteration (Fig. 4-7) (Spector, Simard, Fournier, Sternlicht, & Edgerton, 1982). This, of course, addresses a different, but important question. The question is not, "How do muscles adapt to immobilization?" but rather "How do different muscles adapt to immobilization?" This distinction is important because, as you will see repeatedly, different muscles seem to sense identical stimuli in a way that causes different adaptations. This means that muscles are not generic either in structure, function, or plasticity. Using a rat immobilization model, Spector et al. compared the response of the soleus (SOL), the medial gastrocnemius (MG),

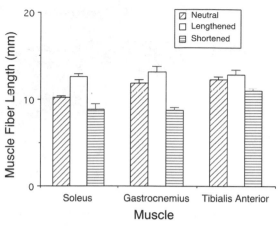

FIGURE 4-7. Change in muscle fiber length for three different rat ankle muscles following chronic length change. For each muscle, a group of animals was immobilized in the shortened (horizontally striped bars), neutral (hatched bars), and lengthened (open bars) position. Note that while all muscles adapted the ankle extensors (soleus and gastrocnemius) were more "adaptable" compared to the ankle flexor (tibialis anterior). (Data from: Spector, S.A., Simard, C.P., Fournier, M., Sternlicht, E., Edgerton, V.R. (1982). Architectural alterations of rat hindlimbs skeletal muscles immobilized at different lengths. *Experimental Neurology, 76*, 94–110.)

and the tibialis anterior (TA) to chronic length change. Recall that the SOL is a monoarticular ankle plantarflexor composed of primarily slow fibers while the MG is a biarticular ankle plantarflexor and, to a lesser extent, a knee flexor composed primarily of fast fibers (Lawrence, Nichols, & English, 1993). The TA is a monoarticular ankle dorsiflexor composed mainly of fast fibers. So here is an experimental paradigm in which the number of joints, fiber type, and function can be tested for their influence on sarcomere number adaptation.

Spector et al. demonstrated that, although the SOL and MG adapted in much the same way as the studies mentioned above (which were all performed on the SOL muscles of other species), the TA was much less responsive (Fig. 4-7). Here is clearly a case in which "all muscles are not created equal"—either with respect to physiological properties or adaptation. Again and again you will see that the muscles that are

often used (*e.g.*, antigravity muscles such as the SOL and MG) are often the most plastic. This differential muscle sensitivity of muscles to adaptation will be encountered again in Chapter 5 as the muscle's response to decreased use is investigated. Overall, however, the distinction between muscles with a postural, antigravity role and those without such a role is probably the best predictor of adaptive tendency.

Sarcomere Type Added During Chronic Stretch

Williams and Goldspink and colleagues (Williams, Watt, Bicik, & Goldspink, 1986) also examined the "type" of sarcomeres added during chronic stretch combined with electrical stimulation. They showed that, regardless of the type of myosin in the sarcomeres of the parent fiber, the sarcomeres added were always of the slow myosin type. (However, this could have been an embryonic myosin, which cross-reacted with the slow myosin antibody.) This observation indicates that, under conditions of increased use, the muscle cell is "programmed" to synthesize slow myosin and create sarcomeres, which are composed of slow myosin. However, these experiments are very difficult technically, since the same fiber must be examined along a very large distance. Therefore, definitive support for this result is not currently available.

These experiments also confirm that the "hot spot" of a muscle fiber in terms of plasticity is the muscle-tendon junction. As stated above, Eisenberg and her colleagues provided supportive data for this concept by demonstrating that muscle fiber ends have a greater concentration of mitochondria, suggesting high metabolic activity (Eisenberg, 1983). Numerous mitochondria provide the ATP required for protein synthesis of contractile proteins and sarcomere assembly. When muscle fiber length is chronically altered, the number of sarcomeres is adjusted to attempt to compensate for the change. The extent of the adaptation is not known, but it is clear, based on our extensive discussion of architecture (Chapters 2 and 3), that fiber length changes will have dramatic functional consequences (see below).

Therapist's Comments

Many therapists have used the sarcomere number adaptation story to claim that these same sarcomere adaptations occur in humans. It may be wise to remind the reader that there is no evidence that these changes occur in humans. There are a set of reports that tried to determine indirectly whether sarcomere number adaptation did occur as a result of stretching exercises. In one case, a mechanical device was used to measure hamstring stiffness during straight leg raising (Halbertsma, et al., 1999) and, in another, an isokinetic device was used (Magnusson, et al., 1998). Both studies provide indirect evidence that sarcomere number does not increase in response to intermittent stretching to gain range of motion. This is important for therapists because, although I would like the animal models to be representative of human sarcomere number changes, I do not think it is appropriate to assume this for patient care purposes.

Effect of Intermittent Stretch on Sarcomere Adaptation

Recently, Dr. Pamela Williams addressed a question directly relevant to physical therapy: How much passive manipulation of the limb is needed to prevent the sarcomere number decrease observed after immobilization in a shortened position? The reason this is so important is that it may turn out that muscle properties can be altered by therapists, but that the amount of time required to produce such changes are not feasible give current clinical restrictions. If so, efforts would have to be directed toward home treatment in which treatment durations on the order of hours are feasible. Williams immobilized mouse soleus muscles in a shortened position as described above, but removed the casts every day to perform passive range of motion exercises

(Williams, 1988). The joints from different experimental groups were manipulated for different amounts of time ranging from 15 min/day to 3 hrs/day (Fig. 4-8). The joint was passed through its entire physiological range of motion at a relatively slow rate. She found that passive stretch for only 30 min/day was suffi-

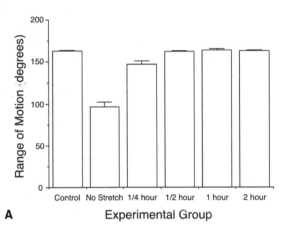

A

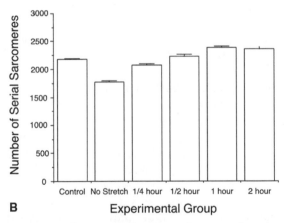

B

FIGURE 4-8. Response of mouse soleus muscle to intermittent stretch during immobilization in a shortened position. At least a 1/2 hour of stretch was required to prevent the fiber shortening seen with no immobilization or with stretch of shorter duration. **(A)** Range of ankle motion after intermittent stretch for time period shown below graph. **(B)** Number of serial sarcomeres following intermittent stretch for the different times shown. (Data from: Williams, P. (1988). Effect of intermittent stretch on immobilised muscle. *Annals of the Rheumatic Diseases, 47*, 1014–1016.)

Box 4-4. How Many Minutes of "Therapy" are Enough to Prevent the Changes Accompanying Immobilization?

While it is a bit dangerous to generalize, in a mouse model that created tremendous muscle atrophy with immobilization, passive range of motion exercises for as little as 15 min/day dramatically decreased the effects of immobilization. With 30 min/day of passive range of motion manipulation, muscles were essentially the same as muscles that were not immobilized.

---

cient to prevent the dramatic decrease in range of motion (Fig. 4-8A) and decrease in sarcomere number (Fig. 4-8B) that was normally observed. Even 15 min/day was significantly better than nothing. The high correlation between serial sarcomere number and range of motion (compare Fig. 4-8A to 4-8B) also illustrated that the change in range of motion was probably because of changes that occurred in the muscle, not just in more commonly studied connective tissues such as ligaments and tendons (Amiel, Frank, Harwood, Fronek, & Akeson, 1984; Amiel, Kuiper, Wallace, Harwood, & VandeBerg, 1991).

Functional Consequences of Altered Fiber Length

What if fiber length adaptation occurs in humans? What would the functional consequences be? The previous discussion regarding the functional significance of fiber length applies here. As stated in Chapter 3, if muscle fiber length increases, muscle velocity and excursion increase (assuming that excursion is not limited by the joint itself). In addition, a muscle's ability to generate force will increase at a given shortening velocity if fiber length increases (Fig. 3-28A). If the fiber length increase is secondary to joint immobilization, when the immobilization is removed, presumably, fiber length will return to normal. However, what if the change in fiber length is due to a surgical procedure? A fairly common surgical procedure is the tendon

transfer, whereby the insertion site of a muscle is moved to a new location to substitute for lost or impaired function. What are the consequences of such a surgical procedure?

There are no experimental data available to define the precise changes that occur after such a transfer so the process has been simulated using the illustrations in Figure 4-9 and Figure 4-10. Figure 4-9 illustrates a "typical" muscle with a "normal" starting fiber length. The muscle is symbolized as a schematic sarcomere. Note that, as the joint rotates from flexion to extension, sarcomere length increases and muscle force changes (Fig. 4-9). The active range of joint motion is thus limited by the active muscle range, which is itself a function of serial sarcomere number. The total active range of motion in this example is 40°. If a surgical procedure moved the muscle insertion site such that muscle fiber length increases by 25%

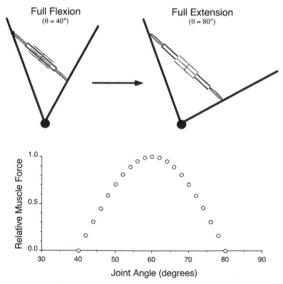

FIGURE 4-9. Schematic illustration of the change in muscle force as a function of joint angle. The muscle (illustrated in the upper panel as a sarcomere) changes from fully shortened to fully lengthened as the joint rotates from extreme flexion to extreme extension. Because of the length-tension relationship, muscle force changes as a function of joint angle (lower panel). This is simulated by the sine function over a 40° range of motion.

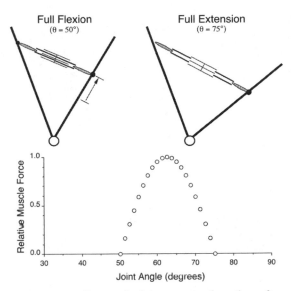

FIGURE 4-10. Change in joint range of motion after simulated surgical tendon transfer. Moment arm is increased (arrow) which causes muscle length to change more for a given rotation (upper panel). As a result of the increased moment arm, muscle active range is "used up" over a smaller joint range, which decreases the active range of this hypothetical muscle from 40° (Fig. 4-9) to only 25° (lower panel).

(Fig. 4-10), what are the changes that would be observed? Immediately postoperatively, the muscle would obviously be at a longer length with the increased moment arm. Now, as the joint rotates, the amount of sarcomere length change per joint angle rotation increases. Thus, muscle force will change over a narrower range of motion, which is 25° in this hypothetical example (Fig. 4-10). Therefore, as a result of increased moment arm, active range decreases and the joint angle at which muscle force is maximum changes (Fig. 4-11). Since the joint angle corresponding to maximum muscle force is now even farther from the angle at which the maximum moment arm occurs (assumed in this case, to be 90°), a torque (strength) decrease would occur simply because the angles at which optimal muscle and joint properties occur are quite different. This is an important point. Weakness can be observed because of a change in muscle fiber length, not just a change in the

muscle's ability to generate tension. This is an extension of our previous discussion, which noted that strength results from the interaction between muscle and joint properties and not either property alone. In this case, weakness resulted from a change in the angle at which muscle generated its maximum muscle force.

To continue to follow the "patient" postoperatively, suppose that, for this muscle, stretch stimulated the fibers to add sarcomeres and compensate for the increased moment arm. As more sarcomeres are added, three things will happen: the subject's active range of motion will increase, torque (strength) will increase, and the joint angle at which maximum strength occurs will shift. At the end of the "experiment" the increase in sarcomere number would compensate for the increase in moment arm and the muscle-joint interaction would return to normal. This scenario would be good news for the surgeon, if it were true. There is still insufficient data available to demonstrate that this process occurs exactly as described here, but it is a reasonable guess based on the experimental data available. This scenario makes several specific predictions that can be experimentally tested. Of course, built into the results of this type of discussion are several assumptions that are probably not true in all cases:

1. All muscles do not adapt to the same extent.
2. Immobilization is not necessarily a realistic adaptation model since muscle length and activity are relatively fixed.
3. There is an age-specific effect that is not yet understood.
4. There are no available analogous data for the upper extremity in which a large number of surgical transpositions are performed (Smith & Hastings, 1993).

Fiber Length Adaptation to Retinaculum Release

To overcome the uncertainties of immobilization models in which it is not clear whether the muscle is adapting to its length, its resting tension, its resting sarcomere length, its sarcomere

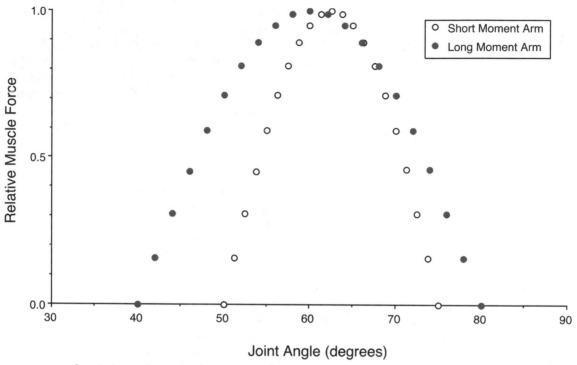

FIGURE 4-11. Comparison of muscle force as a function of joint angle for the short (open circles) and long (filled circles) moment arms. The increased moment arm results in decreased range of motion as illustrated in Figures 4-9 and 4-10.

length range (which equals zero), or a combination of factors, investigators have induced chronic length changes in muscle by transecting the ankle retinacular ligament that is used as a pulley by both the tibialis anterior and extensor digitorum longus muscles. When the retinaculum is released, the ankle dorsiflexion moment arm increases and thus, the range over which the muscle operates also increases. In this relatively simple surgical procedure, animals are permitted unlimited activity, there is no postoperative immobilization which can itself affect results, and neuromuscular activity remains physiological. Such a model permits testing of specific hypotheses regarding the mechanical stimulus to which the muscle adapts. Unfortunately, the literature has produced conflicting results, probably based upon the diversity of models used. However, in spite of the lack of unanimity among investigators, the re-

sults do permit discussion of several potential physiological responses that are still relevant to human patients.

Two recent studies implemented the retinaculum release model and then measured serial sarcomere number after the adaptation had occurred. In the first study, Drs. Walter Herzog and Tim Koh, at the University of Calgary, transected the retinaculum in young rabbits and also implanted a force transducer, similar to that previously described by Gregor et al. (1988) on the tendon to permit measurement of muscle force during various types of locomotion (Koh & Herzog, 1998). The results obtained were as they expected: transection of the ankle retinaculum caused the excursion of the muscle-tendon unit to increase significantly (Fig. 4-12A) and, in response to this increased excursion, serial sarcomere number increased (Fig. 4-12B). Interestingly, maximum muscle

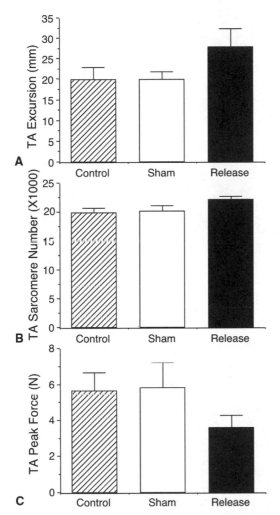

FIGURE 4-12. Muscle properties of the rabbit tibialis anterior in response to release of the ankle pretibial flexor retinaculum. Experimental groups included a control group of normal rabbits (hatched bar), a sham operated group who experienced all surgery except retinaculum transection (open bar) and a group in which the TA was released from the retinaculum (filled bar) **(A)** Muscle-tendon unit excursion measured while rotating the ankle joint from 160° (full plantarflexion) to 40° (full dorsiflexion). **(B)** Serial sarcomere number measured 4 weeks after the surgical procedure. **(C)** Peak muscle force measured during hopping on a motorized treadmill. Muscle PCSA also decreased (not shown). (Data from: Koh, T.J., Herzog, W. (1998). Excursion is important in regulating sarcomere number in the growing rabbit tibialis anterior. *Journal of Physiology (London) 508*, 267–280.)

force during hopping decreased, apparently since a lower force was required to generate the same dorsiflexion torque due to the larger moment arm (Fig. 4-13C). However, a possible complication of the experiment was that these young rabbits were rapidly growing throughout the experimental period. In fact, based on the normal growth of rabbits (Amiel et al., 1991; Frank, McDonald, Lieber, & Sabiston, 1988), the mechanical stimulus given to the muscle by retinaculum release was acting in parallel to a powerful lengthening stimulus provided by bone length increase. This model therefore represents a combination of increased range due to both release and rapid growth. This model may be relevant to the type of adaptation that could occur in children's muscles subjected to stretch during surgical correction of limb length discrepancy. Such experimental models need to be developed to understand physiological adaptation more completely.

In a second retinaculum release study, the ligament was transected in adult mice and their gait and muscle properties were measured 2 and 4 weeks post-transection (Burkholder & Lieber, 1998). Moment arm increased by ~40% due to the surgery which predicted an increase in range of motion of about 20% (Fig. 4-13A). Again, if sarcomere number adaptation were to occur to restore the "normal" range of motion, then the number should have increased due to the surgery. Unexpectedly, it did not. In fact, sarcomere number actually *decreased* by 10% after the surgery. Obviously, the 10% was not a dramatic change, but the most significant factor was that sarcomere number decreased at all. In addition, this was a very robust result that was similar whether a longer duration was studied or whether animals were forced to activate dorsiflexors more strenuously by imposing swimming exercise on them. The final question was how the joints were used after the surgery. One could envision an alteration in muscle properties that would leave the animal with a functional deficit observable by, for example, gait analysis. It turned out that the animals did have an altered gait. Video analysis of gait in

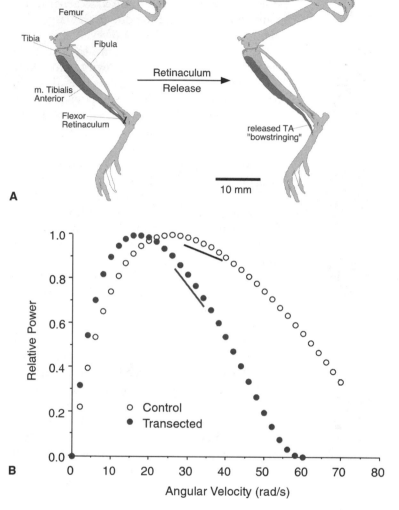

FIGURE 4-13. (A) Schematic diagram of "bowstringing" of the TA as the ankle pretibial flexor retinaculum is released. **(B)** Predicted power-angular velocity diagrams for normal mice and mice that experienced transection of the ankle pretibial flexor retinaculum for two weeks. Note that, after transection, due to decreased serial sarcomere number, muscle power decreased at a given velocity. Gait was measured in these mice from high-speed video and the heavy line over each curve represents that preferred speed. (Data from: Burkholder, T.J., Lieber, R.L. (1998). Sarcomere number adaptation after retinaculum release in adult mice. *Journal of Experimental Biology, 201,* 309–316.)

normal and transected mice revealed that mice with surgical transection preferentially dorsiflexed at slightly slower angular velocities. Unoperated mice dorsiflexed consistently at 2,200 degrees/s which was significantly faster than mice with transected retinacula who dorsiflexed at only 1,900 degrees/s. Despite this 14% decrease in angular velocity after transection, the ~40% increase in moment arm and reduction in serial sarcomere number predicted an approximately 20% increase in velocity of TA shortening during dorsiflexion (Fig. 4-13B). You should be able to predict that such an ad-

aptation would be unfavorable from a muscular force generating point-of-view. This is primarily because the TA muscle fibers shortening at a higher velocity would place them at a lower force level on their force-velocity relationship and require recruitment of more muscle to generate the same absolute force (analogous to the situation shown schematically in Fig. 3-28). This may be why, in this second study, PCSA remained the same even though the moment arm was increased and the muscle could, theoretically, generate a greater torque. Because the animals were not growing during the study, the relative influence of excursion and length on sarcomere number adaptation could be determined. Again, this is in contrast to the numerous reports of sarcomere number adaptation obtained using immobilization models or models that use rapidly growing animals.

Having described the changes that occur after retinaculum release, consider in greater detail the muscle changes that occur using this model: The immediate effect of retinaculum transection was to alter average muscle length as well as its excursion. The average moment arm increase of ~30% had two main effects: the first was to increase muscle excursion by about 25% and the second was to decrease sarcomere length at most joint angles. From a theoretical point of view, the effect that this intervention might have on sarcomere number could be predicted based on assumptions about the mechanical factors that regulate sarcomere number (Herring, Grimm, & Grimm, 1984). For example, if sarcomere length at a particular joint angle was the dominant signal for sarcomere number adjustment, then, after retinaculum transection, sarcomere number would decrease to restore sarcomere length to the identical value as obtained at that joint angle before surgery. On the other hand, if excursion was the dominant signal, then sarcomere number would increase proportional to the increase in moment arm to restore sarcomere excursion to the pre-operative range. Finally, if shortening velocity or power production dominated the signaling, then sarcomere number would increase in proportion to the change in muscle shortening velocity (which need not be the same as the moment arm change). Clearly, since sarcomere number decreased, this does not support the idea that sarcomere number will simply adapt to "reoptimize" the muscle for its new condition. Together, these studies illustrate the complex nature of muscle adaptation to chronic length changes under physiological conditions. Further studies are needed to identify the parameters that cause a muscle to change serial sarcomere number in response to chronic length changes.

The implications of altered serial sarcomere number are obvious for surgery involving muscle. If complete adaptation does not occur for all muscles, it is important to make the surgical transfer of a donor muscle into a new one so that the new muscle is architecturally similar to muscles whose function(s) it is replacing. Inspection of the surgical literature reveals a relatively poor appreciation for this point. The major exception is the excellent treatise by Paul Brand and colleagues (Brand, Beach, & Thompson, 1981) which describes the muscles and joints of the arm and hand, their interaction, and the appropriate surgical procedures for restoration of hand function following disease or injury.

The architectural data presented in Chapter 2 has been used to match the architectural properties of donor muscles to specific functional needs in upper extremity tendon transfer cases (Lieber & Brown, 1992; Lieber, Fazeli, & Botte, 1990). Here, only three cases will be considered. These presentations serve not only to reinforce architectural principles presented in Chapter 2, but also they will illustrate the application of basic muscle physiological information to clinical practice.

SURGICAL RESTORATION OF DIGITAL EXTENSION

In the surgical restoration of digital extension following high radial nerve palsy, described and accepted potential donor muscles (that are transferred to the extensor digitorum communis, EDC) are muscles that are still functional due to their intact innervation by the nerve. These include the flexor carpi radialis (FCR), the flexor carpi ulnaris (FCU), the flexor digitorum superficialis to the middle finger (FDS (M)), and the FDS to the ring finger (FDS (R)). From the standpoint of architecture alone, the FDS (M) most closely resembles the EDC in terms of force generation (i.e., due to a closely-matched physiological cross-sectional area) and excursion (i.e., due to a closely-matched fiber length). This is emphasized by the relatively close position in "architectural space" of the

FDS (M) compared to the EDC (Fig. 4-14A). If one were to compare individual architectural properties, it is clear that the FDS (M) has more than enough excursion to function as an EDC since it has longer fibers whereas the FCU has excessive force-generating potential due to the high PCSA, yet may lack sufficient excursion due to its relatively short fiber length. Thus, if the concern of the reconstructive procedure was sufficient force, the FCU might be chosen whereas if the concern were excursion, the FDS (M) might be chosen. Either way, knowl-

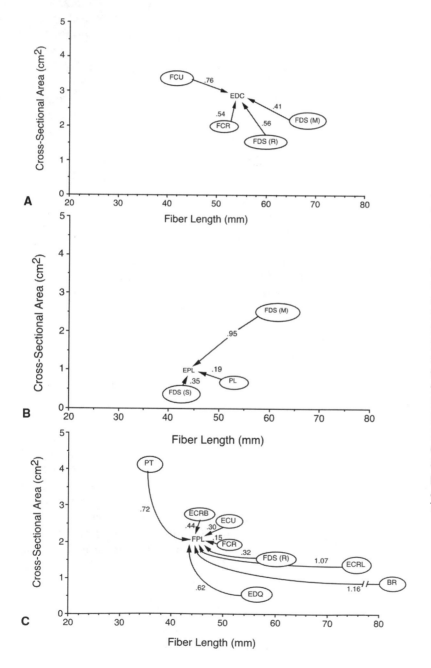

FIGURE 4-14. Graphical representation of tendon transfers from the point of view of skeletal muscle architecture. Each muscle is shown as in Figure 1-18 in terms of its fiber length and PCSA. Circled muscles represent potential donors for the muscle indicated. **(A)** Possible tendon transfers for restoration of digital extension. **(B)** Possible tendon transfers for restoration of thumb extension. **(C)** Possible tendon transfers for restoration of thumb flexion. (Figure modified from: Lieber, R.L., Jacobson, M.D., Fazeli, B.M., Abrams, R.A., Botte, M.J. (1992). Architecture of selected muscles of the arm and forearm: Anatomy and implications for tendon transfer. *Journal of Hand Surgery, 17A,* 787–798.)

edge of muscle architecture permits an informed decision to be made. It should be noted that architectural mismatch between the FCU and EDC has been blamed for the poor clinical result of this transfer (Lieber, Pontén, & Fridén, 1996).

SURGICAL RESTORATION OF
THUMB EXTENSION:

To restore thumb extensor function in high radial nerve palsy, potential donors include the FDS (M), the FDS to the small finger (FDS (S)), and the palmaris longus (PL). Again, in terms of architecture, the FDS (S) and the PL are similar to the extensor pollicis longus (EPL), and therefore should provide the force generation and excursion required to restore lost function (Fig. 4-14B).

SURGICAL RESTORATION OF THUMB FLEXION

As a final example, after high median nerve palsy, anterior interosseus nerve injury, or isolated, irreparable flexor pollicis longus (FPL) muscle injury, multiple potential donors for transfer to restore thumb flexion are available. These donors include the brachioradialis (BR), the extensor carpi radialis brevis (ECRL), the extensor carpi radialis longus (ECRB), the extensor carpi ulnaris (ECU), the extensor digiti quinti (EDQ) or the FDS (R). From an architectural standpoint, the ECRB, the FDS (R) and ECU are most similar to the FPL (Fig. 4-14C). Students interested in a detailed method that enables quantification of architectural differences between pairs of muscles are referred to another source (Lieber & Brown, 1992).

Adaptation to
Compensatory Hypertrophy

Another model that can be used to increase the level of skeletal muscle use is to force a muscle to work harder than normal by using surgical means. Drs. Ken Baldwin and Roland Roy at UCLA and UC Irvine have performed such a series of experiments that defined muscle and fiber responses to this procedure known as compensatory hypertrophy. The term "compensatory hypertrophy" refers to the hypertrophy of one muscle as it compensates for surgical removal of a synergist. Their experimental model was the laboratory rat.

Rat Ankle Extensor Muscle Anatomy

From your anatomical background, recall that the rat soleus, gastrocnemius, and plantaris muscles are the major plantarflexors in rats. (Whereas the human plantaris represents a vestigial muscle, and is even referred to as the "medical student's nerve due to its long "nerve-like" tendon, the rat plantaris muscle is quite sizeable.) The relative proportions of the various muscles that make up the rat ankle extensors are shown in Table 4-1. Note that the medial and lateral gastrocnemius together make up about 80% of the total ankle extensor mass while the plantaris and soleus make up only about 15% and 5% respectively. These muscles also vary with respect to fiber type distribution as shown in Table 4-1. The soleus (SOL) is composed of about 80% type SO fibers and 20% type FOG fibers. The medial gastrocnemius (MG) has two distinct regions that are identifiable based on gross color. The "red" MG is highly oxidative, composed of about 50% FOG fibers and 50% SO fibers. The "white" MG has no SO fibers and is composed of almost all (95%) FG fibers. It is easy to appreciate, therefore, that the MG has many more fast fibers than the soleus. The plantaris muscle is primarily composed of fast fibers (90% FG+FOG). Thus, it is possible to overload any one of the ankle extensors by surgically removing one (or more) of its synergists. After surgery, the remaining muscle(s) are forced to work harder (for 12–14 weeks) because they must replace the lost function of those muscles that were surgically removed. Based on the variety of fiber types, architecture, and muscle sizes available in the rat, it was possible to design experiments that determined the factors important in causing muscle hypertrophy. These investigators were already well aware of the fact that

TABLE 4-1	Relative Mass and Fiber Type Distribution of Rat Ankle Extensors*			
Muscle	Relative Mass of Plantarflexors (%)	Percent SO Fibers (%)	Percent FOG Fibers (%)	Percent FG Fibers (%)
Lateral Gastrocnemius	36	—	—	—
"White" Medial Gastrocnemius	48	—	5	95
"Red" Medial Gastrocnemius		50	50	—
Plantaris	14	10	45	45
Soleus	6	80	20	

*Data from: Roy, R.R., Medows, I.D., Baldwin, K.M., Edgerton, V.R. (1982). Functional significance of compensatory overloaded rat fast muscle. *Journal of Applied Physiology, 52,* 473–478.

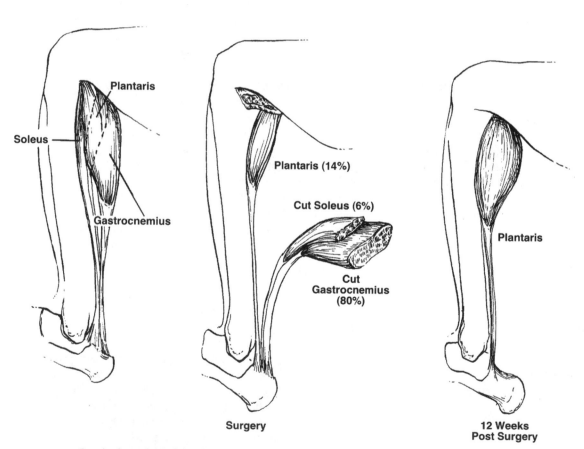

FIGURE 4-15. Surgical manipulation of muscles to perform the compensatory hypertrophy experiment. Muscle overload results from surgical removal or denervation of synergists. Percentage of each muscle contributing to the plantarflexors is shown in parentheses.

muscles with different fiber type proportions may respond differently to altered use and one of the bases for this choice of models was to permit the flexibility of investigation. A useful feature of this model was that the muscles remaining after surgery were subjected to activation by physiological means while the rats were performing their ordinary task of locomotion. Thus, objections to models such as chronic electrical stimulation (that activate an entire nerve trunk in a nonphysiological manner, i.e., synchronous and maximal activation of all axons) cannot be levied against studies with compensatory hypertrophy. Of course, realize that there is always a tradeoff in terms of the type of information to be gleaned. The chronic stimulation model definitely permits precise measurements of "use" dose (such as stimulation time, limb torque, etc.), which may benefit a particular study design. The analogous statement regarding dose cannot be made for the compensatory hypertrophy model.

Effects of Compensatory Hypertrophy on Rat Plantaris

In a series of experiments, these same investigators chose specific ankle extensor muscles that were overloaded and compared to muscles from age-matched animals on which no procedures (or only surgical sham procedures) had been performed. The results provided insights into the process and basis for the adaptation observed.

In the first experiment, the distal gastrocnemius and soleus were removed bilaterally, leaving only the plantaris muscle to perform the plantarflexion function (Fig. 4-15). Only about 15% of the ankle extensor musculature was initially available to the rat after surgery. What adaptations were observed in the plantaris muscle following such a dramatic surgical intervention? Amazingly, the overloaded plantaris muscles nearly doubled in size. They generated a much greater maximum tetanic tension with P_o increasing from about 5 N to 8 N (Fig. 4-16A). V_{max} decreased significantly from

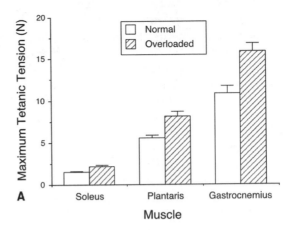

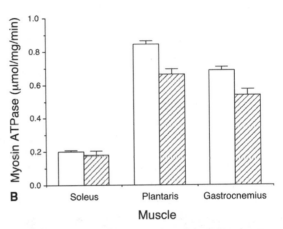

FIGURE 4-16. Muscle changes after compensatory hypertrophy. Properties of the soleus, medial gastrocnemius (red portion) and plantaris are shown. Open bars represent muscles from normal animals while hatched bars represent muscles from overloaded muscles **(A)** Maximum tetanic tension (P_o) of overloaded muscles. **(B)** ATPase activity of muscles subjected to compensatory overload. (Data from: Baldwin, K.M., Valdez, V., Herrick, R.E., MacIntosh, A.M., Roy, R.R. (1982). Biochemical properties of overloaded fast-twitch skeletal muscle. *Journal of Applied Physiology, 52,* 467–472 and Roy, R.R., Medows, I.D., Baldwin, K.M., Edgerton, V.R. (1982). Functional significance of compensatory overloaded rat fast muscle. *Journal of Applied Physiology, 52,* 473–478.)

about 34 mm/s to only 18 mm/s (with no change in fiber length) and myosin ATPase activity decreased from about 0.8 μmoles/mg/min to about 0.6 μmoles/mg/min (Fig. 4-16B). How could that be? Biochemical analysis demonstrated that, although the muscles were nearly twice their original size, the concentration of protein in the two groups of muscles (overloaded versus control) was the same. This indicated that the muscle grew proportional to the increase in protein, which meant that the muscles were probably synthesizing new contractile filaments and not merely "filling up" with inflammatory cells or connective tissue. In addition to the great increase in muscle mass, the calcium transport activity of the overloaded plantaris decreased significantly compared to controls. Finally, the activities of all enzymes associated with glycolysis (phosphofructokinase, phosphorylase, α-glycerophosphate dehydrogenase and lactate dehydrogenase, Chapter 2, decreased significantly).

What caused the change in contractile properties? Examine Figure 4-16 to see if you can determine the theme that is consistent in the adaptation. The astute reader will note that all of the changes in the fast plantaris tended to cause its properties to become more like a "slow" muscle—in fact more like that of the rat soleus. Baldwin et al. (Baldwin, Valdez, Herrick, McIntosh, & Roy, 1982) and Roy et al. (Roy, Medows, Baldwin, & Edgerton, 1982) showed that the overloaded plantaris became more like the normal soleus in every respect and that the magnitude of the "conversion" ranged from about 10% to 70% depending on the property measured. In fact, the proportion of slow fibers in the overloaded plantaris increased from about 15% to about 50% in the deepest muscular region.

In some ways, then, the results of this experiment paralleled the results of the chronic stimulation experiment: increased use tended to cause the muscle to become 'slower' physiologically and biochemically. In addition, at least in the overload model, the plantaris muscles also became significantly stronger. The degree of

> ### Box 4-5. Why Am I Running Faster if My Muscles are Getting Slower?
>
> It is true that strength training such as occurs with sprint training causes muscles to become intrinsically slower. This is true of almost all increased use modes. However, the muscle also becomes stronger because the muscle fibers themselves become larger. Increasing muscle strength can produce more power, which is defined as work produced per unit time. Greater power production by muscles causes faster acceleration of the human body during running in the same way that more horsepower causes greater acceleration of a dragster during a race.

the transformation (which was not complete) depended on the "intensity" of the adaptive stimulus. Perhaps if the overloaded plantaris were left for a year, instead of 12–14 weeks, or if a portion of the plantaris was removed, leaving only a small part of the muscle, it might become composed of 100% slow fibers.

Effects of Compensatory Hypertrophy on Rat Soleus and Medial Gastrocnemius

The plantaris experiments showed that 12 weeks of overloading a fast muscle caused it to become much slower in every respect. What would happen following overload of a muscle which was already slow (*e.g.*, the soleus) or a fast muscle with a greater proportion of slow fibers (*e.g.*, the medial gastrocnemius)? The same group of investigators performed analogous experiments, overloading either the soleus or MG by surgically removing the synergists (similar to Fig. 4-15). The results extended and helped interpret the results from the previous experiments.

Again, the major finding was that functional overload caused the muscles to become stronger and have properties which were more like slow muscles (Fig. 4-16). What was most interesting about the study was the relative degree of adaptation observed in these two muscles compared to the previous studies of the plantaris

(Roy, et al., 1982). The degree of hypertrophy seemed to be related to two major factors: fiber type proportion and the relative fraction of ankle extensor complex represented by the overloaded muscle. The plantaris was the smallest muscle (15% of the ankle extensors) and hypertrophied the most (almost 100%) while the MG was the largest (60% of the ankle extensors) and hypertrophied the least (about 50%), nearly the same amount as the soleus. All fibers within the overloaded muscles hypertrophied, but the SO fibers hypertrophied the most and the FG fibers the least. Based on our discussion of muscle fiber recruitment (Chapters 2 and 3), this finding makes sense: fibers that were activated most often were the SO fibers, and thus it made sense that they would experience the greatest amount of activity and therefore, muscle tension following overload. By increasing muscle tension, muscle fiber strength increases. Perhaps the reason the FG fibers did not hypertrophy to the same extent was that they were not activated as much due to their relatively high threshold to recruitment.

Finally, all overloaded muscles increased their proportion of SO fibers. Note that, in fact, all overloaded muscles increased their proportion of oxidative fibers, whether FOG or SO fibers at the expense of FG fibers. A fiber type conversion in the direction FG → FOG → SO resulted from the overload. Presumably, FG fibers became FOG fibers and, given the appropriate stimulus, FOG fibers became SO fibers.

From the point of view of metabolism, all overloaded muscles demonstrated a decrease in glycolytic enzyme levels. Previously, the complementary relationship between the metabolic and contractile muscle machinery was outlined. This relationship is generally maintained after muscle fiber transformation. It is not clear why low glycolytic activity and low myofibrillar ATPase activity ought to be complementary. However, the data do suggest that there is some advantage to balancing the fiber's ability to deliver ATP under anaerobic conditions with its maximum contractile speed. Often it is observed that an increase in glycolytic potential

parallels an increase in muscle fast fiber percentage. Similarly, when slow fiber percentage increases, glycolytic potential decreases. Overall, the balance between oxidative enzymes, glycolytic enzymes, and myofibrillar ATPase activity appears to be maintained in many different models of adaptation. New methods that allow quantitative determination of enzyme activities in single muscle fibers have been developed and provided insights into this balance. These methods and their results will be discussed as several decreased use models are considered in the next chapter. An example of the use of this method on normal tissue was presented in Chapter 2.

Adaptation to Intermittent Electrical Stimulation

Clinical application of electrical stimulation, and many experimental studies only use intermittently activated muscle, as opposed to the chronic stimulation described above. The purpose of intermittent stimulation basic science experiments has been to determine exactly what the muscle responds to: stimulation pulse number, stimulation frequency, total stimulation time or a combination of one or more of these. Generally, these results are in stark contrast to the chronic stimulation experiments because significant muscle strengthening has been documented. Why the difference?

Intermittent Stimulation With Different Activation Patterns

The Dutch neurophysiologist, Dr. Daniel Kernell attempted to understand what it was about various stimulation patterns that influenced muscle properties by stimulating skeletal muscles using several combinations of stimulation frequency and intensity (Kernell, Donselaar, & Eerbeek, 1987ab). Kernell and his colleagues deafferented cat hindlimb muscles (so that no pain would be felt during stimulation and reflex-mediated effects would be eliminated) and implanted electrical stimulators to activate the peroneal nerve. After 4–8 weeks of stimulation, they measured the contractile properties of the peroneus longus muscle (PerL), which is normally a fast muscle. In addition, they measured dorsiflexion twitch torque noninvasively during the course of the experiment. The stimulation patterns used were designed to provide "physiological" amounts of electrical activity to the muscle (in contrast to chronic stimulation experiments described above) and to mimic the activity of motor nerves normally activating "fast" and "slow" muscles (Fig. 4-17). Recall that, physiologically, motor nerves innervating slow muscles tend to be activated at lower frequencies, and relatively continuously whereas motor nerves innervating fast muscles tend to be activated at higher frequencies and in short bursts.

Kernell et al. designed the stimulation pattern in an ingenious manner to alter the total amount of electrical activity experienced by the muscles and the contractile tension elicited by the electrical impulses. Contractile tension during activation was altered by stimulating muscles at either 10 Hz or 100 Hz. Clearly, the tension reached using 100 Hz stimulation was close to P_o while 10 Hz stimulation would elicit only about 25% P_o. Two experimental groups were stimulated at 100 Hz (Fig. 4-17): one for 5% of the day (72 minutes of 100 ms long trains spread evenly over 24 hours; Group F1) and one for 0.5% of the day (7.2 minutes of 100 ms long trains separated into three separate sessions spaced about 5 hours apart; Group F2). Thus, in both 100 Hz groups, muscles were activated to high tensions but F1 was activated ten times more often than F2. A third group was activated at only 10 Hz for 5% of the day (72 minutes of 1sec long trains separated into three separate sessions spaced about 5 hours apart; Group S1). The final fourth group received a hybrid stimulation protocol consisting of both 10 Hz and 100 Hz stimuli alternately

Stimulation Patterns for Intermittent Muscle Activation

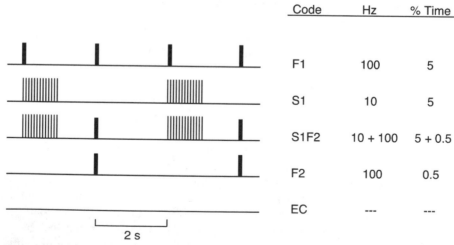

Code	Hz	% Time
F1	100	5
S1	10	5
S1F2	10 + 100	5 + 0.5
F2	100	0.5
EC	---	---

2 s

FIGURE 4-17. Activation patterns of muscles used to study intermittent stimulation. Muscle stimulation treatment was varied by using either 10 Hz for 5% of the day (S1), 100 Hz for 0.5% of the day (F2), 100 Hz for 5.0% of the day (F1), or both 10 Hz and 100 Hz stimulation 5.5% of the day (S1F2). EC represents experimental controls. (Data from: Kernell, D., Eerbeek, O., Verhey, B.A., Donselaar, Y. (1987). Effects of physiological amounts of high- and low-rate chronic stimulation on fast-twitch muscle of the cat hindlimb. I. Speed- and force-related properties. *Journal of Neurophysiology, 58,* 598–613.)

given for a total of 5.5% of the day (superimposing the patterns of the S1 and F2 groups; Group S1F2). What functional changes do you expect would be elicited in the muscles of these different experimental groups?

Maximum Tetanic Tension Resulting From Intermittent Electrical Stimulation

Maximum tetanic tension (P_o) of PerL muscles was measured after 8 weeks. The results demonstrated the importance of stimulation frequency and stimulation amount. In other words, the muscle adaptation was based on the absolute tension reached during stimulation and the total number of muscle contractions during treatment (Fig. 4-18). For example, muscles from the group stimulated only 0.5% of the day at 100 Hz (Group F2) generated the greatest tetanic tension (Fig. 4-18A). Muscles from the group stimulated 5% of the day at 100 Hz (Group F1; ten times more activity but the same type of contraction as F2) generated only about half the tetanic tension compared to F2. "More" was not "better" in terms of strength. In spite of the similar individual contractile events between the F1 and F2 groups (i.e., near maximal contractions), the ultimate muscular adaptation was quite different. Interestingly, there was no difference in P_o between groups F1 and S1 stimulated 5% of the day at 100 Hz or 10 Hz respectively. However, when the F2 pattern was superimposed on S1 (Group S1F2), P_o was significantly increased relative to either F1 or S1. Combine these results plotted in Figure 4-18A with the stimulation conditions and your knowledge of muscle to see if you can "sort out" the way that the muscle was "thinking" in response to the various stimulation protocols.

The first conclusion drawn was that high tensions were required for muscle strengthening. The only groups that demonstrated strengthening were F2 and S1F2. Note that S1 alone did not cause strengthening whereas the addition of F2 did cause the strengthening. The second conclusion drawn from the study was that increasing the amount of muscle activity tended to cause a decrease in P_o. Thus, groups S1 and F1, both activated 5% of the time showed decreased tension relative to the F2 group that was stimulated only 0.5% of the time. However, S1F2 was activated 5.5% of the time and P_o still did not decrease. The fact that F1 did not cause strengthening, but S1F2 did was somewhat paradoxical. It might have been that the F2 contractions, which were farther apart, caused higher tensions than the F1 patterns and thus caused the strengthening. Unfortunately, torque during treatment was not measured so this point could not be explicitly addressed. Incidentally, it would have been interesting to have an "S2" group—a group activated at 10 Hz, but only 0.5% of the day to see if, perhaps, decreasing total stimulation duration alone, with low tension contractions, could cause strengthening. Still there would be no strength increase since the absolute tensions were so low, but this is speculation.

Twitch Kinetics and Fiber Properties Resulting from Intermittent Electrical Stimulation

Interestingly, twitch kinetics (contraction time, CT and half-relaxation time, HRT, see explanation of these parameters in Fig. 2-2) from all muscles in all four experimental groups were significantly slowed. Thus, the experimental PerL muscles all had increased CTs of about 30 ms compared to the normal PerL CT of 17 ms (Fig. 4-18B). This result demonstrated that increased activity (in any "flavor," 10 Hz or 100 Hz) caused muscle slowing. The twitch response slowed after only about 10 days of stimulation and continued at a relatively constant level throughout the 8-week experiment. What was the basis for the increased CT? Since twitch kinetics were primarily determined by the rate at which the muscle can release and uptake calcium (Chapter 2), the data suggested a significant loss in SR calcium transporting ability either due to the loss in the amount and/or activity of the calcium transport ATPase. Again, increased use resulted in muscle slowing. Interestingly, the same observation of increased CT has been made in humans after voluntary exercise training.

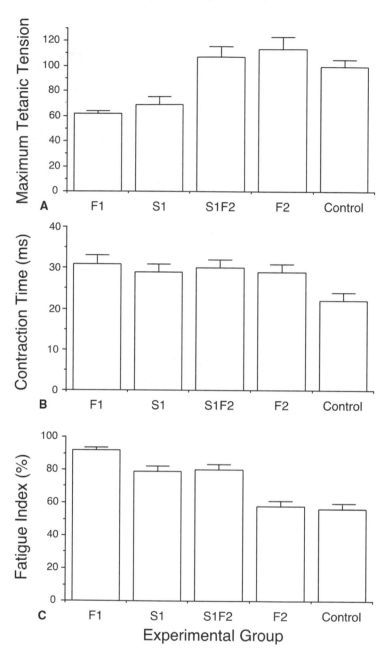

FIGURE 4-18. Contractile properties of peroneus longus muscles following different patterns of intermittent stimulation. The control values of the unstimulated muscle show that it was originally a fast twitch muscle. **(A)** Maximum tetanic tension (P_o) of muscles following stimulation using the parameters shown. Note that P_o was only increased if high-tension contractions were elicited. **(B)** Twitch contraction time (CT) of muscles following stimulation using the parameters shown. Note that CT increased for all groups studied. **(C)** Fatigue index of muscles following stimulation using the parameters shown. Note that fatigue index was only increased if contractions were elicited for at least 5% of the day. (Data from: Kernell, D., Eerbeek, O., Verhey, B.A., Donselaar, Y. (1987). Effects of physiological amounts of high- and low-rate chronic stimulation on fast-twitch muscle of the cat hindlimb. I.Speed- and force-related properties. *Journal of Neurophysiology, 58,* 598–613; Kernell, D., Donselaar, Y., Eerbeek, O. (1987). Effects of physiological amounts of high- and low-rate chronic stimulation on fast-twitch muscle of the cat hindlimb. II. Endurance-related properties. *Journal of Neurophysiology, 58,* 614–627.)

Endurance of Muscles Subjected to Intermittent Electrical Stimulation

In order to determine the endurance level of the PerL muscles after stimulation treatment, a fatigue test was used identical to that previously developed by Burke et al. (Burke, Levine, Tsairis, & Zajac, 1973) for classifying motor units. For the fatigue test, muscles were stimulated at 40 Hz for 330 ms and allowed to rest for 670 ms. This cyclic activation pattern was continued for 2 minutes to determine fatigue index defined as the ending tension divided by the initial tension. During the fatigue test, both tension and electromyographic (EMG) activity were recorded. Again, try to predict the muscle response to the various stimulation treatments.

The results demonstrated that muscle fatigability was dependent only on the amount of stimulation time and not the frequency (Fig. 4-18C). Thus, all three groups that were activated either 5% or 5.5% of the day (groups F1, S1, and S1F2) significantly increased their fatigue index to about 0.8 compared to the normal PerL which has a fatigue index of only about 0.5. The F2 group, stimulated only 0.5% of the day, demonstrated no change in fatigue index relative to control muscles. (Again, it would have been interesting to see the results from an "S2" group, stimulated at 10 Hz only 0.5% of the time. It is possible that there would be a very small, if any, increase in fatigue index.)

The EMGs measured from muscles demonstrated that, during the fatigue test performed on normal muscles, the amplitude of the EMG declined to about 50% of the initial EMG amplitude. In contrast, all experimental groups demonstrated no decline in EMG throughout the test. These results indicated that (1) even 0.5% daily stimulation caused significant adaptations of the nerves and/or neuromuscular junction and (2) that the magnitude of the

EMG was not very closely related to the tension. The latter conclusion was based on the observation that the F2 and control groups had the same fatigue index, but dramatically different EMG amplitudes. Even in normal muscles, EMG may not be very important in determining the magnitude of the contractile tension during fatigue since force decreased with no EMG change. The neuromuscular junction or other parts of the muscle must have a built-in "safety factor" so that moderate EMG changes do not always reflect force deficits (However, see Chapter 6, pages 339–340, for a condition under which EMG decreases due to injury, thus altering muscle force.)

Summary of Intermittent Stimulation Experiments

You learned from these experiments that skeletal muscles respond to both the amount and type of contractile activity imposed. Greater activity is associated with muscle slowing, increased endurance and decreased strength. High-tension contractions are necessary for increased muscle strength. This is a theme which you will see repeatedly as you study muscle adaptation to increased use. These data from animal studies have important implications in physical therapy in which the use of intermittent electrical stimulation is common. The therapist must appreciate that stimulation settings such as frequency and duty cycle, which are easily adjustable on today's commercially-available devices, provide the muscle with specific information to which it then adapts. Importantly, "more" is not "better" when it comes to muscle stimulation. Further implications of this point will be discussed at the chapter's end.

All previous discussions apply to muscles that are innervated appropriately. This is a good time to present the results of a chronic muscle stimulation model performed under conditions in which the muscles were denervated. These results contrast sharply with those presented above. This example provides the first illustration that a denervated muscle is qualitatively different from an innervated muscle in its plasticity.

Box 4-6. Why Shouldn't You Give a Muscle "Mixed Messages" in Therapy?

Muscles are continuously "reading" the amount and type of activity imposed upon them throughout the day. If both "strength" and "endurance" messages are being provided to the muscle, neither adaptation is fully realized. A muscle receiving pure "strength" signals (for example, very intermittent doses of high force contractions) will become stronger compared to the muscle that received the same strengthening stimulus in a background of endurance activity. Similarly, a muscle receiving pure "endurance" signals (for example, frequent doses of low force contractions) will increase endurance more compared with the muscle that received the same stimulus with a few strong contractions in between.

Stimulation of the Denervated Rat Soleus Muscle

Several early studies of chronic stimulation were performed to identify the factors, which controlled the expression of muscle properties. In the classic early experiments, Buller, Eccles, & Eccles (1960) had surgically transferred the proximal portion of a motor nerve from a slow muscle to the distal stump of the motor nerve to a fast muscle. They found that the fast muscle took on the properties of a slow muscle and concluded that the nerve contained some type of chemical—a so-called neurotrophic factor—that determined the muscle's properties. However, others contended that it was the electrical activity of the nerve, not the nerve itself that imparted the specific properties on the muscle. Certainly there was evidence to support both points of view. To test the importance of electrical activity without the "confounding" effect of a neurotrophic factor, the Norwegian neurophysiologist, Dr. Terje Lømo, severed the nerve to the rat soleus muscle and stimulated it with various patterns (similar to the studies above).

After severe muscle atrophy (due to the denervation), Lømo and his colleagues electrically activated the muscle using either low frequency (10 Hz) or high frequency (100 Hz) stimulation for a short time (1 hr/day) or long time (24 hrs/day) over a 4-week period (Lømo, Westgaard, & Dahl, 1974; Lømo, Westgaard, & Engelbretsen, 1980). After the stimulation period, contractile properties were measured and easily interpreted (Fig. 4-19). In all cases in which the muscle was stimulated at 100 Hz, the twitch contraction times were fast and the muscle demonstrated post-tetanic potentiation, as do most fast muscles (independent of stimulation amount). In contrast, after 4 weeks of stimulation at 10 Hz, twitch contraction times were slow (Fig. 4-19B) and muscles demonstrated no post-tetanic potentiation. All muscles stimulated for a long time had much greater endurance than those stimulated for a short time, independent of frequency (Fig. 4-19C). The conclusion was obvious: in the denervated soleus muscle, speed (twitch con-

traction time) and endurance were independently regulated—a nice, clean result. In other words, the muscle's speed was determined only by the frequency at which it was activated while its endurance was determined only by the total amount of muscle activity.

These results were appealing in that they seemed to provide a unifying explanation for speed and endurance regulation by the muscle cell as well as an end to the search for the elusive neurotrophic factor. Unfortunately, these same results could not be obtained for normally-innervated muscle (as in the Kernell et al., 1987ab experiments). This specific, predictable muscle response seemed only to hold true for the denervated soleus muscle. The data demonstrated that the "control" system of a denervated muscle is significantly different than that of a normally-innervated muscle. It should also be noted that, although the denervated muscles adapted to the stimulus pattern imposed, they still generated only about 10% of the force of the normal muscle. These muscles should thus be considered severely atrophic. The denervation model will be considered further in Chapter 5 as a model of decreased use, but remember that denervated muscles are qualitatively different in structure and plasticity compared with normal muscles. Based on the results of some of the other stimulation studies that have been investigated, it would be interesting to know if the force imposed upon the denervated solei was a factor. In other words, what if experiments were performed with the ankles fixed (so the muscles would contract isometrically and generate tension) compared to how the experiments were performed, with the limb free to move and the muscles presumably generating almost no tension?

Comparison Between Animal and Human Studies of Electrical Stimulation

Several hundred human and animal studies of electrical stimulation have been performed. It is fair to say that nearly all stimulation studies, in humans or animals show increased muscle

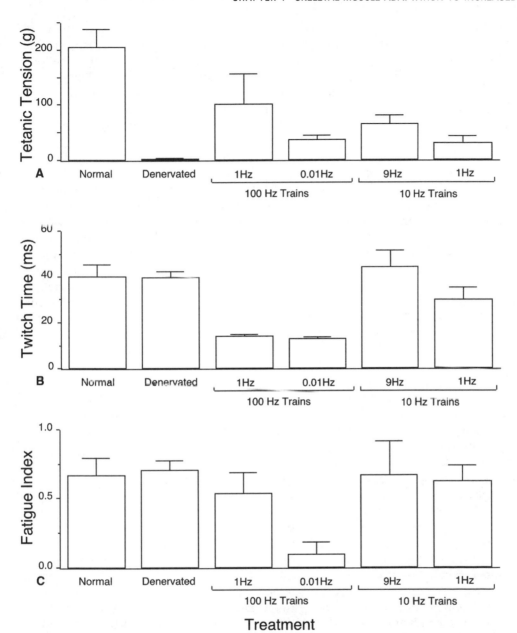

FIGURE 4-19. Effects of chronic stimulation on tetanic tension, twitch time, and fatigue index of the denervated rat soleus muscle. Note that if a large amount of stimulation was used (independent of stimulation frequency), resulting endurance was high, whereas if low amounts of stimulation were used, endurance was low suggesting that stimulation amount alone determines muscle endurance. Similarly, if high frequency stimulation was used (independent of stimulation amount), twitch time was fast, suggesting that stimulation frequency alone determines muscle speed. (Data from: Lømo, T., Westgaard, R.H., Engelbretsen, L. (1980). Different stimulation patterns affect contractile properties of denervated rat soleus muscles. In D. Pette (Ed.), *The plasticity of muscle*, (pp. 297–309). New York: Walter de Gruyter.)

endurance following stimulation. However, although numerous human studies demonstrate muscle strengthening with electrical stimulation, almost all animal basic science studies show just the opposite—muscle weakening with electrical stimulation (Fig. 4-2). Why the difference?

The three major differences between most animal and human studies presented to date are that (1) chronic animal stimulation is usually accomplished using implanted electrode systems whereas most human muscles are stimulated transcutaneously, (2) stimulation "doses" in animal studies are from 10 to 1,000 times greater than the doses used in human studies, and (3) human muscle are usually stimulated isometrically whereas animal limbs are allowed to move freely. Which of these, if any contribute to the disparity of results?

First, the difference is probably not related to the implantation of electrodes. Because motor nerves have a lower threshold to activation than muscle fibers, during electrical activation of a whole muscle, the nerves are first depolarized causing depolarization of the muscle fibers. Thus, even with transcutaneous stimulation, the actual mechanism of muscle fiber activation is probably the same as using implanted electrodes (see below for details). Second, increased stimulation amount causes decreased muscle force in animal studies (Kernell et al., 1987ab), so the fact that human stimulation doses are much lower than animal doses might be responsible for the different degrees of strengthening noted. Finally, consider the mechanical environment of stimulation (*i.e.*, isometric versus free-moving). As you have seen, muscle strengthening depends, to a large degree, on the stress imposed on the muscle. The change in maximum force that occurs as a function of shortening velocity, given by the force-velocity equation, predicts a large difference in force developed under isometric versus free-moving conditions. For example, if a muscle is stimulated isometrically at 10 Hz, the force developed is equivalent to about 30% of its maximum tetanic tension (P_o, as shown in Fig. 2-2 page 50). Now, if the same muscle is allowed to

shorten at a velocity equal to only 10% of its maximum shortening velocity (easily obtainable under physiological conditions), the force developed is only about 18% P_o. Thus, to the extent that muscle stress results in muscle strengthening, the stimulating conditions can influence the results of electrical stimulation training.

In order to reconcile the disparity of animal and human research on NEMS, future research on NMES application to muscle rehabilitation requires an examination of the physiological basis for the muscular response to transcutaneous stimulation. In order to use the available literature on muscle plasticity, experiments must be designed such that muscle treatment force is well defined. It is crucial to understand the tension generated by human muscles during therapeutic stimulation. Numerous values have been reported for human quadriceps NMES ranging from 5% MVC to 120% MVC. Many times the tension levels are simply not reported at all. Obviously, if NMES is to be effective in strengthening skeletal muscle, it must be possible to activate muscles to high tensions.

Human Neuromuscular Electrical Stimulation (NMES)

In light of the discussion presented above, it was of interest to determine the tension generated by the human quadriceps muscles during clinically-applied NMES (Lieber & Kelly, 1991). Knee extension torque was measured in 50 subjects using a specially-designed apparatus which fixed the distal leg to a force transducer (Fig. 4-20). Carbon rubber electrodes were placed on the quadriceps musculature and stimulation intensity was increased to the subject's maximum tolerable level. It was found that it was possible, using young healthy naive subjects, to activate the muscles to about 25% of their MVC. Interestingly, this relatively low fraction of MVC felt like an extremely intense contraction to the subject. These patients felt like their tension levels were much higher. Why were the tensions so low? Several recent studies

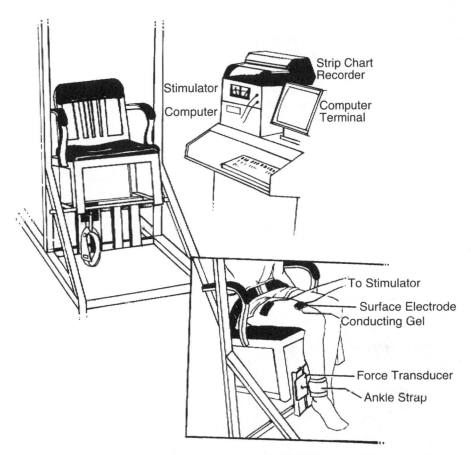

FIGURE 4-20. Experimental apparatus used to study NMES-induced joint torque in humans. Surface electrodes are placed over the quadriceps musculature and the ankle is attached to a strap, which is connected to a strain gauge (inset). Stimulation parameters, timing, and data acquisition are computer controlled. (From: Lieber, R.L., Kelly, J. (1991). Factors influencing quadriceps torque using transcutaneous electrical stimulation. *Physical Therapy, 71*, 715–721.)

have suggested several factors that affect the tension generated during NMES.

Nerve and Muscle Activation with NMES:

To address the mechanism of human muscle activation, Hultman et al. (Hultman, Sjoholm, Jaderholm, & Krynicki, 1983) stimulated the muscles from human subjects who were preparing to have surgery. After informed consent, they first measured the maximum elicited electrically-induced torque from patients under anesthesia so that "pain" would not limit tension levels. Then they "curarized" the pa-

tient (infused curare, a chemical agent which prevents conduction of the neuromuscular junction by binding to the muscle's acetyl choline receptor). Now, the stimulator was again activated and joint torque measured. Muscle force dropped dramatically. In fact, it was nearly impossible to electrically induce a muscle contraction. Why? The interpretation was that, even with NMES applied directly over the muscle, motor nerves were actually activated, which, in turn, activated muscles. Thus, NMES indirectly activated the muscle via the motor nerves. This conjecture was reasonable in light of the fact that nerves were known to have a significantly lower threshold to electrical activation than muscle fibers. (This is one of the reasons why it is so difficult to electrically activate denervated skeletal muscle.) Since motor nerves activate muscles, perhaps the low relative forces achievable with NMES result from the fact that, many motor nerves are anatomically too deep to reach with an electrical stimulator.

Factors Affecting NMES-Induced Torque Production in Humans

The basis for the relatively low muscle activation levels achieved with NMES have been clarified further. The variety and number of stimulators and stimulating electrodes on the market suggested that there was not general agreement on the optimal method for muscle activation. What if very large electrodes were

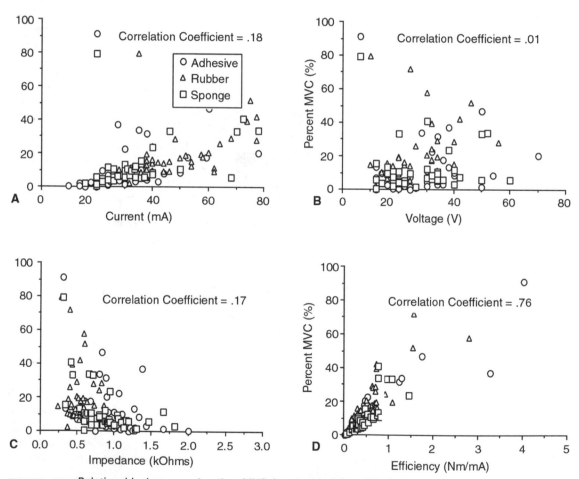

FIGURE 4-21. Relationship between fraction MVC (vertical axis) and individual parameters such as **(A)** stimulation current, **(B)** voltage, **(C)** electrode impedance, and **(D)** efficiency. Each electrode type (which varied in size and material) is represented by a specific symbol. Note that the electrode types do not cluster, suggesting that electrode type alone does not determine the relative percent muscle activation (Data from: Lieber, R.L., Kelly, J. (1991). Factors influencing quadriceps torque using transcutaneous electrical stimulation. *Physical Therapy, 71,* 715–721.)

FIGURE 4-22. Relationship between predicted fraction MVC (vertical axis) and actual measured fraction MVC (horizontal axis) for all 120 tests. Prediction based on multivariate analysis of all parameters in Figure 4-21. Each symbol represents a different electrode type as shown in the legend. Note that all three electrodes are well represented across the entire ranges of relative torque. Note also that the actual data are well-approximated by the predicted data. (Data from: Lieber, R.L., Kelly, J. (1991). Factors influencing quadriceps torque using transcutaneous electrical stimulation. *Physical Therapy, 71,* 715–721.)

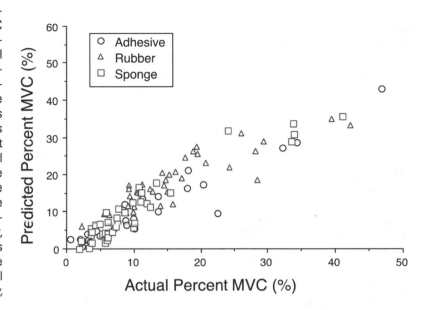

used? Would torque be higher? How about the amount of electrical current? Would that effect the maximum torque elicited by NMES? This question was addressed by using three different electrode types of different sizes and measuring stimulation current, skin resistance, and joint torque associated with the electrical activation. In forty subjects, the order of electrode application was randomly varied, using all electrodes on all subjects (Lieber & Kelly, 1993).

The difficulty of this type of experiment is "sorting out" which of the various parameters measured is important in determining torque. This experimental design is known as a multivariate design (because of the multiple variables). The appropriate analysis of this experimental design requires a stepwise linear regression. Simply stated, the experiment was designed to determine which (if any) of the many experimental variables were important in determining the magnitude of the electrically-induced torque. The analysis also determined the relative importance of each parameter. It was found that, although torque

increased with voltage, current, and electrode size (Fig. 4-21), the most important factor was one that could not be explicitly identified, which was an intrinsic property of the individual (Fig. 4-21D).

A parameter called "efficiency" was defined—the amount of torque produced by an individual for a given amount of electrical current (in units of Nm/mA, *i.e.,* units of torque/current). Some individuals (for reasons still not known) generated a great deal of torque for a given amount of current while others, in spite of high current tolerance, generated relatively low torques. Taken together, all parameters measured accounted for over 90% of the experimental variability (Fig. 4-22). Again, the dominant term was the subject's intrinsic activation ability. Future studies are necessary to clarify this issue further.

In summary, current thoughts are that NMES as typically implemented in most clinics can activate muscle to a relatively low percent of MVC. It is not known whether, in generating 25% MVC, 25% of the muscle fibers are generating maximum tension, if all the fibers are generating 25% of their maximum tension or if some "in-between" combination is occurring. The spatial distribution of the muscle fibers or nerves activated using NMES is also unknown. Are the fibers activated in a superficial "shell" of fibers? Are fibers of a certain type activated throughout the muscle?

Many studies suggest that electrical stimulation, based on proximity to electrodes, activates only a limited portion of the muscle (Knaflitz, Merletti, & De Luca, 1990). Although such an inference is reasonable based on known electrophysiological properties of nerve and muscle, it remains an indirect inference rather than an established fact. New imaging methods have made it possible to test this idea by "imaging" the area of activated muscle during voluntary contraction and electrical stimulation (Jenner, Foley, Cooper, Potchen, & Meyer, 1994; Meyer & Prior, 2000; Yue et al., 1994). Such an experiment was performed at the Kennedy Space Center by Dr. Gary Dudley and colleagues (Adams, Harris, Woodard, & Dudley, 1993), in which healthy subjects first voluntarily exercised and then received electrical stimulation at different torque levels. The authors found, as expected, a roughly linear relationship between the cross-sectional area of quadriceps activated and the torque elicited by electrical stimulation (Fig. 4-23A). However, the actual physical location of the quadriceps activated was highly variable among subjects with some individuals demonstrating more activity superficially in the rectus femoris (*e.g.*, subject #2, Fig. 4-23B) and others demonstrating more activity deeper and laterally in the vastus lateralis (*e.g.*, subject #5, Fig. 4-23B). They concluded that the location of the muscle activated is not simply the closest muscle to the electrodes (which, of course, are always superficial). Rather, the motor nerves that enter the tissue dictate the location of the muscle fibers that will be activated. This is similar to the previous statement that was made regarding the idea of activation "efficiency."

Based on the possibility that electrical stim-ulation resulted in a qualitatively different mechanism of muscle activation, understanding the basic science of electrically-stimulated strengthening treatment was of interest. Obviously, it was not enough to simply stimulate a group and compare it to an exercised group, it was important to compare their effectiveness under identical conditions. In this case, identical conditions meant identical forces. Therefore, to control for the effect of force on strengthening of human quadriceps muscles an experiment in which muscle tension was tightly controlled was performed (Lieber, Silva, & Daniel, 1996). In 40 patients recovering from anterior cruciate ligament reconstruction, the patients were randomly placed into either a voluntary exercise group or a stimulated group. While this type of experiment had been performed many times before, the novel aspect of this experiment was that it nearly matched the tension imposed upon the muscles between the two groups based on measurement of each muscle contraction (Fig. 4-24A). The stimulated group was allowed to receive maximum-tolerable intensity and the exercise group was matched to their tension. For the voluntary group, this was almost always less than they could have performed. Even in spite of the effort to match force between groups, the exercise group still generated more tension over the 4-week treatment period (Fig. 4-24A). Both groups of subjects dramatically increased their strength over the 4-week treatment period (Fig. 4-24B). Interestingly, there was no significant difference in relative strengthening under these conditions in which treatment tensions were tightly controlled even one year later (Fig. 4-25). Of course more work is required in this area but our provisional interpretation is that muscle strengthening with electrical stimulation is equally as effective as voluntary exercise provided the tension levels are equivalent. The caveat is that most individuals can perform higher force contractions with voluntary activation and, thus, often in the literature, voluntary exercise appears more effective.

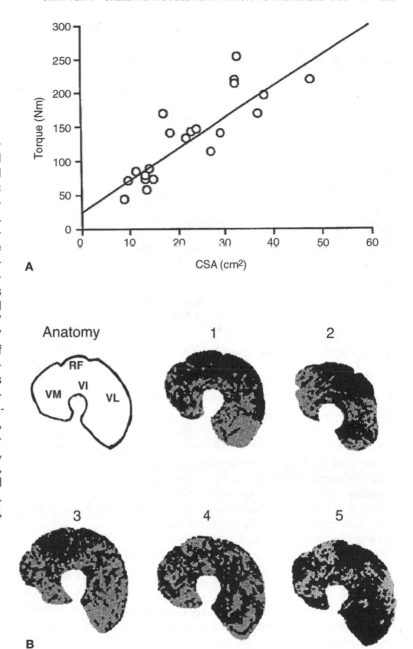

FIGURE 4-23. **(A)** Relationship between knee extension torque and the total area of muscle activated as measured from the magnetic resonance image (MRI) in the human quadriceps femoris muscle. As expected, torque and activated muscle cross-section are roughly linearly related. **(B)** Sample single slice maps of activated quadriceps. Black portions represent "active" muscle and gray portions represent "relaxed" muscle. Upper left "anatomy" drawing illustrates the location of the vasti, rectus femoris, and femur. Note the variation in regions activated between subjects (#1-#5). Abbreviations: VM, vastus medialis; VI, vastus intermedius; VL, vastus lateralis; RF, rectus femoris. (Adapted from: Adams, G.R., Harris, R.T., Woodard, D., Dudley, G.A. (1993). Mapping of electrical muscle stimulation using MRI. *Journal of Applied Physiology, 74,* 532–537.)

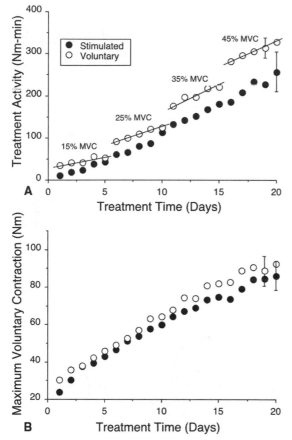

FIGURE 4-24. (A) Time course of neuromuscular activity (measured in Nm-min) for two study groups. Voluntary contraction group (open circles) was paced at the intensity shown above the symbols. Note that exercise intensity increased during the treatment period. Stimulation group (filled circles) was exercised at the maximum tolerable level. At the end of the treatment period, there was no difference between groups in the total treatment activity (symbols are mean ± SEM for n=20 subjects). Abbreviation: MVC, maximum voluntary contraction. **(B)** Maximum voluntary contraction level (in Nm) for experimental subjects during the time course of treatment. Note that both groups gained strength at the same rate and to the same extent. (Data from: Lieber, R.L., Silva, P.D., Daniel, D.M. (1996). Equal effectiveness of electrical and volitional strength training in quadriceps femoris muscles after anterior cruciate surgery. *Journal of Orthopaedic Research, 14,* 131–138.)

Adaptation to Exercise

All of the models presented above are just that—models. This means that they have the advantage of being well controlled, but they are not necessarily realistic or representative of how muscles are normally used. Of course, muscle adaptation occurs simply as a result of exercise. The literature (and magazines) are replete with examples of the many exercises that can increase strength and stamina. Is it possible to apply the principles that you just learned to the more physiological types of increased use normally experienced by muscle? The answer is, fortunately, yes. In fact, based on what you already know, you can probably predict the themes that will be reiterated in the context of exercise. What are they? The answer: The tension that a muscle experiences and its total activity dictate the nature and extent of the adaptation seen in exercise. This section will investigate the changes that occur in muscle and in performance in response to exercise. It will reinforce the concept that skeletal muscle responds to the amount and type of activity, which is imposed upon it. The added nuance of training studies is that muscle fiber recruitment is an important variable. For example, in sprint training, a greater fraction of the quadriceps muscles are activated compared to slow running or swimming. The response of the muscles as a whole might be quite different between the two training protocols. However, much of the difference can be ascribed to differences in recruitment, not to differences in an individual fiber's response to training. This is one of the most difficult aspects of studying human muscle response to exercise—the fact that it is rarely possible to measure the detailed properties of the muscle fibers that cause the response observed.

Definition of Exercise Intensity

Comparisons among various exercises often distinguish between "endurance" exercises and "strengthening" exercises. However, this can be largely a matter of semantics. In most exercise studies (as opposed to the studies described using the model systems above), it is very difficult to define precisely the muscular conditions that cause the adaptation. Thus, the type of exercise is generally referred to in terms of the amount of exercise (minutes per day × days per week × total weeks), and makes some reference to exercise intensity (percent of maximum voluntary contraction, for example, in an isometric exercise). The disclaimer must also be made that it might not really be known what is happening at the muscle fiber level but the study on the idea that most people perform the exercise in a similar manner.

Ideally, it would be helpful to know the force and length history of a muscle during exercise, and the number of fibers recruited, to attempt to provide a mechanistic explanation for any adaptations seen. Chapter 2 showed that knowledge of muscle length and velocity allows prediction of muscle tension. It would also be good to know which of the various fiber types are activated at which particular frequency and for how much time. However, in most human exercise studies, such information is simply not available.

Exercise Intensity in Terms of the Maximal Rate of Oxygen Consumption

One index that describes exercise intensity is the maximal rate of oxygen consumption (the chemical abbreviation for the oxygen molecule is O_2), which is abbreviated as VO_{2max}. VO_{2max} can be expressed in absolute units of liters of oxygen consumed per minute (l/min or $l \cdot min^{-1}$) or in units that are normalized to the size of the person as milliliters of oxygen consumed per kilogram body mass per minute (ml/kg/min or $ml \cdot kg^{-1} min^{-1}$). Because metabolic rate during exercise is primarily determined by muscle metabolism, VO_{2max} represents the maximum rate at which oxygen can be used by the muscles of the individual. Clearly, it says nothing about the anaerobic capacity of an individual, and therefore should not necessarily be closely linked with performances not requir-

ing oxygen such are a brief power lift or short sprint. However, the greater the aerobic capacity of the individual's muscles and the greater the ability for the cardiovascular system to deliver oxygen, the greater will be VO_{2max}.

It is not possible to exercise near VO_{2max} for very long. In fact, the relationship between exercise intensity (in terms of VO_{2max}) and exercise duration is well-established. For example, if an individual exercises at an intensity of

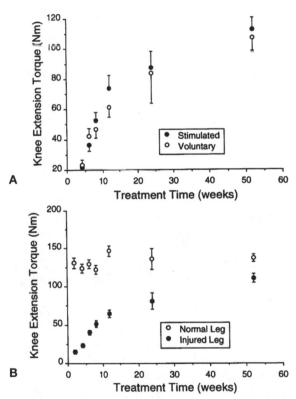

FIGURE 4-25. (A) Long-term maximum knee extension torque of the injured leg vs. time for voluntary (open circles) and electrically stimulated (filled circles) patients. **(B)** Difference between injured leg of both voluntary and electrically stimulated patients (filled circles) and contralateral control legs' (open circles) strength during study. Note that after one year, injured knee extension strength is approximately 80% of contralateral values. The electrical stimulation treatment period was four weeks.

about 80% VO_{2max} (very intense exercise), they will only be able to exercise for about 10 minutes before exhaustion. However, if the exercise intensity is relatively low (20–30% VO_{2max}) the exercise can last much longer.

Exercise Intensity in Terms of Maximum Voluntary Contraction

A second index that is often used as a "standard" for exercise intensity is the percent effort compared to a maximum voluntary contraction (MVC). The MVC is usually performed at a standardized fixed joint angle to prevent complications having to do with uncertainties in muscle length, muscle velocity, limb inertia, and joint kinetics. The important (and unlikely) assumption in using the MVC is that there exists such a measurable entity as MVC in humans that can be measured. In fact, there is excellent evidence that the MVC, in contrast to VO_{2max} is not at all a measurable entity. In the first place, there is a great deal of histochemical and electrophysiological evidence that, when a person voluntarily activates their muscles to "maximum," that not all muscle fibers are activated (Enoka & Fuglevand, 1993). Current estimates regarding the fraction of muscle fibers activated during an MVC range from 50% to 80%. It is also likely that training affects this percentage. Future studies are required to determine the exact nature of physiological muscle activation. Suffice it to say that, although MVC is used as a "standard" by which to compare intensities between individuals, it is not an absolute standard that provides a reliable indicator of a muscle's maximum contractile ability.

Muscle Fiber Activation During Exercise at Varying Intensities

Which muscle fibers are activated under different exercise conditions? Technically, it is difficult to quantify muscle fiber activation during exercise. Even if muscle biopsies are taken immediately after exercise, only a small portion of the muscle is sampled and it is not possible to sample repeatedly the same region of the same individual. However, using methods similar to those used in motor unit identification, exercise physiologists have demonstrated, as expected, that different muscle fiber types are activated at different exercise intensities and durations.

For example, Drs. Phil Gollnick, Bengt Saltin and their colleagues performed a series of studies in which they obtained small muscle biopsies from different subject's vastus lateralis muscles after exercise of various intensities and durations (Fig. 4-26; see summary in Saltin & Gollnick, 1983). By staining the biopsies for glycogen, they identified the muscle fibers that were activated during exercise. (As with motor unit identification, the potential problem was that they might not have been able to deplete the SO muscle fibers of glycogen since they relied primarily on aerobic metabolism.) Using a bicycle ergometer, they exercised subjects at intensities ranging from 31 to 85% VO_{2max} for durations ranging from 12 to 180 minutes (of course, long durations could only be accomplished at low intensities). They found that, at an exercise intensity of about 30% VO_{2max}, mostly SO fibers were used to perform the exercise. Only after about 3 hours, did FOG fibers begin to be used significantly at this low intensity (Fig. 4-26). However, at a higher intensity of 75% VO_{2max}, after 20 minutes, SO fibers and some FOG fibers were recruited, and after 2 hours of exercise at 75% VO_{2max}, all three fiber types were recruited. At 85% VO_{2max}, all three fiber types were recruited after only 12 minutes. These studies support (but do not prove) the orderly recruitment of muscle fibers during exercise and demonstrate increased fiber recruitment at longer durations and higher exercise intensities.

Recall that the spike-triggered averaging method was also used in humans to measure motor unit tension as a function of recruitment order. At low voluntary exertion levels, motor units with small twitch forces were recruited. At higher exertion levels, high force motor units were recruited. If these results are combined with the observation that slow motor units tend to develop lower tensions than

FIGURE 4-26. Illustration of muscle fiber recruitment as a function of exercise intensity and duration. Shading patterns represent the amount of glycogen contained in the various muscle fibers grouped by physiological type. Filled bars represent fibers full of glycogen while open bars represent glycogen-depleted fibers. Other bars represent intermediate glycogen contents. Note that, only as exercise intensity and duration increase, are fast oxidative glycolytic and fast glycolytic fibers depleted of glycogen. These data are interpreted to indicate that muscle fibers are recruited in the order SO → FOG → FG which is consistent with the motor unit data presented in Figure 2-26. (Data from: Saltin, B., Gollnick, P.D. (1983). Skeletal muscle adaptability: Significance for metabolism and performance. In *Handbook of Physiology* (pp. 539–554). Baltimore, MD: American Physiological Society.)

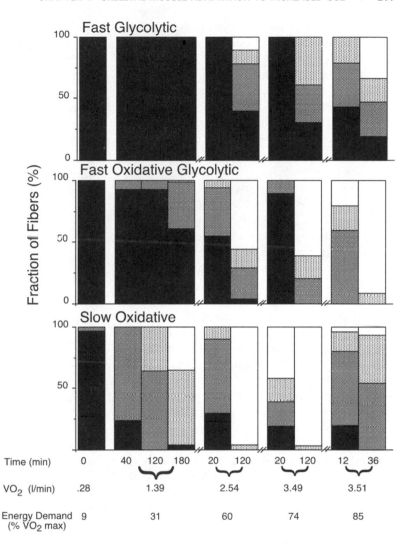

fast motor units, the implication is that, even in humans, motor unit recruitment occurs in an orderly fashion as originally proposed by Henneman et al. (Henneman, Somjen, & Carpenter, 1965) with slow motor units being recruited at low exertion levels and faster motor units being recruited at higher exertion levels.

Having given the disclaimers regarding the difficulties in measuring exercise intensity and muscle activation mechanism, what are some of the muscular changes that have been demonstrated during exercise? You will see that, in many ways, these adaptations represent special cases of the experiments discussed above: Exercise causes muscle "slowing," increased endurance, and, given the appropriate tensions, muscle strengthening.

Oxidative Enzyme Adaptation to Exercise

One lesson learned was that early muscular changes in response to increased use are increased oxidative metabolism. Does this also occur in humans? The Swedish physiologists Drs. Jan Henriksson and Jan Reitman (Henriksson & Reitman, 1977) demonstrated that it does. They trained 15 college males in bicycle ergometry for 1 hour/day × 3 days/week at 45% VO_{2max} × 8 weeks. They then allowed the subjects to "detrain" for an additional 6 weeks. At weekly intervals, muscle biopsies were removed from the subject's vastus lateralis and the enzyme activity of succinate dehydrogenase and cytochrome oxidase (two oxidative enzymes, Chapter 2) were measured along with the subject's new VO_{2max}. They found that oxidative enzyme activity increased significantly within about 3 weeks and was paralleled by increases in VO_{2max} (Fig. 4-27). For the next 5 weeks of training, muscle enzyme activity continued to increase but VO_{2max} increased at a much slower rate. The authors interpreted the data as saying that, while VO_{2max} and muscle oxidative enzyme activity are correlated, they are not causally related. Clearly, in spite of a great capacity for oxidative metabolism in the subject's muscles after 3 weeks of training, the body did not use this entire capacity. Perhaps VO_{2max} was limited by the cardiovascular system's ability to deliver oxygen or perhaps muscle oxidative enzyme activity was not simply responding to the tissue oxygen debt.

This experiment again cautions one from making performance statements based only on muscle properties. The cardiovascular system, nervous system, and musculoskeletal system are all involved in performance. Coordination and complementation are generally the rule; however, it is unwise to make global performance statements based on analysis of only one of these systems.

In detraining, when the subjects stopped exercising, oxidative enzyme levels dropped precipitously—almost twice as fast as they had increased. This is bad news for those who attempt to "stay in shape" in that getting out of shape happens about twice as fast as getting into shape.

Glycolytic Enzyme Adaptation to Exercise

In contrast to increases in muscle oxidative capacity, training does not appear to increase muscle glycolytic capacity (if anything, it tends

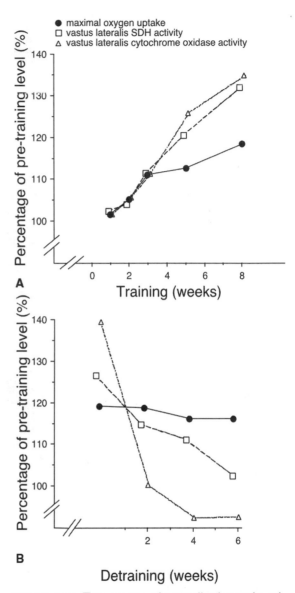

FIGURE 4-27. Time course of normalized muscle oxidative enzyme and whole-body VO_{2max} change after exercise and detraining. Note that, early in the training period, VO_{2max} and oxidative enzyme activity increase at similar rates. After about 3 weeks, enzyme activity increase faster than VO_{2max}. Also note that detraining occurs faster than training. (Data from: Henriksson, J., Reitman, J. (1977). Time course of changes in human skeletal muscle succinate dehydrogenase and cytochrome oxidase activities and maximal oxygen uptake with physical activity and inactivity. *Acta Physiologica Scandinavica, 99,* 91–97.)

to decrease). For example, Gollnick et al. (Gollnick, Armstrong, Saubert, Piehl, & Saltin, 1972) trained young males for 5 months by pedaling a bicycle ergometer for 1 hr/day × 4 days/week at an intensity of about 75% VO_{2max} (of course, initially, the subjects could not pedal this long at this intensity, but by the study's end, they were pedaling for 1 hour at 85–90% of their VO_{2max}). After 5 months, the subjects increased their VO_{2max} by 13%. As in the previous example, SDH activity increased much more—by almost 100%—while glycolytic activity (using phosphofructokinase, PFK, as the indicator) also increased by about 100%. Inspection of biopsies from the various subjects revealed that, while both fast and slow muscle fibers appeared to increase their SDH activity, only fast fibers increased their PFK activity. This coincided with an increased muscle glycogen content.

More recent quantitative studies of muscle metabolic activity during different models of transformation have shown that muscle metabolic enzymes generally maintain a certain relationship to each other even after adaptation. This concept will be discussed further in the next chapter while discussing muscle adaptation to spinal cord isolation.

Fiber Type Changes After Exercise

You know already that, given the appropriate stimulus, muscle fiber type transformation can occur. Numerous exercise studies have claimed emphatically that muscle fiber type cannot change and just as many, just as emphatically, have claimed that fiber type transformation does occur. Neither set of reports should surprise you based on your understanding of the way in which muscle fibers adapt. If the exercise stimulus is relatively low, increased oxidative capacity will occur with no change in fiber type. However, at very intense exercise levels, you would not be surprised to observe a fast-to-slow muscle fiber type transformation. Such transformations have been reported/debated in the literature and precise definitions for the conditions under which it occurs are lacking.

However, even if such transformation does occur, its influence on performance is relatively small compared to intrinsic architectural and kinematic musculoskeletal properties. Muscle fiber types are clearly related to performance, but are not the cause for performance at a particular level.

Muscle Strength Changes After Exercise

Changes in muscle strength are easily documented after many types of exercise. Although changes in the nervous system can also account for performance changes (see below), true changes in muscle strength are a direct result of muscle fiber hypertrophy—fibers themselves get larger and thus, generate higher tension. Although selected cases of muscle fiber "splitting" have been documented in the literature, primarily in chicken muscle (Alway, Gonyea, & Davis, 1990), by far the main mechanism for increasing muscle strength is increasing fiber size (hypertrophy) not fiber number (hyperplasia).

Which muscle fibers increase in size following exercise? To answer this question, remember that, for a fiber to increase in size, the tension imposed upon it must be high. Therefore, any time fiber tension is high, it will hypertrophy. Whether or not a given fiber type will hypertrophy will depend on whether it is recruited during the particular training regimen and to what tension.

For example, "endurance training" protocols are usually performed at low intensities during which mostly SO and FOG fibers are used. Since the tensions are relatively low, fiber hypertrophy is small, and no strength increase is detected. With power lifting, on the other hand, most fibers are recruited and tension levels are very high. As a result, muscle fibers hypertrophy and muscle strength increases. It is obvious, therefore, that exercise prescriptions ought to be considered in terms of muscle fiber recruitment and muscle fiber tension. In this way, specific adaptations can be more easily predicted. A reminder from the chronic stimulation model results presented above is that "more" is not necessarily "better" when it comes to strengthening. High forces imposed upon fibers for a relatively short duration seem to provide the most potent strengthening stimulus.

Evidence for Exercise Specificity

Having documented muscular changes occurring during exercise, consider once again, performance changes following exercise. A number of exercise training studies, taken together, support the idea of exercise specificity, which states that exercise benefits are specific to the method and quality of training.

Cross-sectional studies (studies performed across different populations of individuals) allude to the concept of training specificity—that measures of performance are specific to training mode. Stromme et al. (Stromme, Ingjer, & Meen, 1977), in a study of specifically trained athletes, demonstrated that the highest VO_{2max} measured for each athlete was measured in the sport for which that athlete was specifically trained. For example, elite cross-country skiers yielded a ski-VO_{2max} that was significantly higher than their VO_{2max} measured during running. Similarly, rowers and cyclists attained significantly higher VO_{2max} values while rowing or cycling compared with treadmill running.

In addition to the information gathered from cross-sectional studies, several investigators have addressed the phenomenon of training specificity by studying the performance of a group of individuals before and after exercise training (a longitudinal study since the same group is tested before and after training). In a study involving young male swimmers, Magel et al. used interval swim-training for 1 hr/day × 3 days/week × 10 weeks. Swim- and run-VO_{2max} were measured before and after training (Magel et al., 1975). While the swim-trained individuals significantly increased their swim-VO_{2max}, there was no significant change in run-VO_{2max}. Similarly, in a study from the same laboratory, Magel et al. (Magel, McArdle, Toner, & Delio, 1978) found that 10 weeks of arm training significantly increased VO_{2max} measured during arm-crank ergometry, but had no effect on VO_{2max} measured during treadmill running. How can these results be explained based on the concept of muscular training previously presented?

Physiological Basis of Exercise Specificity

It appears that support for the concept of training specificity occurs when peripheral (muscular) adaptations occur without significant accompanying central (cardiovascular) adaptations. Keep in mind that performance is based on complex interaction between systems and cannot be attributed to one system alone. Differential peripheral versus central adaptation arises when a relatively small muscle mass is trained and, therefore, total metabolic demand is insufficient to cause significant central cardiovascular adaptation. For example, in the study cited above, Magel et al. (1978) trained subjects in one-arm ergometry at about 85% of each subjects one-arm ergometry-VO_{2max}. They then measured a significant increase in one-arm ergometry-VO_{2max} but no significant increase in treadmill-VO_{2max}. This means that the one-arm ergometry training was insufficient to elicit a significant central cardiovascular training adaptation. Thus, it is apparent that exercise training can result in significant adaptations, which occur at the peripheral level alone. Under these conditions, testing in the mode that imposes exercise on the trained peripheral

---

Box 4-7. Why Can't I Become a Better Swimmer by Run-Training?

Numerous studies have shown that training effects are usually specific to the type of exercise used during the training. Thus, run-training may increase aerobic capacity measured during running, but aerobic capacity measured during swimming, even after significant training would remain unchanged. This is because the training effects occur specifically in the muscles being activated. This concept of exercise specificity is one reason that therapy routines should match, as closely as possible, the activities of daily living needed by the individual.

musculature will yield significant performance improvements. However, testing in modes that do not exercise the trained musculature or that exercise the trained musculature as a small fraction of the overall muscle mass activated will show less improvement owing to the lack of central cardiovascular adaptation. Presumably, if the exercising muscle mass were to provide sufficient cardiovascular stress, adaptation would be expected to occur at both the peripheral and the central levels.

The difficulty in not demonstrating exercise specificity comes from the fact that, in different exercise modes, oxygen consumption values differ. Thus, the relative cardiovascular stresses between exercise modes (for instance, running versus swimming) differ, resulting in specificity demonstration. If absolute exercise intensities could be made to be exactly equivalent, presumably specificity would not be required.

Support for the lack of specificity was reported in a study comparing run-training and swim-training at the same absolute intensity (Lieber, Lieber, & Adams, 1989). Runners and swimmers were forced to exercise at the same absolute intensity (for example, it is well-known that swimming can cause heart-rate variations simply due to body angle and facial immersion in water). After correcting for these factors, and exercising 20 young men for 1 hr/day $\times$ 3 days/week $\times$ 12 weeks at an intensity equivalent to 75% of their treadmill VO_{2max}, both swimmers and runners increased their treadmill VO_{2max} to the same extent, by about 25%.

This study leads to the hypothesis that if different groups of subjects are trained in different exercise modes at a identical absolute intensities and in modes (or at intensities) sufficient to cause central cardiovascular adaptation, and then tested in a mode that elicits sufficient cardiovascular demands, training specificity will not be demonstrated. This notion does not deny the existence of training specificity but, instead, merely places numerous restrictions on the conditions under which training specificity will not be demonstrated. In addition, it emphasizes the importance of choice of training mode, training intensity, and testing mode on the interpretation of results from training studies.

Thus, specificity is not a "magical" feature of exercise, but a reaffirmation that performance results from interaction between numerous physiological systems and not a single system alone.

Neural Adaptation to Exercise

It is clear that exercise training does alter cardiovascular and muscular properties. Consider now the final component of the "performance" system—the nervous system. Obviously, performance indices such as strength depend on the level of neural activation. Is it actually possible for the nervous system to adapt to exercise? If it occurs, is it significant?

An illustrative experiment was performed by Moritani and DeVries (1979) who trained young men and women in elbow flexion. Elbows were maintained at a joint angle of 90° and subjects were asked to perform the following isometric elbow flexion protocol: 10 repetitions at an intensity of 2/3 maximum voluntary contraction (MVC) $\times$ 2 times/day $\times$ 3 times/week $\times$ 8 weeks. Note that this was not an extraordinarily long nor intense training protocol.

At 2-week intervals during the training period, subject MVC and electromyogram (EMG) were measured. At the end of 8 weeks of training, the trained arms increased strength almost 25% (from 58 to 79 lb.). However, the untrained contralateral limb also increased in strength by about 15% (from 54 to 67 lb.). How could these results be explained? How could the untrained muscle, which was never exercised, increase in strength?

In order to investigate the basis for the strength change in both trained and untrained arms, Moritani and DeVries developed a method to determine whether strength changes were due to muscular and/or neural factors. These methods could easily be used today in strength evaluation and will be explained before proceeding with the experimental results.

Method for Evaluating Neural and Muscular Components of Strength Change

By measuring both EMG and MVC, it is possible to "decompose" strength changes into neural and muscular factors. Figure 4-28 presents the scheme used to perform the decomposition. If strength increase is due only to increased level of neural activation, this will be manifest as an increased force, which is directly proportional to the increased EMG (Fig. 4-28A). If, however, the strength increase is due only to muscle hypertrophy, this will be manifest as an increased force with no increase in EMG (Fig. 4-28B). Finally, if the strength increase is due to a combination of neural and muscular factors, the relative proportion of each can be determined algebraically as shown in Figure 4-28C. The beauty of this method is that strength changes can be ascribed totally or in part to muscular and/or neural changes.

This method was used in the study described above to document the time course of strength change in the study as well as the time course of the relative contributions of neural and muscular components to the strength change.

Time Course of Muscular and Neural Components to Strength Change

After 2 weeks of training, about 80% of the strength change of the trained arm was due to increased muscle activation (neural factors) and only 20% was due to changes in the muscle itself. In the remainder of the study, the relative proportion of neural contribution decreased while the relative muscular contribution increased until, after 8 weeks, over 95% of the strength change was due to muscular factors while only about 5% could be ascribed to neural factors (Fig. 4-29). Thus, early strength changes were primarily neural in basis while later, the strength changes were almost all muscular.

In the untrained arm, the relative contributions of muscular and neural factors were relatively constant throughout the study (Fig. 4-29). Almost all of the strength increase seen in the untrained arm at all time points was due to changes in neural activation level.

In summary, isometric joint strength was increased by about 25% in the trained arm and 15% in the untrained arm. The trained arm increased strength early on by increasing neural activation (increased muscle fiber recruitment) while later on strength increased because of muscle changes. Finally, strength increases in the untrained arm were due to increased EMG activity. The significance of these findings was the demonstration of the neural plasticity demonstrated in normal subjects following training. How much more might these factors be involved in rehabilitation of disabled patients? A pressing need is to perform these types of studies in the rehabilitative setting to determine the physiological basis of recovery. If recovery is due primarily to neural factors, emphasis should be placed on treatments, which emphasize muscle activation. If, however, recovery is due primarily to muscular factors, emphasis should be placed on treatments which strengthen muscle.

(As a side note, a recent study should be mentioned that demonstrated that myosin changes can occur in contralateral limbs from rats who had one leg electrically stimulated while the other was allowed to rest. This study suggested that, indeed, muscle changes in contralateral limbs might be due to systemic effects such as altered hormone levels. Not all contralateral changes observed are necessarily due to neural changes. Future research will provide insights into the mechanism of these observed results.)

Neural Adaptations to "Imaginary" Exercise

A particular striking example of neural adaptation was reported by Yue and Cole who trained a very small muscle of the hand with a specialized protocol (Yue & Cole, 1992). The hypothenar muscles were studied because they are small and there is evidence they can be fully activated (Enoka & Fuglevand, 1991). Subjects trained using one of three protocols: exercise subjects performed active abduction of the fifth (pinky)

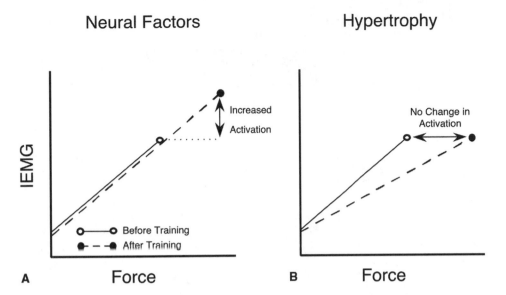

Percent of Neural vs. Hypertrophy

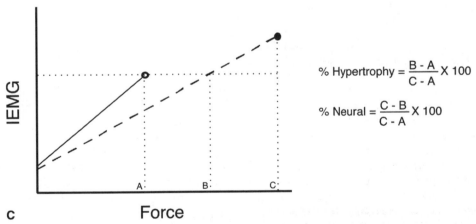

$$\% \text{ Hypertrophy} = \frac{B - A}{C - A} \times 100$$

$$\% \text{ Neural} = \frac{C - B}{C - A} \times 100$$

FIGURE 4-28. Theoretical presentation of an experimental method for determination of neural and muscular factors which are responsible for strength increase. **(A)** Situation in which all strength increase is due to neural factors since strength increase is directly proportional to EMG increase. **(B)** Situation in which all strength increase is due to muscular factors since strength increase occurs with no change in EMG. **(C)** Situation in which both neural and muscular factors are involved in strength increase along with method for calculation of the relative component of each. (Adapted from: Moritani, T., DeVries, H.A. (1979). Neural factors versus hypertrophy in the time course of muscle strength gain. *American Journal of Physical Medicine, 58*, 115–130.)

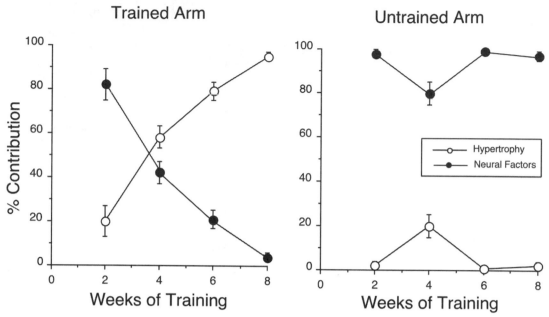

FIGURE 4-29. Time course of neural and muscular contribution to strength gain in men and women. Note that, for the untrained arm (right panel), strength increase was due to neural factors whereas for the trained arm (left panel) strength change was more complex. Early in training, the trained arm strength increased due to neural factors whereas later in training strength increased due to muscular factors. (Data from: Moritani, T., DeVries, H.A. (1979). Neural factors versus hypertrophy in the time course of muscle strength gain. *American Journal of Physical Medicine, 58*, 115–130.)

Box 4-8. How Much Can You "Train" the Nervous System?

No question that the nervous system can be trained as much or more than the muscular system. Repeated voluntary activation is a very powerful method that can improve an individual's ability to activate their muscles. In fact, even the thought of exercise can be enough to cause neural training effects to occur. This powerful effect must be incorporated into physical therapy routines to train affected and contralateral limbs in patients with neuromuscular disorders.

finger, control subjects came into the laboratory for the same amount of time and were simply tested, and "imaginary" exercise subjects came into the lab, were strapped into the small exercise device and "imagined" the entire repetitive exercise protocol but did not actually activate the muscle (as evidence by zero EMG signal and zero muscle force). The results of the study were impressive: The voluntary exercise subjects increased abduction strength by 30% over a 4- week period, the control subjects increased MVC by 3.6%, simply due to "learning" the testing procedure and becoming familiar with the task of muscle activation, and the imagined exercise group increased MVC by 22% (Fig. 4-30). This was significantly greater than controls but not quite as much as the voluntary exercise group. Clearly, the "thought" of exercising had some effect on the nervous system that made it more capable of performing the exercise. As a means of investigating the physiological basis for the adaptation, the authors tested the abduction strength of the contralateral untrained hand and found significant increases for both the imagined and exercise groups, but not the controls, consistent with "neural training" that is often observed in contralateral limbs (Fig. 4-30). They also demonstrated, by supramaximal stimulation of the ulnar nerve yielding no change in force, that the muscle had not hypertrophied and that the maximal force of the great toe extensors did not increase, suggesting no change in effort level—very provocative results. Clearly, the precise basis for this type of adaptation is not known although current studies are underway to measure the responses in the brain to this type of training using the noninvasive functional MRI method (Ashe & Ugurbil, 1994; Karni et al., 1995; Karni et al., 1998).

Therapist Exploitation of Neural Plasticity

Since neural changes can occur, it seems logical to exploit the nervous system's plasticity in rehabilitation after injury, disuse, or disease. However, a review of the therapeutic literature reveals a paucity of work in this area. Because of the great promise of such therapeutic approaches, below are a few suggested therapeutic applications of neural training that could be implemented in the future (of course, such suggestions must be clinically validated before routine use):

1. "Imaginary" exercise of an injured extremity during the recovery period when active exercise is contraindicated due to instability, trauma, or other factors.
2. "Imaginary" exercise of an affected extremity in a stroke or head injury patient prior to recovery of use of the limb.

Therapist's Comments

A fairly common clinical example of application of the "neural training" theories is in anterior cruciate ligament (ACL) rehabilitation. During the initial stages of rehabilitation, it is possible that the uninvolved extremity could be exercised vigorously in an attempt to strengthen the involved side. Such an approach could also be taken in patients after total knee and hip replacement, fracture repair, or any other unilateral surgical procedure.

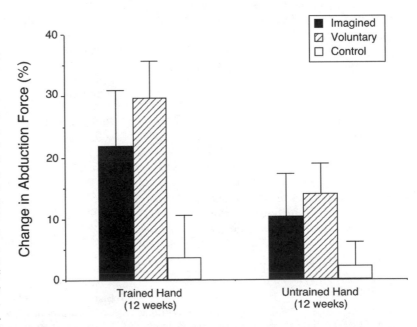

FIGURE 4-30. Increase in abduction force of trained (left) and untrained (right) hands subjected to different experimental protocols. Note that both voluntary (hatched bars) and imagined (solid bars) exercise training resulted in significant strength increases while control subjects (open bars), who simply experienced repetitive testing, did not increase in strength. Changes in the untrained hand for voluntary and imagined exercise groups were consistent with a neural basis for the change. (Data from: Yue, G., Cole, K.J. (1992). Strength increases from the motor program: Comparison of training with maximal voluntary and imagined muscle contractions. *Journal of Neurophysiology, 67,* 1114–1123.)

3. "Imaginary" or active exercise of a contra-lateral, unaffected limb in a stroke or head injury patient to improve the condition of the affected limb (presumably by neural pathways).

While these may sound far-fetched, the plasticity of the nervous system has not been exploited anywhere near the degree to which the plasticity of the muscular system has been. The concept of muscle exercise is a familiar one now, so it is a logical extension to develop the methods for "neural" exercise as well. This represents a rich area for future study and application.

■ Chapter Summary

The stereotypic response of muscle to increased use was detailed in this chapter. The main lesson, aside from the almost-unbelievable capacity of a muscle to adapt, is that muscle responds to increased used by becoming "slower" with increased endurance capacity. The extent to which this adaptation occurs depends on the intensity of the increased used: In chronic stimulation, complete fast-to-slow fiber type transformation is observed, whereas in voluntary exercise training the specific results depend on the exercise duration and intensity. You saw that metabolic adaptation of muscle occurs more readily than change in myosin type. Muscle fibers appear to maintain a balance between oxidative, glycolytic, and contractile enzyme activities. Finally, using the examples of exercise specificity and neural adaptation, you saw that external performance indices such as strength cannot be uniquely ascribed to muscle properties alone, but represent the interaction between the body's various physiological systems. In the next chapter, the reverse stimulus—decreased use—will be considered and again some generalized conclusions made.

REFERENCES

Adams, G.R., Harris, R.T., Woodard, D., Dudley, G.A. (1993). Mapping of electrical muscle stimu-lation using MRI. *Journal of Applied Physiology, 74*, 532–537.

Alway, S.E., Gonyea, W.J., Davis, M.E. (1990). Muscle fiber formation and fiber hypertrophy during the onset of stretch-overload. *American Journal of Physiology, 259*, C92–C102.

Amiel, D., Frank, C., Harwood, F., Fronek, J., Akeson, W. (1984). Tendons and ligaments: A morphological and biochemical comparison. *Journal of Orthopaedic Research, 1*, 257–265.

Amiel, D., Kuiper, S.D., Wallace, C.D., Harwood, F.L., VandeBerg, J.S. (1991). Age-related properties of medial collateral ligament and anterior cruciate ligament: a morphologic and collagen maturation study in the rabbit. *Journal of Gerontology, 46*, B159–B165.

Ashe, J., Ugurbil, K. (1994). Functional imaging of the motor system. *Current Opinion in Neurobiology, 4*, 832–839.

Baldwin, K.M., Valdez, V., Herrick, R.E., MacIntosh, A.M., Roy, R.R. (1982). Biochemical properties of overloaded fast-twitch skeletal muscle. *Journal of Applied Physiology, 52*, 467–472.

Bottinelli, R., Betto, R., Schiaffino, S., Reggiani, C. (1994a). Maximum shortening velocity and coexistence of myosin heavy chain isoforms in single skinned fast fibres of rat skeletal muscle. *Journal of Muscle Research and Cell Motility, 15*, 413–419.

Bottinelli, R., Betto, R., Schiaffino, S., Reggiani, C. (1994b). Unloaded shortening velocity and myosin heavy chain and alkali light chain isoform composition in rat skeletal muscle fibres. *Journal of Physiology (London), 478*, 341–349.

Brand, P.W., Beach, R.B., Thompson, D.E. (1981). Relative tension and potential excursion of muscles in the forearm and hand. *Journal of Hand Surgery, 3A*, 209–219.

Buller, A.J., Eccles, J.C., Eccles, R.M. (1960). Interactions between motorneurons and muscles in respect to the characteristic speeds of their responses. *Journal of Physiology, 150*, 417–439.

Burke, R.E., Levine, D.N., Tsairis, P., Zajac, F.E. (1973). Physiological types and histochemical profiles in motor units of the cat gastrocnemius. *Journal of Physiology (London), 234*, 723–748.

Burkholder, T.J., Lieber, R.L. (1998). Sarcomere number adaptation after retinaculum release in adult mice. *Journal of Experimental Biology, 201*, 309–316.

Eisenberg, B.R. (1983). Quantitative ultrastructure of mammalian skeletal muscle. In L. D. Peachey, Adrian, R.H. and Geiger, S.R., (Eds.) *Skeletal Mus-*

cle. *Vol. 10* (pp. 73–112). Baltimore, MD: American Physiological Society.

Eisenberg, B.R., Brown, J., Salmons, S. (1984). Restoration of fast muscle characteristics following cessation of chronic stimulation. *Cell and Tissue Research, 238,* 221–230.

Eisenberg, B.R., Milton, R. (1984). Muscle fiber termination at the tendon in the frog's sartorius: A stereological study. *American Journal of Anatomy, 171,* 273–284.

Eisenberg, B.R., Salmons, S. (1981). The reorganization of subcellular structure in muscle undergoing fast-to-slow type transformation. A stereological study. *Cell and Tissue Research, 220,* 449–471.

Enoka, R.M., Fuglevand, A.J. (1993). Neuromuscular basis of the maximum voluntary force capacity of muscle. In M.D. Grabiner (Ed.), *Current Issues in Biomechanics* (pp. 215–235). Champaign, IL: Human Kinetics.

Frank, C., McDonald, D., Lieber, R., Sabiston, P. (1988). Biochemical heterogeneity within the maturing rabbit medial collateral ligament. *Clinical Orthopaedics and Related Research, 236,* 279–285.

Goldspink, G. (1983). Alterations in myofibril size and structure during growth, exercise, and changes in environmental temperature. In L.D. Peachey, (Ed.), *Handbook of Physiology* (pp. 539–554). Baltimore, MD: American Physiological Society.

Gollnick, P.D., Armstrong, R., Saubert, C., Piehl, K., Saltin, B. (1972). Enzyme activity and fiber composition in skeletal muscle of untrained and trained men. *Journal of Applied Physiology, 333,* 312–319.

Gregor, R.J., Roy, R.R., Whiting, W.C., Lovely, R.G., Hodgson, J.A., Edgerton, V.R. (1988). Mechanical output of the cat soleus during treadmill locomotion: In vivo vs. in situ characteristics. *Journal of Biomechanics, 21,* 721–732.

Halbertsma, J.P., Mulder, I., Goeken, L.N., Eisma, W.H. (1999). Repeated passive stretching: Acute effect on the passive muscle moment and extensibility of short hamstrings. *Archives of Physical Medicine and Rehabilitation, 80,* 407–414.

Henneman, E., Somjen, G., Carpenter, D.O. (1965). Functional significance of cell size in spinal motorneurons. *Journal of Neurophysiology, 28,* 560–580.

Henriksson, J., Reitman, J. (1977). Time course of changes in human skeletal muscle succinate dehydrogenase and cytochrome oxidase activities and maximal oxygen uptake with physical activity and inactivity. *Acta Physiologica Scandinavica, 99,* 91–97.

Herring, S.W., Grimm, A.F., Grimm, B.R. (1984). Regulation of sarcomere number in skeletal muscle: A comparison of hypotheses. *Muscle and Nerve, 7,* 161–173.

Hultman, E., Sjoholm, H., Jaderholm, E.I., Krynicki, J. (1983). Evaluation of methods for electrical stimulation of human skeletal muscle in situ. *Pflugers Archiv. European Journal of Physiology (Berlin), 398,* 139–141.

Jenner, G., Foley, J.M., Cooper, T.G., Potchen, E.J., Meyer, R.A. (1994). Changes in magnetic resonance images of muscle depend on exercise intensity and duration, not work. *Journal of Applied Physiology, 76,* 2119–2124.

Karni, A., Meyer, G., Jezzard, P., Adams, M.M., Turner, R., Ungerleider, L.G. (1995). Functional MRI evidence for adult motor cortex plasticity during motor skill learning. *Nature, 377,* 155–158.

Karni, A., Meyer, G., Rey-Hipolito, C., Jezzard, P., Adams, M.M., Turner, R., Ungerleider, L.G. (1998). The acquisition of skilled motor performance: Fast and slow experience-driven changes in primary motor cortex. *Proceedings of the National Academy of Sciences of the United States of America, 95,* 861–868.

Kernell, D., Donselaar, Y., Eerbeek, O. (1987a). Effects of physiological amounts of high- and low-rate chronic stimulation on fast-twitch muscle of the cat hindlimb. II. Endurance-related properties. *Journal of Neurophysiology, 58,* 614–627.

Kernell, D., Eerbeek, O., Verhey, B,A., Donselaar, Y. (1987b). Effects of physiological amounts of high- and low-rate chronic stimulation on fast-twitch muscle of the cat hindlimb. I. Speed- and force-related properties. *Journal of Neurophysiology, 58,* 598–613.

Knaflitz, M., Merletti, R., De Luca, C.J. (1990). Inference of motor unit recruitment order in voluntary and electrically elicited contractions. *Journal of Applied Physiology, 68,*1657–1667.

Koh, T.J., Herzog, W. (1998). Excursion is important in regulating sarcomere number in the growing rabbit tibialis anterior. *Journal of Physiology (London), 508,* 267–280.

Lawrence, J.H., Nichols, T.R., English, A.W. (1993). Cat hindlimb muscles exert substantial torques outside the sagittal plane. *Journal of Neurophysiology, 69,* 282–285.

Lieber, R.L. (1986). Skeletal muscle adaptability iii: Muscle properties following chronic electrical stimulation. *Developmental Medicine and Child Neurology, 28*, 662–670.

Lieber, R.L. (1988). Time course and cellular control of muscle fiber type transformation following chronic stimulation. *ISI Atlas of Science, 1*, 189–194.

Lieber, D.C., Lieber, R.L., Adams, W.C. (1989). Effects of run-training and swim-training at similar absolute intensities on treadmill VO$_2$ max. *Medicine and Science in Sports and Exercise, 21*, 655–661.

Lieber, R.L., Brown, C.C. (1992). Quantitative method for comparison of skeletal muscle architectural properties. *Journal of Biomechanics, 25*, 557–560.

Lieber, R.L., Fazeli, B.M., Botte, M.J. (1990). Architecture of selected wrist flexor and extensor muscles. *Journal of Hand Surgery, 15A*, 244–250.

Lieber, R.L., Kelly, J. (1991). Factors influencing quadriceps torque using transcutaneous electrical stimulation. *Physical Therapy, 71*, 715–721.

Lieber, R.L., Kelly, M.J. (1993). Torque history of electrically stimulated human quadriceps: Implications for stimulation therapy. *Journal of Orthopaedic Research,11*, 131–141.

Lieber, R.L., Pontén, E., Fridén, J. (1996). Sarcomere length changes after flexor carpi ulnaris-to-extensor digitorum communis tendon transfer. *Journal of Hand Surgery, 21A*, 612–618.

Lieber, R.L., Silva, P.D., Daniel, D.M. (1996). Equal effectiveness of electrical and volitional strength training in quadriceps femoris muscles after anterior cruciate surgery. *Journal of Orthopaedic Research, 14*, 131–138.

Lømo, T., Westgaard, R.H., Dahl, H.A. (1974). Contractile properties of muscle: Control by pattern of muscle activity in the rat. *Proceedings of the Royal Society of London Series B: Biological Sciences (London), 187*, 99–103.

Lømo, T., Westgaard, R.H., Engelbretsen, L. (1980). Different stimulation patterns affect contractile properties of denervated rat soleus muscles. In D. Pette (Ed.), *The Plasticity of Muscle* (pp. 297–309). New York: Walter de Gruyter.

Lutz, G.J., Cuizon, D.B., Ryan, A.F., Lieber, R.L. (1998). Four novel myosin heavy chain transcripts in Rana pipiens single muscle fibres define a molecular basis for muscle fibre types in the frog. *Journal of Physiology (London), 508*, 667–680.

Magel, J.R., Foglia, G.F., McArdle, W.D., Gutin, B., Pechar, G.S., Katch, F.I. (1975). Specificity of swim training on maximum oxygen uptake. *Journal of Applied Physiology, 38*, 151–155.

Magel, J.R., McArdle, W.D., Toner, M., Delio, D.J. (1978). Metabolic and cardiovascular adjustment to arm training. *Journal of Applied Physiology, 45*, 75–79.

Magnusson, S.P., Aagard, P., Simonsen, E., Bojsen-Moller, F. (1998). A biomechanical evaluation of cyclic and static stretch in human skeletal muscle. *International Journal of Sports Medicine, 19*, 310–316.

Meyer, R.A., Prior, B.M. (2000). Functional magnetic resonance imaging of muscle. *Exercise and Sport Sciences Reviews, 28*, 89–92.

Moritani, T., DeVries, H.A. (1979). Neural factors versus hypertrophy in the time course of muscle strength gain. *American Journal of Physical Medicine, 58*, 115–130.

Pette, D. (1990). *The Dynamic State of Muscle Fibers*, (pp. 729). Berlin: Walter de Gruyter & Company.

Roy, R.R., Medows, I.D., Baldwin, K.M., Edgerton, V.R. (1982). Functional significance of compensatory overloaded rat fast muscle. *Journal of Applied Physiology, 52*, 473–478.

Salmons, S., Henriksson, J. (1981). The adaptive response of skeletal muscle to increased use. *Muscle and Nerve, 4*, 94–105.

Salmons, S., Vrbova, G. (1969). The influence of activity on some contractile characteristics of mammalian fast and slow muscles. *Journal of Physiology (London), 201*, 535–549.

Saltin, B., Gollnick, P.D. (1983). Skeletal muscle adaptability: significance for metabolism and performance. In *Handbook of Physiology*, (pp. 539–554). Baltimore: American Physiological Society.

Schiaffino, S., Reggiani, C. (1996). Molecular diversity of myofibrillar proteins: Gene regulation and functional significance. *Physiological Review, 76*, 371–423.

Smith, R.J., Hastings, H. (1993). Principles of tendon transfers to the hand. *AAOS Instructional Course Lectures, 21*, 129–149.

Spector, S.A., Simard, C.P., Fournier, M., Sternlicht, E., Edgerton, V.R. (1982). Architectural alterations of rat hindlimbs skeletal muscles immobilized at different lengths. *Experimental Neurology, 76*, 94–110.

Stromme, S.B., Ingjer, F., Meen, H.D. (1977). Assessment of maximal aerobic power in specifically trained athletes. *Journal of Applied Physiology, 42,* 833–837.

Tabary, J.C., Tabary, C., Tardieu, C., Tardieu, G., Goldspink, G. (1972). Physiological and structural changes in the cat's soleus muscle due to immobilization at different lengths by plaster casts. *Journal of Physiology (London), 224,* 231–244.

Williams, P. (1988). Effect of intermittent stretch on immobilized muscle. *Annals of the Rheumatic Diseases, 47,* 1014–1016.

Williams, P.E., Goldspink, G. (1971). Longitudinal growth of striated muscle fibres. *Journal of Cell Science, 9,* 751–767.

Williams, P., Goldspink, G. (1973). The effect of immobilization on the longitudinal growth of striated muscle fibers. *Journal of Anatomy, 116,* 45–55.

Williams, P., Watt, P., Bicik, V., Goldspink, G. (1986). Effect of stretch combined with electrical stimulation on the type of sarcomeres produced at the ends of muscle fibers. *Experimental Neurology, 93,* 500–509.

Williams, R.S., Salmons, S., Newsholme, E.A., Kaufman, R.E., Mellor, J. (1986). Regulation of nuclear and mitochondrial gene expression by contractile activity in skeletal muscle. *Journal of Biological Chemistry, 261,* 376–380.

Yue, G., Alexander, A.L., Laidlaw, D.H., Gmitro, A.F., Unger, E.C., Enoka, R.M. (1994). Sensitivity of muscle proton spin-spin relaxation time as an index of muscle activation. *Journal of Applied Physiology, 77,* 84–92.

Yue, G., Cole, K.J. (1992). Strength increases from the motor program: comparison of training with maximal voluntary and imagined muscle contractions. *Journal of Neurophysiology, 67,* 1114–1123.

CHAPTER 5

Skeletal Muscle Adaptation to Decreased Use

Chapter Overview

Having laid the foundation in the previous chapter of muscle's response to increased use, this chapter will consider muscle's response to decreased use. As in previous chapters, the response to decreased use will be illustrated by considering various experimental models. This chapter will begin with the "simplest" model (at least from the point of view of creating it)—immobilization; it will then consider various spinal cord interruption models, followed by simulated weightlessness (such as that which occurs in spaceflight). In recent years, a tremendous boom in understanding muscle's response to aging has been achieved and this is presented as one of the final models. Finally, the denervation model is presented to demonstrate its uniqueness. Again, patterns emerge as each model adds to an understanding of muscle adaptation. The description of many of these abnormal states also clarifies an understanding of many aspects of normal structure-function relationships in neuromuscular units.

Educational Objectives

- To be able to describe the basic experimental "models" of adaptation to decreased use.
- To be able to explain the strengths and weaknesses of each model in its ability to provide an understanding of adaptation to decreased use.
- To be able to define the factors that cause adaptation to decreased use.

- To provide clinical examples that parallel the experimental models of decreased use.
- To be able to predict changes in muscles that occur after experimental and clinical examples of decreased use.

Introduction

The investigation of muscle adaptation continues with a detailed view of a muscle's response to decreased use. In contrast to the previous chapter, which began by presenting a very "clean" model of *increased use* by chronic stimulation, there is no equivalently clean model of *decreased use* that results in uniform results across all fiber types. In other words, there is no chronic decreased use model because a "dramatic" decrease in use is sometimes difficult to elicit. Some muscle fibers are so rarely used that immobilization may not have much influence on them. As a result, investigators have developed various models that cause a decrease in muscle use, although in different ways. One of the models that is the easiest to understand is immobilization. This one will be used as the starting point. However, for each model, as in the previous chapter, always consider the relevance of that model to your area of interest. Some models are very "clean" in terms of creating a reproducible response but are not very relevant to real clinical problems. Others are very relevant, but so complex that they are difficult to decipher. Ideally, information from all types of models can be synthesized to permit a general understanding of neuromuscular plasticity to decreased use. I apologize in advance for the numerous types of models presented as long as the detailed response of the neuromuscular system to each model. Don't just read this as a list of treatments and changes. Rather, try to first predict the response of muscle to the treatment and then try to predict the underlying muscular changes that could occur to explain the functional responses measured. Use the discussion of these models to reinforce your understanding of neuromuscular structure and function.

Adaptation to Immobilization

Limb immobilization has been used since the turn of the century to protect fractured bones and injured tissues from repeated injury. The most common complication of immobilization as used clinically is the muscle wasting that occurs secondary to decreased muscle use. However, you probably already have some concerns about immobilization as a decreased use model since, as seen in the previous chapter, immobilization *per se* does not necessarily cause atrophy. Strictly speaking, atrophy-inducing models using immobilization, implement immobilization in a shortened position. In this and other models, the model will first be pre-

sented, followed by experimental data that describe the muscle changes resulting from the treatment.

The Immobilization Model
Immobilization models have long been used to study muscle adaptation. In addition to their obvious clinical relevance, immobilization models are relatively noninvasive—no surgery is necessary. In Chapter 4, you saw that a muscle responds to the tension level imposed upon it. (To date, muscle tension during immobilization has not been experimentally measured directly.) Immobilization should not be viewed as placing a muscle in a state of "suspended animation" since electrical activity, tension, and motion can still occur within the cast (Fig. 5-1). Do not consider immobilization as a "disuse" model either, in the sense that the muscle is completely unused. Rather, it is more appropriate to consider immobilization a "reduced-use" model.

Electromyographic Changes During Immobilization
Since direct measurement of muscle tension within the cast is technically difficult, an indirect "measure" of muscle activity during immobilization was made by quantifying the electro-

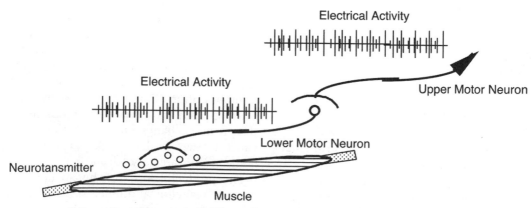

FIGURE 5-1. Schematic representation of the immobilization model. Each portion of the neuromuscular system is shown. Note that muscle electrical activity and even some degree of loading are present and, therefore, it is not appropriate to term this model "disuse," but rather decreased use.

myographic (EMG) activity. Experimentally, this was performed by implanting fine wire electrodes into a muscle and routing the leads to an external connector. Then, at various time intervals after electrode implantation and immobilization, muscle EMG activity was recorded to determine the long-term activity changes following immobilization.

Dr. Reggie Edgerton and colleagues implanted electrodes in both the fast-contracting medial gastrocnemius (MG) muscle and the slow-contracting soleus (SOL) muscle of the rat (Fournier, Roy, Perham, Simard, & Edgerton, 1983). Their purpose was to determine the extent to which immobilization resulted in muscle "disuse." EMG activity was measured for several days after the electrodes were first implanted, to determine whether the implantation procedure itself affected muscle activity (fortunately, it did not). Next, EMG activity was measured continuously for 15 minutes every hour, for 24 hours on days 7, 17, and 28 post-immobilization. To produce varying degrees of atrophy, joints were immobilized such that the SOL and MG muscles were either shortened, at neutral length, or in a lengthened position. At these same time intervals, the muscle mass of animals was measured as an index of "atrophy" (you will see below that wet muscle mass was probably not the best index of atrophy, but for the purposes of this study, it was probably adequate. Since skeletal muscle fibers may contain

over 80% protein, protein content and muscle fiber size are the most common index of muscle atrophy.)

Fournier et al. demonstrated that the total EMG activity of both the SOL and MG muscles decreased markedly after only 1 week of immobilization with the muscle in a shortened position. The SOL EMG activity decreased to a greater extent than did the MG. EMG activity continued to remain low throughout the remainder of the experiment such that, after 28 days, SOL EMG had decreased by 77% while MG EMG had decreased by 50%. With the muscle immobilized in the neutral position, no change was seen in MG EMG activity whereas only a 50% decrease in SOL EMG was measured.

The interesting aspect of the study was that the atrophic muscle response was not closely related to the magnitude of the EMG change (Fig. 5-2). For example, when the MG was immobilized in a neutral position, EMG did not change appreciably (Fig. 5-2A) but the muscle atrophied dramatically (black arrow, Fig. 5-2B). Also, in spite of the fact that the EMG response of the MG initially, in the neutral position and lengthened, was nearly identical, the magnitude of the atrophic response was different. The immobilization model decreased the level of MG "use" (by decreasing EMG and thus the electrical activity of the muscle fibers), but this change in "use" was not proportional to the magnitude of the resulting muscle atrophy. Similarly, for the SOL muscle, the EMG decreased to the same extent, whether the muscle was immobilized in the neutral or fully lengthened position (decreasing to about 50% of control values). However, the SOL muscle immobilized in the neutral position decreased in mass by about 50% while the SOL muscle immobilized in the lengthened position showed no decrease at all (white arrow, Fig. 5-2B). Again, the change in level of "use" as measured by EMG was not related to the magnitude of the atrophic response.

The take-home lesson of this study was that the change in muscle electrical activity was not the *cause* of muscle atrophy. It is also obviously inappropriate to refer to atrophy that occurs

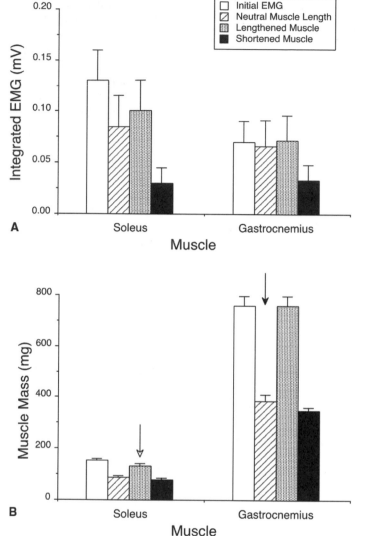

FIGURE 5-2. (A) Change in EMG activity from the rat soleus and medial gastrocnemius immobilized in the different positions denoted by different shading patterns. **(B)** Change in muscle mass from the rat soleus and medial gastrocnemius immobilized in different positions. Note that EMG changes are not paralleled by mass changes (arrows). (Data from: Fournier, M., Roy, R.R., Perham, H., Simard, C.P., Edgerton, V.R. (1983). Is limb immobilization a model of muscle disuse? *Experimental Neurology, 80,* 147–156.)

secondary to immobilization as "disuse" atrophy since neural activity to muscles remained throughout the entire immobilization period.

Dog Quadriceps Immobilization Model

To determine the nature of muscle's response to immobilization, literally thousands of experiments have been performed using practically every conceivable muscle group and animal or human model. There is general agreement among studies that muscles composed mainly of slow fibers atrophy to a greater extent than

muscles composed mainly of fast fibers (as seen above). It also appears that antigravity muscles atrophy to a greater extent than their antagonists. Thus the "fast" gastrocnemius atrophies to a greater extent than its "fast" tibialis anterior antagonist. However, there are numerous exceptions to these generalizations. One reason for this lack of agreement is the lack of control of muscle length during immobilization. If, for example, the ankle joint is immobilized with the ankle plantarflexed, the soleus will dramatically atrophy (due to the lack of tension) while the tibialis anterior may actually hypertrophy (due to stretch). Should it therefore be concluded that muscles composed primarily of slow fibers (such as the soleus) atrophy after immobilization while muscles composed primarily of fast fibers (such as the tibialis anterior) actually hypertrophy? No. It is important, therefore to control for muscle length and other factors in order to properly generalize regarding the effects of immobilization on fast and slow skeletal muscles. In fact, as you review the literature on immobilization, be sure to define the relative degree of stretch placed upon a muscle since this will affect its atrophic response greatly. For example, human plantarflexors immobilized with the ankle joint in a neutral position would be expected to atrophy less compared to plantarflexors immobilized with the ankle joint in a plantarflexed position.

A study of muscle immobilization was performed using as our experimental model, three heads of the dog quadriceps muscles: the rectus femoris (RF), vastus lateralis (VL), and vastus medialis (VM) (Lieber, Fridén, Hargens, Danzig, & Gershuni, 1988). These three muscles contain nearly identical architectures and fiber lengths but differ in fiber type percentage and number of joints crossed. For example, the RF acts both as a knee extensor and hip flexor and is composed of about 50% slow fibers. The VM and VL both function only as knee extensors, but the VL contains only about 20% slow fibers while the VM contains about 50% slow fibers. This model thus allowed comparison between the VM and VL, which could be immobilized at precisely the same length but contain different percentages of slow and fast fibers. Similarly, comparisons between the RF and VM could be made since they have similar fiber type percentages but cross different joints. Thus, comparison of the vasti tests for the effects of fiber type whereas comparison between the VM and RF tests for the effects of architecture.

Note that the dog muscle fibers have simply been referred to as "fast" and "slow" in spite of our relatively lengthy muscle fiber types discussion presented in Chapter 2. Why? Fortunately, dog muscles contain no type FG fibers (Armstrong, Saubert, Seeherman, & Taylor, 1982). Therefore all fast fibers in dogs are of the FOG type and all slow fibers are of the SO type. Unequivocal fiber type identification can thus be made from a single histochemical stain for myofibrillar ATPase activity (remember that this type of statement is only valid having first experimentally determined that dog muscle contains no FG fibers).

DOG QUADRICEPS IMMOBILIZATION METHOD

To assure that muscle lengths were held constant during the immobilization period, a custom external skeletal fixator, designed by the orthopedic surgeon Dr. David Gershuni, was used to fix the knee joint angle at 90° (Fig. 5-3). One leg was immobilized while the other leg was left as a control. However, note that contralateral legs from experimental animals are not truly "normal" for a variety of reasons. First, they probably bear more weight since the immobilized leg is raised. Second, systemic effects might affect all muscles differentially. In this particular study, control experiments were performed which demonstrated no differences between truly normal muscles, taken from untreated animals, and contralateral muscles from those used in this study.

After 10 weeks of immobilization, small biopsies were taken from the VL, VM, and RF and prepared for histochemical analysis as described in Chapter 2 (Fig. 5-4). An added point, which should be mentioned here is that the biopsies were always kept under some tension since fiber shortening will cause an apparent increase in fiber cross-sectional area. After staining muscles for myofibrillar ATPase activity, and classifying each fiber as fast or slow, muscle fiber areas were measured using well-defined stereological methods (Weibel, 1980). It is important to sample muscle fibers across the entire section so that representative areas are obtained. As a result of this approach, the following simple experimental data set was obtained for each muscle

1. Type 1 fiber area (μm^2)
2. Type 2 fiber area (μm^2)

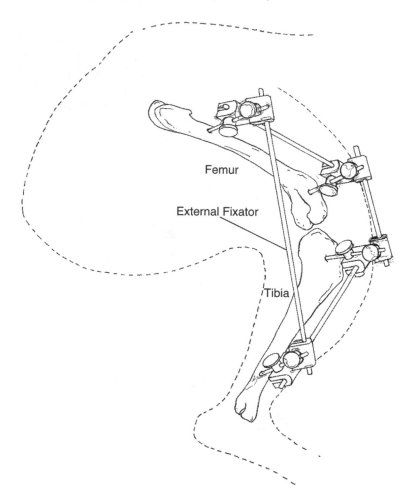

FIGURE 5-3. Experimental method for immobilization of the dog quadriceps muscles. An external skeletal fixator was used to maintain the knee angle at 90° of flexion. In this way, muscle length could be carefully controlled. (Modified from: Lieber, R.L., Fridén, J.O., Hargens, A.R., Danzig, L.A., Gershuni, D.H. (1988). Differential response of the dog quadriceps muscle to external skeletal fixation of the knee. *Muscle Nerve, 11*, 193–201.)

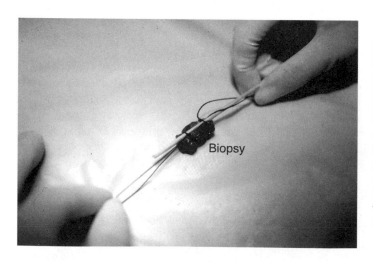

FIGURE 5-4. Photograph of a muscle biopsy obtained from a vastus lateralis muscle. Note that, to obtain excellent muscle fiber morphology, the biopsy is securely attached to a wooden stick with sutures. Since muscle fibers contract with a constant volume, muscle fiber shortening will erroneously be interpreted as fiber size increase while muscle fiber lengthening will erroneously be interpreted as fiber size decrease. It is thus important to preserve muscle fiber length when obtaining a biopsy.

3. Percentage of each fiber type
4. Area fraction of endomysial/perimysial connective tissue (%)

Clearly, fiber area relates to the force generating capacity of the fiber. If muscle fiber number does not change with immobilization, fiber area ought to be a good predictor of muscle force. The greater the fiber area, the greater the number of myofibrils arranged in parallel within the fiber. Thus, when muscle fiber atrophy is discussed, strictly speaking, myofibrillar number or a parameter that is closely related to it (such as fiber area) must be considered. As myofibrillar number decreases, the force generated by the fiber also decreases. Fiber area (as an index of myofibrillar number) is compared from control and immobilized muscles to determine their responses to immobilization. In the increased-use models, fiber type percentage provided insights into the degree of use experienced by the muscle. Recall in the chronic stimulation model that the fast-to-slow fiber type conversion resulted from the dramatically increased level of fiber activity compared to normal. In the same way, a muscle's normal fiber type distribution is probably related to the amount of normal activity experienced by the muscle. In Chapter 1, during development, differentiation past the secondary myotube required innervation (Miller & Stockdale, 1987). Infer from this that, during maturation, muscle fibers receiving a great deal of neural activity have a greater likelihood of becoming slow fibers. The take-home lesson is that a muscle's normal fiber type distribution provides insights into its normal level of use and, as you will see, its response to decreased use.

Muscle Fiber Response to Immobilization

The most obvious response of the immobilized dog quadriceps was the sizable fast and slow muscle fiber atrophy (Fig. 5-5). However, although all micrographs were taken at the same magnification, it was obvious that the magnitude of the atrophy was different for the three different muscles. Using stereometric

---

> **Box 5-2. Don't All Muscles Atrophy the Same?**
>
> Absolutely not. Some muscles (primarily anti-gravity muscles) atrophy tremendously while their antagonists do not atrophy much at all. Thus, different muscles are more vulnerable to immobilization-induced atrophy. In fact, even the same muscle fiber type within different muscles may atrophy to different extents and the different types of the same fibers within the same muscles may atrophy to different extents. This seems to be related to each muscle's and perhaps even each fiber's "set point" regarding the level of activity that will maintain its mass constant.

---

techniques developed in Switzerland by Professor Weibel (1979) it was found that there was no difference in fast or slow muscle fiber area between any of the muscles on the control side. Yet 10 weeks of immobilization caused significant decreases in both fast (Fig. 5-6) and slow (Fig. 5-7) muscle fiber area. Clearly this would result in decreased muscle force generating capacity. However, the most interesting result was not that muscle fiber areas decreased in response to immobilization (a result that had already been demonstrated by numerous scientists), it was that the amount of muscle fiber atrophy was *different* for each of the three muscles. Specifically, the fast fiber area of the immobilized VM and VL was less than the fast fiber area of the immobilized RF (Fig. 5-6). Similarly, in an even more dramatic differential response, slow fiber area of the VM muscles was much less than that of the VL, which was much less than that of the RF (Fig. 5-7). The atrophic response for slow fibers was thus, in order from most to least atrophied: VM > VL > RF, while for fast fibers the corresponding order was VM = VL > RF. This difference was even more dramatic on inspection of the actual micrographs. Compare, for example, the fiber sizes in the micrographs of Figure 5-5, photographed at the same magnification. In addition

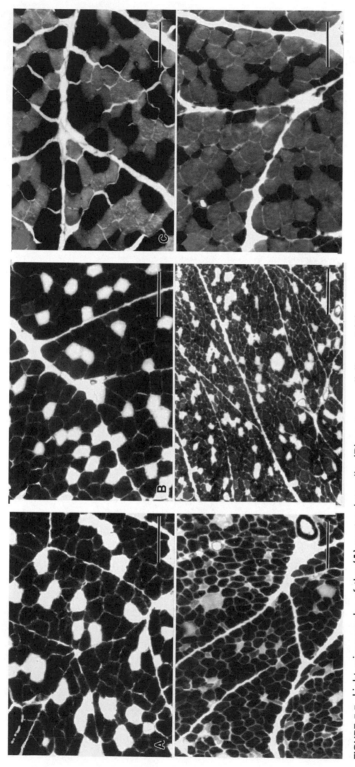

FIGURE 5-5. Light micrographs of the **(A)** vastus lateralis, **(B)** vastus medialis, and **(C)** rectus femoris muscles. The top panel represents micrographs from normal muscles and the bottom panel represents micrographs from immobilized muscles. All micrographs were taken at the same magnification. Fast fibers appear dark and slow fibers appear light. Calibration bars = 100 μm. (From Lieber, R.L., Fridén, J.O., Hargens. A.R., Danzig, L.A., Gershuni, D.H. (1988). Differential response of the dog quadriceps muscle to external skeletal fixation of the knee. *Muscle Nerve, 11,* 193–201.)

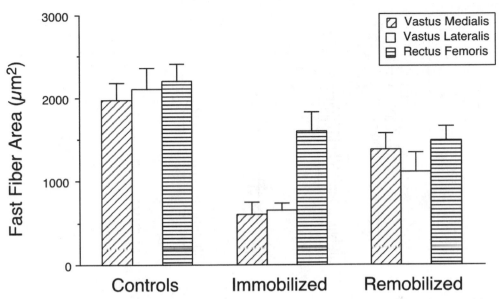

FIGURE 5-6. Graph of fast fiber area from control, immobilized, and remobilized dog quadriceps muscles. Note that the magnitude of atrophy was muscle specific. Upon remobilization, muscles returned to parity. (From Lieber, R.L., Fridén, J.O., Hargens, A.R., Danzig, L.A., Gershuni, D.H. (1988). Differential response of the dog quadriceps muscle to external skeletal fixation of the knee. *Muscle Nerve, 11*, 193–201 and Lieber, R.L., McKee-Woodburn, T., Fridén, J., Gershuni, D.H. (1989). Recovery of the dog quadriceps after ten weeks of immobilization followed by four weeks of remobilization. *Journal of Orthopaedic Research, 7*, 408–412.)

to these changes in fiber area, a significant increase in fast fiber percentage following immobilization was observed in the VM. You may have already experienced firsthand the differential atrophy observed in human quadriceps after immobilization. One patient population in which this is common is the relatively young patient who is recovering from injury and reconstruction of their anterior cruciate ligament (ACL). The "caving in" of the distal portion of the vastus lateralis (known as the vastus medialis obliques, or VMO, based on the oblique pennation angle of the fibers in this region of the VM) is easily appreciated in these patients and represents a challenge to the therapist who must treat this severe muscle atrophy.

Immobilization also caused proliferation of endomysial and perimysial connective tissue relative to control legs with a significantly greater increase in the immobilized VM and VL muscles compared with immobilized RF muscles.

Proposed Explanation for Differential Muscle Fiber Response

How can the differences between these muscles be accounted for based on our understanding of muscle plasticity? Why would slow fibers in one muscle dramatically atrophy while slow fibers in another muscle atrophy only slightly? Consider each muscle sequentially . . .

The differences observed between the VM and VL could not simply be explained by differences in immobilization length. Immobilization length strongly influences the atrophic response as we have seen (Fig. 5-2), but the VL and VM were fixed at identical lengths. Using a similar argument, differences observed between the VM and RF could not be explained by differences in fiber type distribution since they both

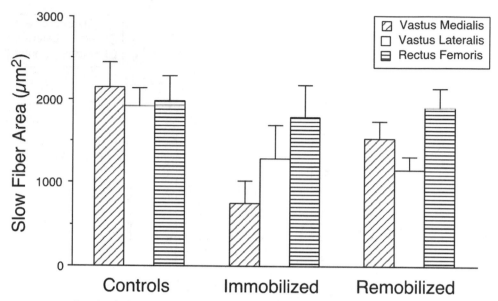

FIGURE 5-7. Graph of slow fiber area from control, immobilized, and remobilized dog quadriceps muscles. (From Lieber, R.L., Fridén, J.O., Hargens, A.R., Danzig, L.A., Gershuni, D.H. (1988). Differential response of the dog quadriceps muscle to external skeletal fixation of the knee. *Muscle Nerve, 11*, 193–201 and Lieber, R.L., McKee-Woodburn, T., Fridén J, Gershuni DH. (1989). Recovery of the dog quadriceps after ten weeks of immobilization followed by four weeks of remobilization. *Journal of Orthopaedic Research, 7*, 408–412.)

began with about 50% fast and 50% slow fibers. The architecture of all three muscles is similar. The ratio of fiber length/muscle length has been studied in humans and guinea pigs and approximates 0.2 for all three muscles and thus, architecture differences could not account for the differences observed. In order to explain the differential atrophy of the VM, VL, and RF, other factors must be considered.

The RF demonstrated the smallest degree of atrophy of the three muscles studied. Conversely, the most severe atrophy was observed in the VM. This is interesting in light of the fact that the two muscles initially contained nearly identical fiber type distributions. Therefore, initial fiber type distribution alone does not dictate the magnitude of the atrophic response. However, the RF crosses both the hip and knee functioning both as a knee extensor and hip flexor while the VM and VL cross the knee functioning as knee extensors. The RF is there-

fore less rigidly immobilized than either of the vasti, probably explaining the small atrophic response.

The slow fibers of the VM atrophied to a greater extent than those of the VL. Both the VM and VL were immobilized at the same length since they both arise from the proximal femur and insert together with the rectus tendon onto the patella. It seems unlikely then, that the small difference in anatomical location could account for the markedly different response. The VM initially contained a much larger proportion of slow fibers than the VL, which indicates that the VM was probably used more since muscle fiber type distributions provide insights into muscle activation history. Therefore, after immobilization, the change in the amount of VM activation was probably greater than the change for the VL even though the absolute levels following immobilization may have been similar. This provides support for the idea that immobilization represented a model of decreased but not disuse.

Fiber Type Transformation After Immobilization

Perhaps this large change in VM activation level could also account for the slow-to-fast transformation. This is our first exposure to the idea that, in contrast to increased-use models, that were shown to routinely cause a fast-to-slow transformation, decreased-use models cause the opposite—a slow-to-fast transformation. This type of transformation has been observed clinically. For example, Haggmark and co-workers observed a significant increase in vastus lateralis type 2-fiber percentage after surgical reconstruction of the anterior cruciate ligament (Haggmark & Eriksson, 1979). Interestingly, the magnitude of the transformation seemed to be correlated with the change in use since elite athletes (whose muscles were most "used" to high activity levels) demonstrated the greatest degree of slow-to-fast transformation. Similarly, Dr. Gunnar Grimby, the Swedish rehabilitation physician, observed dramatic slow-to-fast fiber type transformations in patients recovering from traumatic spinal cord lesions (Grimby, Broberg, Krotkiewska, & Krotkiewski, 1976).

Muscle fiber type transformation after decreased use may have functional implications. First, recall that faster muscles only generate smooth tetanic contractions at the higher stimulation frequencies (Fig. 2-2). Thus, if contraction and relaxation speed increase, higher neural drive frequencies will be required to maintain steady tension levels. This may result in decreased neuromotor control in these patients, many of whom retain significant residual function.

Generalizations of Muscle Fiber Atrophy

This study established the relative influence of two factors that contribute to immobilization-induced atrophy. The most significant factor was the degree of immobilization (number of joints crossed), and next was the change in use

relative to normal function. The initial percentage of slow muscles fibers was a fair indicator of the normal muscle use level and was a good predictor of the relative degree of atrophy.

These data indicate that a blanket concept of "slow fiber atrophy" cannot apply to all muscles. Rather, it is a combination of factors that determines the muscular response to decreased use. Given the structure and fiber type distributions of the various human muscles, it is possible to predict those that are most vulnerable to immobilization-induced atrophy, i.e., those that function as antigravity muscles, cross a single joint and contain a relatively large proportion of slow fibers. This description fits the soleus, multifidus, vastus medialis, and vastus intermedius muscles. The next class of muscles that are susceptible to immobilization-induced atrophy would be antigravity muscles, predominantly slow that cross multiple joints, namely the longissimus and transversospinalis (erector spinae), gastrocnemius, and rectus fe-

---

Therapist's Comments

If I might speculate a bit about the functional significance of fiber type transformation and implications for therapy . . . Since the fiber type change with disuse is to the fast fiber type, perhaps rehabilitation should focus on exercises that impose a constant low level of activity (higher repetition and lower weight) to encourage transformation back to the slow fiber type. This type of exercise protocol may initially shift fiber type back to the "normal" fiber type distribution and then the therapist could follow with higher weight/lower repetition strengthening to increase fiber size. The problem with trying to apply some of this information is that there is not enough analogous information from humans to say that exercising in a particular way will change the muscle in the way that you might suspect.

moris. These muscle groups should be immobilized conservatively to avoid severe strength loss. Conversely, phasically activated, predominantly fast muscles (*e.g.,* tibialis anterior, extensor digitorum longus, biceps) can be immobilized with less loss of strength.

This hierarchy of susceptibility to immobilization is supported by the data of Dr. Edgerton and colleagues, who measured morphological, biochemical, and physiological properties of immobilized hindlimb muscles from *Galego senegalensis* (a small primate commonly known as the bushbaby) and found that muscles atrophied in the order (most to least atrophy): soleus > plantaris > vastus intermedius = vastus lateralis > gastrocnemius > tibialis anterior = rectus femoris, agreeing well with the principles stated above (Edgerton, Barnard, Peter, Maier, & Simpson, 1975). Remember, increased atrophy is observed upon immobili-

---

Therapist's Comments

Another clinical example related to joint position is the typical rehabilitation after ankle sprain injury (Safran, et al., 1999). The typical acute phase of rehabilitation focuses on ice, compression, and immobilization. The immobilization can be of various forms from some kind of cast to an Aircast that allows some motion in plantarflexion and dorsiflexion. It is stated that the immobilization should be in as much dorsiflexion as possible to help to lengthen the soleus. However, because of the swelling in the joint, the ankle will most likely be in a position of plantarflexion during the first week which means that soleus atrophy and fiber type changes will occur to a greater degree. The therapist must be aware of this and progress to controlled movement as soon as possible to limit the detrimental effects of immobilization on the soleus that is shortened secondary to plantarflexion.

---

zation in muscles which are normally used a great deal. These tend to be muscles that contain a relatively high percentage of slow fibers.

Descriptors of Muscle Atrophy

Numerous immobilizations studies have documented differing degrees of atrophy following different types of immobilization treatment. How should the magnitude of the atrophic response be calculated? Is the atrophy directly related to the change in muscle force? Muscle mass? In order to describe appropriate measures of atrophy, return to the immobilization study performed in Edgerton's laboratory that was discussed in the Chapter 4.

Recall that muscles were immobilized at different lengths after which time architectural (Spector, Simard, Fournier, Sternlicht, & Edgerton, 1982) and contractile (Simard, Spector, & Edgerton, 1982) properties were measured. Compare the conclusions that would be reach using muscle mass as a measure of atrophy compared to maximum tetanic tension as a measure of atrophy. The soleus and medial gastrocnemius will be considered. The normal rat MG weighs about 800 mg. After immobilization in the lengthened position, mass dropped to 635 mg, while in the shortened position, mass decreased dramatically to 350 mg (Fig. 5-8A). In terms of mass, therefore, the stretched MG atrophied by only 15% while the shortened MG atrophied by over 50%. These represent impressive and quite different changes. Unfortunately, these changes in mass had almost no relation to the actual muscle performance following the immobilization period. While the shortened MG decreased in mass by 50%, MG, P_o decreased by over 75% (Fig. 5-8B). The lengthened MG decreased in mass by 15% while MG P_o decreased by over 40%—quite a disparity. Using a similar argument for the soleus, the results were quite different. Following immobilization in the lengthened position, soleus mass dropped from 150 mg to 132 mg, while in the shortened position, mass decreased dramatically to 79 mg (Fig. 5-8A). In terms of mass, therefore, the stretched soleus atrophied by only 12% while

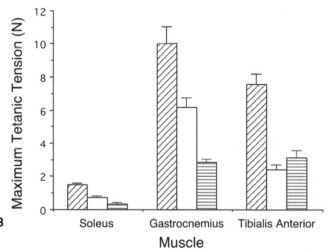

FIGURE 5-8. (A) Muscle mass and **(B)** P_o from normal and immobilized rat skeletal muscles. Note that mass and P_o changes are not uniquely correlated. Mass is thus a poor predictor of muscle tension. Note also that immobilization in a lengthened position spares the muscle of mass and tension losses which accompany immobilization in the shortened position. (Data from: Simard, C.P., Spector, S.A., Edgerton, V.R. (1982). Contractile properties of rat hindlimb muscles immobilized at different lengths. *Experimental Neurology, 77,* 467–482.)

the shortened soleus atrophied by 50%. In terms of contractile tension, the stretched soleus atrophied by 50% and the shortened soleus atrophied by 80%. Again, quite different results—12% mass versus 50% P_o and 50% mass versus 80% P_o. More "atrophy" if P_o is considered instead of mass. Why the disparity? Think about what you have already learned about the relationship between muscle force and muscle mass. This is a good test of your understanding of the relationship between PCSA, as defined in Chapter 1 (Equation 1-1, page 31) abd Muscle force generation.

The reason mass and performance were not closely related was that performance was a direct function of architecture whereas mass was simply proportional to the total amount of contractile material in the muscle. These immobilization treatments resulted in a change in muscle fiber length, as discussed in Chapter 4 (Fig. 4-8), which strongly affected the PCSA calculations. The explanation for the disparity between the results using mass or P_o was due to the changes in fiber length that occurred after immobilization. For example, immobilization in the shortened position resulted in decreased fiber length. This will show up as a decrease in mass, but fiber length changes alone will not affect contractile tension. The functional effects of fiber length change would be seen in measures of V_{max} or muscle excursion, neither of which were explicitly measured in the previous study. Therefore, the only conditions under which mass, or protein content, provide a reli-

---

Box 5-3. Why Does Muscle Strength Not Decrease to the Same Extent as Muscle Mass?

Strictly speaking, muscle strength is proportional to the muscle's physiological cross-sectional area (PCSA). Since PCSA is a calculated value, it is almost never seen on any type of "scan" such as an MRI or even a CT scan. Sometimes, immobilization results in muscle shortening which results in a decrease in mass but not necessary the same effect on PCSA. Thus, this immobilization would have no effect on maximum strength. One must be careful to measure the correct parameter from a patient in order to describe muscle's response to atrophy.

---

able index of tension decrease are those in which no architectural adaptations are seen. To reiterate, knowledge of muscle mass change following immobilization provided little information as to the functional consequence without some knowledge of the concomitant architectural changes.

Incidentally, Edgerton and his colleagues also demonstrated that the decrease in P_o was nearly proportional to the decrease in muscle fiber area. It thus appears that atrophy of muscle fiber cross-section truly is the primary cause for decreased muscle force—the muscle fibers themselves generate less force. This relationship between muscle fiber area and torque was recently directly demonstrated using the dog immobilization model (Fig. 5-9) (Lieber et al., 1997). Small biopsies were removed from the muscles during a functional testing protocol in which maximum quadriceps extension torque was also measured. Taken together, these animal studies provide strong support for the use of muscle fiber area from biopsies to infer functional properties of human muscles after immobilization. The biggest problem with such stud-

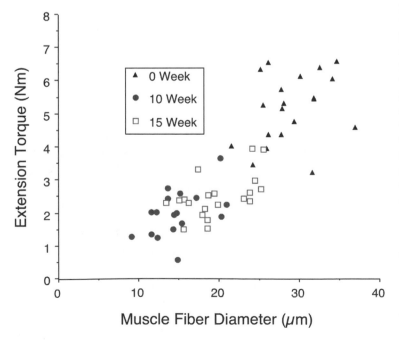

FIGURE 5-9. Relationship between fiber size and joint torque in the dog immobilization model. Each symbol obtained at different times after immobilization from 0 (filled triangles) to 10 weeks (filled circles) and after 5 weeks of remobilization (open squares). The fact that the relationship between fiber area and torque is maintained during immobilization and remobilization indicates that torque changes are due to changes in muscle fiber size. (Data from: Lieber, R.L., Jacks, T.M., Mohler, R.L., Schleim, K., Haven, M., Cuizon, D., Gershuni, D.H., Lopez, M.A., Hora, D., Nargund, R., Feeney, W., G.J. H. (1997). Growth hormone secretagogue increases muscle strength during remobilization after canine hindlimb immobilization. *Journal of Orthopaedic Research, 15,* 519–527.)

ies in humans is that the biopsies obtained represent a small area of the entire muscle and may not be representative since not all fibers within the muscle will be equally represented in a muscle biopsy.

Remobilization After Immobilization

How long does it take to recover from immobilization-induced atrophy? Interestingly, very few remobilization studies have been performed. The few that have been performed suggest that it takes longer to recover from immobilization than to elicit the initial response. This is a similar finding that was seen in which muscle "detraining" was about twice as fast as muscle "training" to endurance exercise (Fig. 4-27).

The dog study described above was essentially repeated by remobilizing canine quadriceps for 4 weeks after 10 weeks of immobilization (Lieber, McKee-Woodburn, Fridén, & Gershuni, 1989). During this 4- week remobilization period, normal activity was permitted, and daily 1-hour walking/running outings were encouraged. Normal weight-bearing resumed spontaneously within about 1 week.

As in the initial study, no difference in slow or fast fiber area was observed among any of the control muscles. However, 10 weeks of immobilization followed by 4 weeks of remobilization still resulted in about a 30% decrease (or not full recovery) of both slow and fast fiber areas (Figs. 5-6 and 5-7) relative to control. However, in contrast to the study of immobilization, no difference between immobilized muscle fiber areas was seen. While immobilization-induced atrophy was muscle and fiber type specific, recovery following immobilization was neither a function of muscle nor of fiber type. The fiber type transformation that occurred with immobilization had also returned to normal following remobilization.

A second difference between the immobilization and remobilization was that, while a large increase in the amount of extracellular connective tissue was seen after 4 weeks of immobilization, no difference was seen be-

tween control and remobilized muscles in the amount of extracellular connective tissue. Thus, the previously elevated area fraction of connective tissue (about 20%) observed after immobilization, returned to control levels (about 10%) after the remobilization period. Since connective tissue may be associated with passive muscle stiffness, these data may imply that muscle stiffness, which had increased due to the immobilization process, returned to normal after remobilization. Joint stiffness after immobilization is a significant clinical problem. Most previous experimental models of such stiffness have focused on changes that occur in the affected joint capsules and ligaments (Akeson, Amiel, Abel, Garfin, & Woo, 1987). However, these studies show that the muscle itself may represent a source of increased joint stiffness after immobilization.

The muscle response to remobilization may also be interpreted in light of the level of use experienced by each muscle following remobilization. Recall that the differential immobilization-induced atrophy based on the change in level of use relative to normal was explained. Now, during remobilization, it is presumed that the normal "use" levels returned and brought fiber area back to parity. Detailed confirmation of this hypothesis will await future experiments. However, quantifying "use" in terms of EMG, force, or movement is difficult technically, and excellent studies using these methods areas are lacking.

Adaptation to Spinal Cord Transection

Decreased use models have also been developed that induce either an upper- or lower-motor neuron lesion. As you will see, lower motor neuron disruption (denervation) induces numerous changes in muscle that are quite distinct from other decreased use models. (For example, a denervated muscle responds in a qualitatively different manner to chronic stimulation than a normal muscle.) This difficulty has been overcome by developing a model that interrupts the upper motor neuron pathway by transecting the spinal cord (*i.e.,* cordotomy; Fig. 5-10). This procedure has been performed in several animal models. Again, muscle contractile, histochemical, and biochemical alterations will be discussed after cordotomy.

Experimental Method of Rat Cordotomy

In a previous study, Lieber et al. were interested in the extent of muscle adaptation which could occur following long-term spinal cordotomy (Lieber, Johansson, Vahlsing, Hargens, & Feringa, 1986a). The rat was chosen as the experimental model since they live only 2–3 years and 1 year of cordotomy would represent about one-half a lifetime of chronic disuse.

Two groups of rats were studied. Control rats were permitted normal growth for 1 year after entry into the study at age 6 weeks. At age 6 weeks (about 2 weeks after the muscle fiber types were differentiated) experimental rats were anesthetized and, after laminectomy, the spinal cord and its coverings were completely transected.

Postoperative care of the cordotomized rats required special cage bedding to prevent pressure sores. Initially, there was a flaccid paraplegia with the limbs dragging behind the rats as they crawled about in the cage. They were able to move using their forelimbs, and had no difficulty reaching food and water. At approximately 3 to 4 weeks, the paralyzed hind limbs of the animals changed from flaccid to spastic. After spasticity developed, the limbs were almost always held in extension and no recovery of voluntary activity was ever observed. At first, it was exciting in that we thought this model could mimic the spasticity that is often observed in patients after stroke or head injury. However, this spasticity was qualitatively different from that observed in humans. Unfortunately, it cannot be explained why the rat spastic phase is transient and not reflective of the condition observed in humans. In fact, there is no adequate animal model for the type of spasticity seen in humans, which severely impairs our ability to understand and treat this debilitating condition.

Contractile Properties of Muscles After Long-Term Cordotomy

Two muscles were chosen for study—the soleus and the extensor digitorum longus (EDL). The two muscles differ in fiber type percentage (80% slow fibers in the soleus and 5% in the EDL). In this way, it would be possible to determine whether any observed effects of cordot-

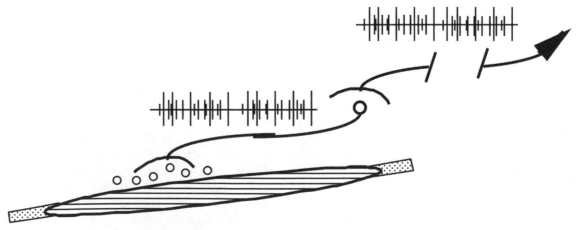

FIGURE 5-10. Schematic representation of the cordotomy model. The upper motor neuron pathway has been interrupted, but muscle EMG activity remains due to segmental influences. Muscle tension is low since the limbs are not used for locomotion.

Box 5-4. How Does Spinal Cord Injury Change Muscle Properties?

Spinal cord injury, as a typical decreased-use model, causes muscle to become weaker, due to muscle fiber atrophy, and faster, due to slow-to-fast fiber type conversion. In addition, there is evidence that, after chronic spinal cord injury, muscles become much more easily fatigued. Loss of strength, increased speed, and increased fatigability affect the patient's ability to perform normal activities of daily living. The good news is that all of these properties can be affected by the therapeutic interventions described in this book.

omy were fiber type- or muscle-specific. The contractile properties of the soleus and EDL muscles were tested in both groups of rats at age 58 weeks. The distal muscle insertion was carefully dissected free and attached to a force transducer. The peripheral nerve innervating the muscle was also carefully isolated and electrically activated using an artificial stimulator. Note that in spite of a year of cordotomy, the lower motor neuron was completely intact and able to be activated. Paralyzed muscle may still be quite functional.

The responses of the soleus from normal and transected rats stimulated at 5 and 10 Hz are shown in the upper and lower panels of Figure 5-11 respectively. Note that at 10 Hz, the transected soleus developed a greater force and was less fused than the soleus, implying faster contraction and/or relaxation. Unfused tetani of the EDL stimulated at 10, 20, and 30 Hz are shown in Figure 5-12. The differences between the normal EDL (upper panel) and transected EDL (lower panel) were clearly much less dramatic than those observed for the soleus.

Analysis of the averaged contractile responses showed that no differences were observed between normal and transected EDLs (Fig. 5-13). In contrast, for the soleus muscle, dramatic changes were observed in all contrac-

tile properties measured. For example, time to peak tension decreased by about 50% (Fig. 5-13A), suggesting a change in the properties of the sarcoplasmic reticulum. The change was probably due to an increase in the calcium transporting ability of the SR. Supporting this hypothesis, the soleus fusion frequency increased by 100% (Fig. 5-13B). Absolute maximum tetanic tension (in N) did not change significantly following transection. However, since the soleus muscle cross-sectional area decreased by about 50% (Fig. 5-13C), specific tension (in N/cm²) of the soleus significantly increased by over 100% one year following transection. Thus, the soleus muscle was half the cross-sectional area, but still generating the same tension (Fig. 5-13D)—How (See below, page 242)? To summarize, after transection,

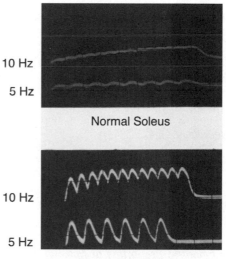

FIGURE 5-11. Unfused tetani from rat soleus muscles. Upper panel: records from control animals. Lower panel: records from transected animals. Note that the upper records demonstrate greater fusion than the lower records implying increased calcium transport kinetics following cordotomy. (From Lieber, R.L., Johansson, C.B., Vahlsing, H.L., Hargens, A.R., Feringa, E.R. (1986). Long-term effects of spinal cord transection on fast and slow rat skeletal muscle. I. Contractile properties. *Experimental Neurology, 91,* 423–434.)

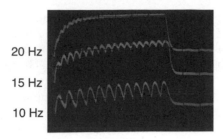

Normal EDL

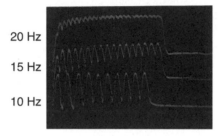

Transected EDL

FIGURE 5-12. Unfused tetani from rat extensor digitorum longus muscles Upper panel: records from control animals. Lower panel: records from transected animals. Very little difference is observed between records. (From Lieber, R.L., Johansson, C.B., Vahlsing, H.L., Hargens, A.R., Feringa, E.R. (1986). Long-term effects of spinal cord transection on fast and slow rat skeletal muscle. I. Contractile properties. *Experimental Neurology, 91*, 423–434.)

the soleus muscle increased in contractile speed and specific tension while no significant contractile changes were seen in the EDL.

Morphometric Properties of Muscles After Long-Term Cordotomy

To try to understand the contractile results, the fiber type and fiber size distributions were measured within the soleus and EDL using methods similar to those previously described (Lieber, Fridén, Hargens, & Feringa, 1986).

Low magnification cross-sections of normal soleus and EDL muscles stained for myofibrillar ATPase are presented in the upper panels of Figures 5-14 and 5-15, respectively. Note that in the normal soleus, fast fibers are scattered

throughout the muscle while the transected soleus (lower panel of Fig. 5-14) is composed almost entirely of fast fibers. This represents a dramatic slow-to-fast muscle fiber type conversion (the opposite type of conversion which we observed with chronic stimulation). The SOL at higher magnification (Fig. 5-16) showed a decreased size of both the slow and fast fibers. While fiber type transformation occurred in the EDL also (lower panel of Figure 5-15), the magnitude of the effect was small. The normal EDL contains only a few slow fibers (light staining) in the anterior superficial region of the muscle. After transection, even fewer slow fibers were visible.

Quantitative changes observed following transection were similar for both muscles although the magnitude of the changes were greater for the SOL compared to the EDL. As can be appreciated from the micrographs, the percentage of slow muscle fibers decreased significantly for both muscles. The average slow fiber area decreased significantly by about 50% for the SOL but not for the EDL. The percentage of fast fibers increased significantly for both muscles. Again, the magnitude of the increase was greater for the SOL. Fast fiber area decreased by about 25% in both muscles. The percentage of extracellular connective tissue increased significantly for both muscles by about the same amount. Thus, both muscles demonstrated fiber atrophy, a slow-to-fast fiber type transformation, and a significant increase in connective tissue. However, since the EDL is normally composed of about 95% fast fibers, these changes had no effect on contractile properties. Clearly such a transformation had much more profound consequences for the normally 80% slow soleus muscle. Finally, since the SOL muscle generated the same absolute contractile force in spite of its smaller muscle fibers, the force per unit area of muscle fiber (i.e., the specific tension) must have increased. Since most of the fibers in the SOL following cordotomy, it was concluded that the fast fibers of the rat have a higher specific tension than the slow fibers.

The Importance Of Tension In Determining Muscle Properties After Cordotomy

What factors contribute to the dramatic changes observed following cordotomy? What can be done to prevent these changes or to ameliorate recovery from such changes?

In yet another interesting plasticity study, Dr. Reggie Edgerton and his colleagues exercised adult cats that had been spinalized (Roy et al., 1998). After transection at the midthoracic level and 1 month of postoperative recovery, animals were exercised on a treadmill for 30 min/day for 6 months. Measurement of EMG activity after spinalization had shown the reduction similar to that seen in the immobilization models. In addition, using the implanted force transducers (such as those shown in Color Plate C-5A), direct measurement of muscle force during locomotion confirmed that significant weight bearing was induced by the exercise training procedure.

One of the goals of their study was to understand the role that muscle force played during rehabilitation of these severely atrophic

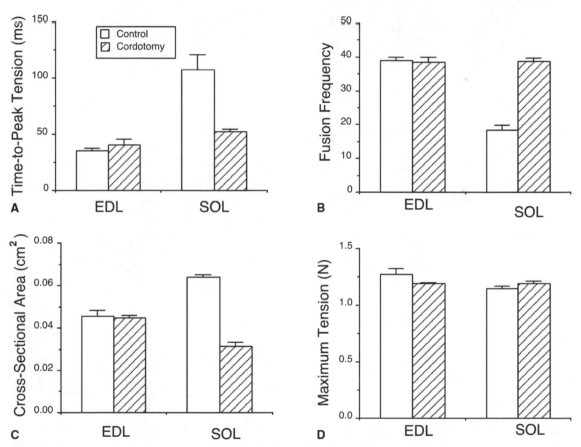

FIGURE 5-13. Contractile properties from normal (open bars) and cordotomized (hatched bars) rat skeletal muscles. **(A)** Time-to-peak twitch tension, **(B)** fusion frequency, **(C)** muscle cross-sectional area, and **(D)** maximum tetanic tension. Note that the soleus contractile properties changed dramatically while EDL properties show little change. (From Lieber, R.L., Johansson, C.B., Vahlsing, H.L., Hargens, A.R., Feringa, E.R. (1986). Long-term effects of spinal cord transection on fast and slow rat skeletal muscle. I. Contractile properties. *Experimental Neurology, 91*, 423–434.)

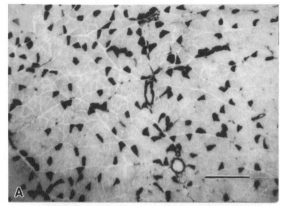

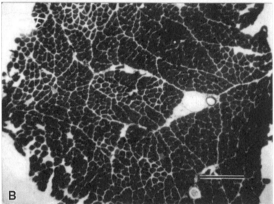

FIGURE 5-14. Low magnification micrographs from soleus muscle **(A)** before and **(B)** after cordotomy. Muscle sections stained for myofibrillar ATPase activity. Fast fibers are dark. Calibration bar represents 500 μm. Note the increase in fast fiber percentage following cordotomy. Right panel of micrographs represent higher magnification views of same muscles. Note the modest fiber atrophy. Calibration bars represent 100 μm. (From Lieber, R.L., Fridén, J.O., Hargens, A.R., Feringa, E.R. (1986). Long-term effects of spinal cord transection of fast and slow rat skeletal muscle. II. Morphometric properties. *Experimental Neurology, 91,* 435–448.)

planning this study, it was not even clear that it would be possible for a cat, with a transected spinal cord to "walk" on a treadmill. Edgerton, Roy, and colleagues published a sequence of fantastic electromyograms from these spinalized animals demonstrating tremendous, and nearly normal rhythmic activity of the locomotory muscles (Fig. 5-17) demonstrating that the spinal cord itself could be "trained" to recover the stepping pattern! This clearly indicated that

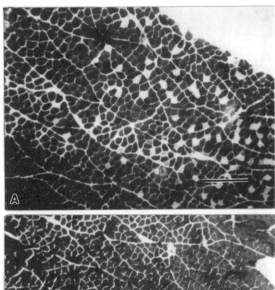

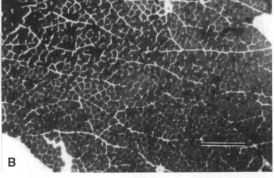

FIGURE 5-15. Low magnification micrographs from EDL muscle **(A)** before and **(B)** after cordotomy. Muscle sections stained for myofibrillar ATPase activity. Fast fibers stain darkly. Calibration bar represents 500 μm. Note the increase in fast fiber percentage following cordotomy which is more modest than the soleus. (From Lieber, R.L., Fridén, J.O., Hargens, A.R., Feringa, E.R. (1986). Long-term effects of spinal cord transection of fast and slow rat skeletal muscle. II. Morphometric properties. *Experimental Neurology, 91,* 435–448.)

muscles. To provide different muscle forces to the muscles, they compared training that involved standing alone with training that involved stepping along a treadmill with weight-bearing (De Leon, Hodgson, Roy, & Edgerton, 1998, 1999; Roy et al., 1998). Standing involves lower loads that are relatively constant while step training involves higher, more intermittent loading patterns to the muscles. In the reciprocal activation of limbs, phasic muscular activity, and amplitude of muscle activation are all parameters that could be initiated and controlled by the spinal cord.

After the 6 month training period, soleus muscle fiber histochemical properties were measured which demonstrated the expected slow-to-fast fiber type transformation. Not only were the usual qualitative histochemical stains implemented, but quantitative measurement of myosin ATPase activity (MATPase), succinate dehydrogenase activity

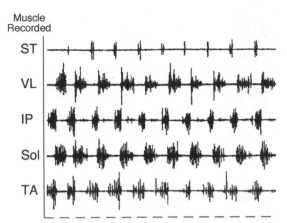

Muscle Recorded

FIGURE 5-17. Raw electromyogram record from hindlimb muscles of a spinalized cat during treadmill walking at 0.4 meters/s after step training had been performed. Note the rhythmic muscle activity and reciprocal activation of hip and ankle flexors and extensors. This indicates that the spinal cord can "learn" such properties in the absence of influence from higher centers. (Figure used with permission from De Leon, R.D., Hodgson, J.A., Roy, R.R., Edgerton, V.R. (1999). Retention of hindlimb stepping ability in adult spinal cats after the cessation of step training. *Journal of Neurophysiology, 81*, 85–94.)

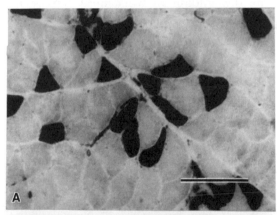

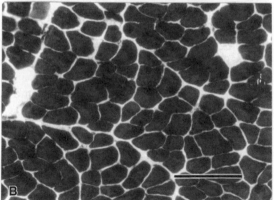

FIGURE 5-16. Higher magnification micrographs from soleus muscle **(A)** before and **(B)** after cordotomy. Muscle sections stained for myofibrillar ATPase activity. Fast fibers stain darkly. Note the modest fiber atrophy. Calibration bars represent 100 μm. (From Lieber, R.L., Fridén, J.O., Hargens, A.R., Feringa, E.R. (1986). Long-term effects of spinal cord transection of fast and slow rat skeletal muscle. II. Morphometric properties. *Experimental Neurology, 91*, 435–448.)

(SDH), and α-glycerophosphate dehydrogenase activity (αGP) were also measured which enabled detailed description of the fiber metabolic properties themselves. Six months of exercise caused muscle fiber size to be somewhat larger compared with spinalization without exercise. For example, while the normal SOL muscle fiber area was about 4200 μm^2, the spinalized slow fibers were about 2700 μm^2 and the spinalized+exercised slow fibers were about 3000 μm^2. The prevention of fiber atrophy by exercise was not complete, but the data suggest that the added muscle tension due to exercise improved muscle strength.

What about the functional changes that occurred in the muscles? The usual structural, functional, and biochemical properties were measured revealing not only the influence of spinalization but of training. First, compared to control subjects, the spinalized cats demonstrated significant loss in maximum tetanic tension (Fig. 5-18A), increase in V_{max} (Fig. 5-18B)

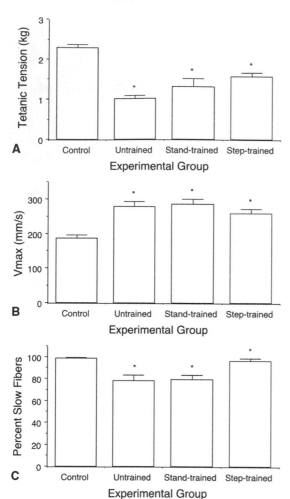

FIGURE 5-18. Functional and structural properties of soleus muscles from control and spinalized cats. **(A)** Maximum tetanic tension, **(B)** Maximum contraction velocity, and **(C)** Percentage of slow fibers. Note that in all cases, spinalization causes muscles to become weaker and faster whereas training tends to reverse these effects toward normal. If anything, step training is more effective than stand training in this regard. (Data plotted from: Roy, R.R., Talmadge, R.J., Hodgson, J.A., Zhong, H., Baldwin, K.M., Edgerton, V.R. (1998). Training effects on soleus of cats spinal cord transected (T12-13) as adults. *Muscle & Nerve, 21*, 63–71.)

and decrease in slow fiber percentage (Fig. 5-18C). Thus, the expected muscle atrophy and velocity increase expected by decreased use is observed. Interestingly, step training was much more effective in bringing muscle properties closer to "normal" compared with standing alone in terms of maximum force, muscle speed, and fiber type percentages. The authors suggested that, not only was the load important in determining muscle properties, but that the *rhythmic activity* of the motor nerves also caused muscle properties to be altered. These data may indicate that the muscle senses not only the amount of mechanical activity imposed upon it, but also the pattern of the activity itself. Although this is a highly speculative statement, it would not be surprising if muscles "tune" their structural and functional properties to fairly specific signals provided to them via the neuromuscular junction.

As has been seen repeatedly, the soleus is a highly responsive muscle that often shows atrophic and hypertrophic changes that are not "typical" of all muscles. To determine whether more typical muscles demonstrate the same response to spinalization and exercise, Dr. Roland Roy and colleagues performed similar studies on the faster muscles of the hindlimb and showed trends that were in the same direction but of a smaller magnitude (Roy et al., 1999). In fact, as you have already seen, a differential effect was demonstrated on the antigravity medial gastrocnemius (MG), a plantarflexor, compared to the tibialis anterior (TA), a dorsiflexor. As you might guess, the TA was much less responsive compared with the MG to spinalization and to the effects of exercise on the muscles. Again, all muscles are "not created equal" with regard to response to altered use. Muscles that demonstrate the greatest response to changes in use are those that are most often used (*e.g.*, antigravity muscles) such as the soleus, vastus intermedius and, to a lesser extent, quadriceps and gastrocnemius muscles.

In terms of metabolic properties, muscle oxidative capacity, as indicated by SDH activity did not change following spinalization, and even increased with exercise. Because the SOL muscles also demonstrated a significant slow-to-fast fiber type conversion, this increase in oxidative capacity probably reflected the increased SDH activity of the FOG fibers relative to SO fibers. This study illustrates that, while increases in SDH activity can occur relatively rapidly and to a large extent following increased use, the converse does not occur following decreased use. It appears that skeletal muscle fiber "baseline" oxidative capacity is not easily changed.

Application of Training to Humans

The obvious question one asks after reviewing the fantastic results reported by Edgerton, Roy, and colleagues obtained in cats is, "Can these therapeutic approaches to rehabilitation of the spinal cord injured subject be applied to humans?" In the face of tremendous scientific and clinical disbelief, Edgerton and colleagues showed tremendous leadership by repeating their experiments on human spinal cord injured patients. In effect, they basically achieved the same fantastic results—demonstrations of rhythmic locomotor activity, manifestations of weight-bearing, and presumably, improved muscle properties (Harkema et al., 1997). One clear lesson here is, do not be too quick to dismiss animal models while in search of answers to questions regarding human patients. In fact, it is difficult to define a result from animal muscle structure, function, or plasticity studies that, when repeated in humans, have not provided essentially the same result. This is good news for those interested in the physiological basis of therapy.

Clinical Relevance

The main result of these studies is that, after spinal cord injury, a slow-to-fast muscle fiber type transformation can occur. The consequences are that a dramatic change occurs in muscle contractile properties that have a large proportion of slow fibers. This clearly happens in a number of animal models as seen above and has been reported to occur in human pa-

tients as well (Grimby et al., 1976). As a result of this increased contraction and relaxation speed, these "slow" muscles become less able to generate low-level, prolonged contractions, as is required of predominantly slow muscles (e.g., soleus and vastus intermedius). If the specific tension of fast and slow muscle fibers differ, slow-to-fast transformation may result in increased (or, at least not decreased) muscle strength, causing an imbalance of muscle forces about the joint. The joints would thus tend to remain extended as most of the "antigravity" muscles contain a larger proportion of slow fibers. This concept may explain the observation that, after transection, the rat hindlimbs remained fully extended. However, this observation, even in animal models, is not universal.

This study suggests that paraplegia is not necessarily associated with muscular weakness, especially after a relatively long period. While neuromuscular weakness follows injury, muscle strength is not necessarily compromised. This is not to say that muscle strength cannot decrease, only that it is not necessarily decreased.

These data also show that modalities that increase muscle tension are effective in reducing the atrophy seen with spinalization alone. Thus far, it has not been possible to completely reverse the effects of spinalization, but perhaps future treatments might include greater exercise duration or intense muscle contractions (eccentric contractions? see Chapter 6).

Electrical Stimulation After Spinal Cord Injury in Humans

An obvious clinical intervention that could be used to prevent or at least minimize the effects of spinal cord injury is electrical stimulation. You have already seen that chronic electrical stimulation causes dramatic and persistent changes in mammalian skeletal muscle (Chapter 4, pages 174 to 179) and, when used clinically, can assist in strength recovery after disuse or injury (Chapter 4, pages 202 to 208). However, there are little physiological data available from the muscles of spinal cord injured patients that would make the application of a therapeutic intervention more rational. As a result of this void, using a transcutaneous electrical stimulation model (similar to that shown in Fig. 4-20), Dr. Rick Shields and colleagues studied the human soleus muscle by determining its fatigue properties in patients with complete spinal cord transection accompanied by complete sensory and motor paralysis. Two groups of patients were studied, those with acute paralysis (defined as less than 5 weeks from injury) and those with chronic paralysis (defined as more than 3 years since injury). Muscles were "fatigued" by activating the tibial nerve in the popliteal fossa using electrical stimulation. The pattern consisted of 20 Hz stimulation pulses delivered for 300 ms every 1.5 seconds over a total period of 3 minutes (Shields, Law, Reiling, Sass, & Wilwert, 1997). By design, this protocol was similar to that used by Dr. Bob Burke and colleagues who defined the fatigability of motor units (Chapter 2, page 92). (Burke, Levine, Tsairis, & Zajac, 1973). Shields et al. measured only about a 10% drop in torque generated by soleus muscles from the acute patients over the 3 minute stimulation period, but about an 80% drop in torque generated by the chronic patients (Fig. 5-19). Just as in the

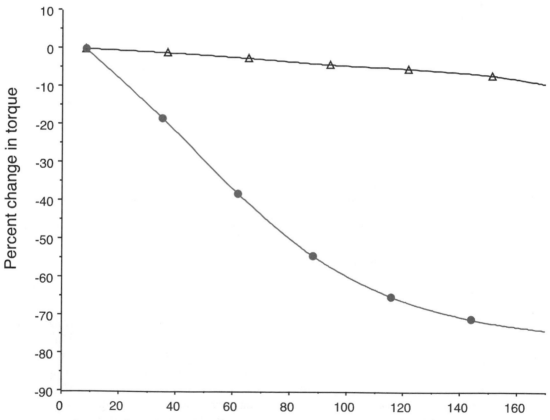

FIGURE 5-19. Increase in muscle fatigability after spinal cord injury. Quadriceps femoris muscles were electrically stimulated and torque measured as a function of time. Acutely injured patients (open triangles) showed muscle less drop in force compared to chronically injured (>2 years after injury) patients. (Data from: Shields, R.K., Law, L.F., Reiling, B., Sass, K., Wilwert, J. (1997). Effects of electrically induced fatigue on the twitch and tetanus of paralyzed soleus muscle in humans. *Journal of Applied Physiology, 82,* 1499–1507.)

discussion of fatigue, part of the question regarding the mechanism of this change relies on an understanding of the site of the fatigue measured. In a subsequent study, these authors demonstrated that, in response to electrical stimulation, the fatigued muscle actually generated near normal EMG activity in spite of the large drop in torque. This means that the fibers themselves were still being activated, but the force they generated was severely compromised (Shields, Chang, & Ross, 1998). Future studies are necessary to define, more precisely, the muscle fiber defects that cause the decreased performance observed.

The fact that the fatigability of these muscles is altered after injury is actually a bit promising in that it is a fairly straightforward task to change the endurance properties of skeletal muscle—presumably even paralyzed skeletal muscle. There is evidence that the endurance properties of muscles from spinal cord injured patients can be changed with electrical stimulation treatment. For example, increased vastus lateralis muscle fiber size (23%) and increased number of capillaries (40%) was reported by Chilibeck et al. who trained six patients for 30 min/day × 3 days/week × 8 weeks (Chilibeck, Jeon, Weiss, Bell, & Burnham, 1999). Similarly, an increase in the percentage of type 2A myosin heavy chain and decrease in percentage of type 2B myosin heavy chain was reported by Anderson et al., who trained vastus lateralis muscles for 30 min/day × 3 days/week for 6 and 12 months (Anderson, Mohr, Biering-Sorensen, Galbo, & Kjaer, 1996). There is thus no doubt that the muscles are able to adapt. Of course, the key issue is defining the mechanical conditions and "dose" of electrical stimulation necessary to elicit the appropriate functional changes (Baldi & Reiser, 1995).

Adaptation to Hindlimb Unloading

Recently, a new model for studying muscle fiber atrophy was developed. In cooperation with the National Aeronautics and Space Administration (NASA), Dr. Emily Morey developed the hindlimb unloading model for simulating the weightless environment (Morey, Sabelman, Turner, & Baylink, 1979). It is well known that space flight results in muscle atrophy and loss of bone mineral content. Astronauts who return from space are significantly weaker and more vulnerable to bone fracture. Such changes are similar to those observed with other decreased use models and thus, there is great interest in discovering the factors that cause them. In addition, because there is a good deal of support from NASA to study the problem of muscle atrophy, many muscle physiologists have decided to "specialize" in the problem of muscle atrophy secondary to weightlessness (Edgerton & Roy, 2000). Because it is extremely costly and logistically difficult to perform scientific research in space, this "ground-based" experimental model, the so-called "hindlimb unloading" model was developed (Fig. 5-20).

The Hindlimb Unloading Model

To mimic the effects of space flight, Morey and her colleagues removed the weight-bearing function of the rat hindlimbs. Connectors were secured to the base of the rat tail and were attached to a revolving gimbal mount at the top of the cage. The rats could easily navigate about the cage using their forelimbs to explore the cage and to feed themselves. Early experimental results using this model were promising: after hindlimb unloading, rats demonstrated many of the physical changes that had been documented in space flight: muscle atrophy, bone mineral loss, interstitial fluid shifts, and decreased growth. From the point of view of studying muscle plasticity, the hindlimb unloading model also provided a unique opportunity to study a "decreased use" model in which the lower motor neuron was intact and muscle tension was extremely low. (Incidentally, it was shown that the model itself caused a small degree of transient stress in the rats, based on measurement of a small increase in adrenal gland mass and transiently increased plasma corticosterone levels. These levels were very similar to other treatments in which the animal

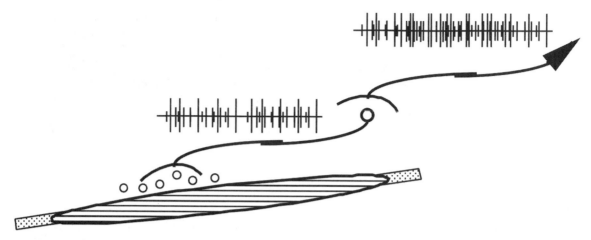

FIGURE 5-20. Schematic view of the hindlimb unloading model. Muscles experience little tension and a decreased (but finite) EMG activity.

Box 5-5. What Does Sending Animals and Humans into Space Have to Do with Physical Therapy?

Space flight produces repeatable changes in muscle unloading patterns that result in muscle fiber atrophy, fiber type transformation, and neuromuscular weakness. These are all very similar to the problems that human patients experience after surgery, prolonged disuse, or injury. To the extent that we understand these phenomena in space and can develop ways to prevent atrophy or recover from it, we can assist our patients here on earth.

---

was manipulated in some way, for example, applying a cast.)

Skeletal Muscle Activity During Hindlimb Unloading

In a manner similar to that described for their prior study of muscle immobilization, Alford et al. measured the chronic EMG activity from both the tibialis anterior ankle flexor and the soleus and medial gastrocnemius ankle extensors in order to better understand the level of muscle "use" that actually occurred during hindlimb unloading (Alford, Roy, Hodgson, & Edgerton, 1987). These investigators

showed that the extensor activity of the soleus and gastrocnemius muscles decreased initially and then returned to control levels after about 4 weeks (Fig. 5-21). However, the TA, which was slightly loaded because of gravity-induced ankle extension, actually increased electrical activity by 2–4 times. Thus, as with most experimental models, the hindlimb unloading model did not cause complete disuse (since the muscles retained some EMG activity).

Changes in Muscle Contractile Properties Following Hindlimb Unloading

Interestingly, in spite of the unremarkable changes in muscle EMG after hindlimb unloading, dramatic changes in muscle mass and muscle contractile forces have been reported by numerous investigators. The nature of these changes was as expected based on the previous immobilization studies. For example, Dr. Don Thomason, working in Dr. Ken Baldwin's laboratory, showed that the mass of both the plantaris and soleus muscles decreased continually throughout the unloading period (Fig. 5-22). This provided a nice comparison of two extensor muscles, one primarily composed of slow fibers (the soleus) and the other primarily composed of fast fibers (the medial gastrocnemius). Soon after unloading began, muscle mass of both muscles rapidly decreased. For the next 30 days, mass decreased at an increasingly slower rate until after about 30 days, mass stayed relatively constant.

The properties of other muscles subjected to unloading had also been measured in other

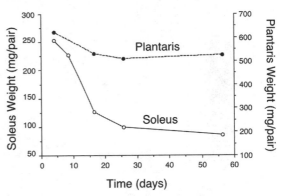

FIGURE 5-22. Change in muscle mass over an 8-week hindlimb unloading experiment. Muscle mass decreases quickly and then "levels off." The effect is more dramatic for the antigravity soleus muscle compared with the plantaris muscle, which has a greater percentage of fast fibers. (Data from: Thomason, D.B., Herrick, R.E., Surdyka, D., Baldwin, K.M. (1987). Time course of soleus muscle myosin expression during hindlimb unloading and recovery. *Journal of Applied Physiology, 63,* 130–137.)

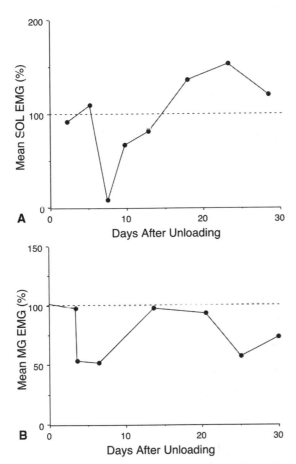

FIGURE 5-21. Skeletal muscle EMG following hindlimb unloading. Muscle EMG was measured continuously over 30 days after hindlimb unloading using indwelling electrodes. This graph shows that soleus (circles) and medial gastronemius (squares) EMG activity initially decreases and then returns to near normal levels after 7–10 days. Thus, hindlimb unloading is clearly not a "disuse" plasticity model. (Data from: Alford, E.K., Roy, R.R., Hodgson, J.A., Edgerton, V.A. (1987). Electromyography of rat soleus, medial gastrocnemius, and tibialis anterior during hindlimb suspension. *Experimental Neurology, 96,* 635–649.)

laboratories. Consistent with the change in mass, contractile tension of both muscle types decreased by about 50% during the same time period. Again, consistent with other decreased-use models, the soleus muscle demonstrated an increased muscle speed, as manifest by a decrease in both contraction and half-relaxation times and shift in fiber type percentage from slower to faster isoforms. Interestingly, Dr. Bob Fitts has reported that rat soleus muscle single fibers, subjected to hindlimb unloading can demonstrate an increase in V_{max} in the absence of a shift in myosin heavy chain. This indicates that V_{max} itself is determined by more than just the myosin isoform (McDonald, Blaser, & Fitts, 1994). These authors also demonstrated that, not only do all of the muscles not change properties to the same extent, the fibers, even of the same type, isolated from different muscles do not adapt identically. For example, slow fibers from the soleus decreased size, specific tension and increased their V_{max} values (Fig. 5-23A) whereas slow fibers from the medial gastrocne-

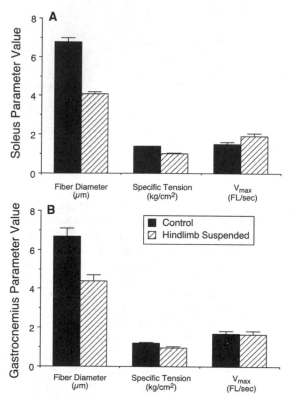

FIGURE 5-23. Change in fiber diameter, specific tension and V_{max} in single fibers from **(A)** rat soleus single fibers or **(B)** rat medial gastrocnemius single fibers. Note that fiber diameters are divided by 10 for display on the same axes as the other parameters. (Data from: Gardetto, P.R., Schluter, J.M., Fitts, R.H. (1989). Contractile function of single muscle fibers after hindlimb suspension. *Journal of Applied Physiology, 66,* 2739–2749.)

mius muscle decreased size, specific tension and yet showed no change in V_{max} (Fig. 5-23B). Again, this is a situation in which not only muscles, but also muscle fibers may have different susceptibilities to adaptation under altered use conditions.

Changes in Fast and Slow Muscle Fibers Following Hindlimb Unloading

Using quantitative analysis of muscle fiber area and muscle fiber enzyme activity, Drs. Edgerton and Roy demonstrated that the lower limb plantarflexors and dorsiflexors adapted differently

to the unloading (Hauschka, Roy, & Edgerton, 1987; Roy, Bello, Bouissou, & Edgerton, 1987). Whereas the fast and slow fibers within the gastrocnemius muscle atrophied by about 25%, the TA muscle fibers showed no atrophy whatsoever (Fig. 5-24). Part of the TA response was probably due to the slight stretch placed on the TA during unloading, but most of the change was probably attributable to the low responsiveness of the pretibial ankle flexor to decreased

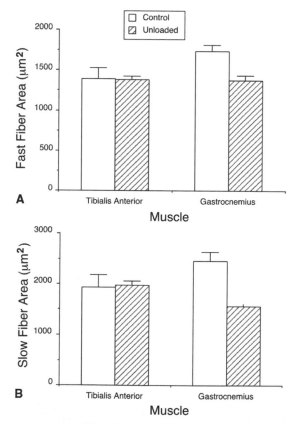

FIGURE 5-24. Muscle fiber area following hindlimb unloading. **(A)** Fast fiber area. **(B)** Slow fiber area. Note significant atrophy of the medial gastrocnemius but no atrophy of the tibialis anterior. These data indicate that not all muscles atrophy to the same extent. (Data from: Roy, R., Bello, M., Bouissou, P., Edgerton, R. (1987). Size and metabolic properties of fibers in rat fast-twitch muscles after hindlimb suspension. *Journal of Applied Physiology, 62,* 2348–2357.)

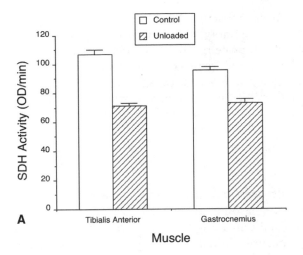

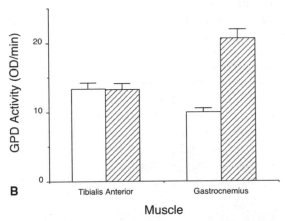

FIGURE 5-25. Muscle fiber enzyme activity following hindlimb unloading. **(A)** Muscle fiber oxidative capacity as indicated by succinate dehydrogenase (SDH) activity. **(B)** Muscle fiber glycolytic capacity as indicated by glycerol phosphate dehydrogenase (GPD) activity. Note the decrease in oxidative capacity is correlated with an increase in glycolytic capacity (Data from: Roy, R., Bello, M., Bouissou, P., Edgerton, R. (1987). Size and metabolic properties of fibers in rat fast-twitch muscles after hindlimb suspension. *Journal of Applied Physiology, 62,* 2348–2357.)

use. This is the same story that was seen with the immobilization and cordotomy models.

In terms of metabolic activity, the single fibers of both the MG and TA dramatically decreased in SDH activity while only the MG dramatically increased in α-GP activity (Fig.

5-25). This actually represented a departure from the norm in which decreased use models usually showed no change in muscle oxidative capacity. The increased α-GP activity was interpreted as before: glycolytic capacity appears to be matched to muscle fiber type. Thus, muscles that increase their proportion of fast fibers also increase their glycolytic capacity. (Incidentally, the same investigators demonstrated that 1.5 hours of exercise/day on a 30% grade at relatively high speeds could partially ameliorate these deleterious effects—further evidence that muscle tension can modulate the atrophic response.)

Mechanism of Muscle Fiber Atrophy

Introduction to Muscle Protein Turnover

You know already that the muscle fiber size is related to the number of myofibrils that are arranged in parallel within the fiber, and that myofibrils comprise 70%–80% of the total protein within the muscle cell. Thus, it follows that muscle force would be related to the total amount of myofibrillar protein within the fiber.

It may not be obvious, but all proteins (indeed, all cellular components) eventually "wear out" and die. The rate at which these different components are replaced depends on their location and function. The control center of the cell (the nucleus) is responsible for synthesizing new muscle proteins and repairing the portions of the cell that have been damaged or that have aged. If protein synthesis is completely blocked, the cell cannot repair itself and eventually dies (this is the basis for use of some chemotherapeutic drugs).

Protein synthesis and protein degradation are always occurring within the muscle cell, or any cell for that matter. In this way, cells retain the ability to adapt to a new environment. If proteins were permanently in place after synthesis, there would be no way to change them. Thus, proteins are constantly "turning over" to yield to the current cellular demands. It is this study of protein turnover in atrophying muscle that has provided new insights into the atrophy mechanism. To study these phenomena, it is not enough to simply know how much contractile material is present (*e.g.*, by measuring muscle mass) since the instantaneous amount of tissue mass present represents a balance between the amount of protein being made (synthesis) compared with the amount of protein being lost (degradation) (Fig. 5-26).

Protein Turnover During Hindlimb Unloading

Studies of protein turnover in muscle were pioneered in the muscle research laboratories of Drs. Ken Baldwin and Frank Booth. These investigators measured rates of synthesis and degradation in muscles following various "altered-use" models and have "painted a picture" of muscle mass regulation following altered used. Specifically, hindlimb unloading was studied by Dr. Don Thomason working in both laboratories (Thomason, Herrick, Surdyka, & Baldwin, 1987). Recall the data demonstrating that both plantaris and soleus muscle mass decreased continually throughout the unloading period. For about the first 30 days of unloading, mass decreased at an increasingly slower rate (Fig. 5-22). After about 30 days, mass stayed rela-

tively constant. Muscle mass (or change in mass) simply represents the net balance between protein synthesis and degradation. This means that mass could decrease even if degradation rate decreased, so long as synthesis rate decreased more. Similarly, mass could increase even if synthesis rate decreased, as long as degradation rate decreased even more. What was the explanation for muscle mass changes following hindlimb unloading?

Changes in Synthesis and Degradation

Thomason et al. showed that, soon after hindlimb unloading (within a day), soleus muscles decreased their protein synthetic rate by about 50% and this rate remained relatively constant for the remainder of the unloading period (up to 7 days have been measured) (Thomason, Biggs, & Booth, 1989). The protein synthesis rate decrease occurred in spite of the fact that soleus EMG activity continued to increase (another lesson demonstrating that increased electrical "activity" does not translate into increased strength). Since muscle mass continued to decrease during this rate of constant protein synthesis, the data predicted that protein degradation rate must have increased from the

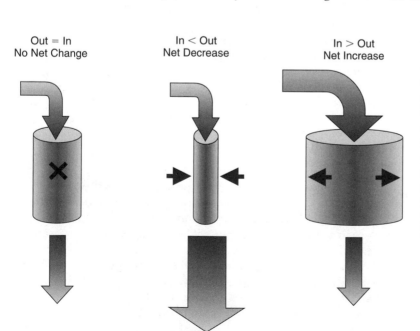

Out = In
No Net Change

In < Out
Net Decrease

In > Out
Net Increase

FIGURE 5-26. Schematic figure illustrating the balance between synthesis and degradation and its effect on "mass." **(A)** Equal inflow to and outflow from the tank so that the net volume of water (analogous to mass) remains the same. **(B)** Inflow to tank is less than outflow from tank so that net volume decreases. **(C)** Inflow to tank is greater than outflow from tank so that net volume increases.

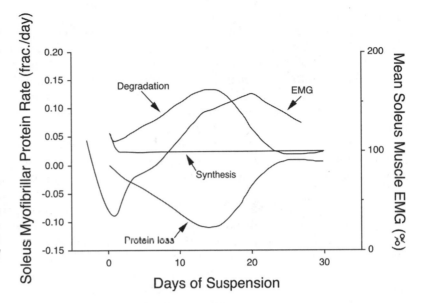

FIGURE 5-27. Time course of muscle mass and protein synthesis and degradation during rat hindlimb unloading. Initially, the electromyogram (EMG) activity decreases, resulting in an increase protein degradation and decreased protein synthesis rate. Subsequently, EMG increases. (Figure redrawn from: Thomason, D.B., Herrick, R.E., Surdyka, D., Baldwin, K.M. (1987). Time course of soleus muscle myosin expression during hindlimb suspension and recovery. *Journal of Applied Physiology, 63,* 130–137.)

4th to 14th day of unloading, then degradation decreased to a value less than control at which time degradation must have become relatively constant (Fig. 5-27). All of these calculations are based on the fact that total muscle mass always represents the net balance between synthesis and degradation.

The take-home lesson from these experiments is that, in hindlimb unloading, it took about 30 days for the muscle to reach a new state of homeostasis even under constant unloading conditions. The phenomenon must be even more complicated under conditions when muscle state changes continually (*e.g.*, exercise, immobilization, continuous passive motion).

Cellular Control of Synthesis and Degradation After Unloading

What are the factors that caused the synthetic and degradation rates observed? Clearly, electrical activity was not the cause of either the synthetic or degradation rates (compare Figure 5-21 with Figure 5-27). Take a step back from measuring the rates of protein synthesis and look at the earlier events that precede protein synthesis, namely, mRNA formation. This is the trend of many adaptation studies being performed today. Instead of measuring protein levels, most investigators are studying mRNA lev-

els because, by looking at earlier events, it is possible to look at the immediate effects of the treatment rather than events that happen much later.

Recall that the central dogma of molecular biology is that DNA is produced by replication, DNA single strands are encoded into mRNA by transcription, and mRNA single strands are used to make protein by the process of translation. Thus, potentially replication, transcription, or translation can all be used to change the level of any cellular protein. Booth and his colleagues have looked at several different mRNAs and have found very small decreases in mRNA coding for either α-actin (measured after 1 day of unloading) or the β-myosin heavy chain (measured after 7 days of unloading) (Babij & Booth, 1988a). This small change was measured even though the synthesis rates of both proteins had decreased precipitously during these time periods. Specifically, after 7 days, α-actin mRNA concentration decreased by only 30% but synthetic rate decreased by about 60%. Finally, administration of clenbuterol abolished the 30% decrease in α-actin mRNA, but had no effect on protein synthetic rate.

They concluded that, while hindlimb unloading resulted in downregulation of both transcription and translation, the dramatic synthesis rate decrease was primarily due to the downregulation of translation. Apparently, there was more than enough mRNA in the muscle cell such that α-actin mRNA concentrations did not limit the synthetic rate. Recently, Booth reviewed other plasticity models and showed that regulation can occur (and does occur) at many different levels within the cell. The unifying principles that explain why regulation should occur at one point or another remain to be elucidated (Booth & Thomason, 1991).

In an attempt to address the molecular basis of muscle adaptation to unloading, Dr. Baldwin and his colleagues developed a model in which they directly transferred DNA fragments into rat soleus muscles and used "reporter genes" (*i.e.*, genes that code for a visible or measurable protein) to determine which portions of the DNA were active. In most genes, the portion of the DNA that precedes the actual coding region determines the conditions under which the gene is transcribed and is termed the "promoter." To identify the specific region of the DNA sequence that was responsible for activating the soleus muscle myosin heavy chain gene, they inserted different "constructs" (pieces of DNA created with specific regions of the upstream region inserted into a plasmid) into the muscle and measured reporter gene activity. Three constructs were investigated—those containing the 3500, 914, or 408 base pairs (bp) of DNA that were normally observed before the coding region (expressed as negative numbers since the DNA is "upstream" of the coding region) (Fig. 5-28). They found that, for the −3500, −914, and −408 bp constructs, reporter gene activity decreases by about 40% with hindlimb unloading indicating that the constructs still contained the "load-sensitive" portion of the gene while with the −215 bp construct, there was no significant change in reporter gene activity. Thus, the muscle's ability to "sense" unloading was contained in the DNA sequence between 215 and 408 base pairs upstream of the myosin heavy chain gene (Fig. 5-28). You can probably anticipate that the next series of experiments will be to identify the spe-

cific DNA binding regions and even DNA sequences that affect the mechanical and biological response to unloading. You have already seen that there are many DNA binding proteins that affect muscle development (the so-called myogenic regulatory factors or MRFs). It is highly likely that similar transcription factors are at work in regulating muscle response to load. Since muscle atrophy is the "problem" that is addressed by these studies, there is the intriguing possibility that, in the future, gene therapy could be used to cause muscle hypertrophy in postoperative or injured patients or that it could be used to prevent atrophy in the first place. Picture this: a small piece of DNA is delivered to the muscle in a patient with severe muscle atrophy. The gene contains the promoter region to "turn on" the muscle hypertrophy program. After delivery of the gene to the muscle, it is "turned on" using a simple antibiotic such as Tetracycline because the piece of DNA contained a Tetracycline-sensitive region. The patient could cause muscle hypertrophy as long as necessary to recover their function. A bit far-fetched to be sure, but not out of the question.

Adaptation to Aging

One could argue that aging represents a chronic increased use model since the changes that occur in aged muscle occur after many decades of activity. However, current experimental evidence suggests that the changes observed are actually due to the low level of use experienced by muscles as an individual ages. The literature in this area is fairly new and extremely relevant since the aged population is the fastest growing subgroup in the world (2000). Experimental data obtained from the aging model in both humans and animals offers the NIA working group the unique opportunity to test much of the muscle knowledge gained elsewhere in this textbook. As the data are presented, think about the underlying structural bases that could explain the observations and see if you can come up with the next experiment.

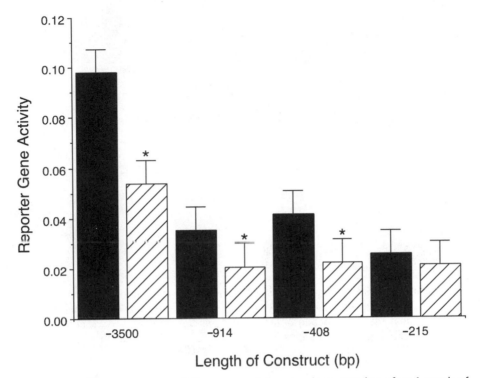

FIGURE 5-28. Reporter gene activity measured in rat soleus muscles after 1 week of hindlimb unloading. Filled bars represent activity of control rats while hatched bars represent activity of hindlimb suspended rats. Note that for the −3500, −914, and −408 bp constructs, activity decreases by about 40% with hindlimb unloading (asterisks) whereas with the −215 bp construct, there is no significant change in activity. This suggests that the portion of the promoter region sensitive to hindlimb unloading lies between 215 and 408 bp upstream of the myosin heavy chain gene. (Data from: Giger, J.M., Haddad, F., Qin, A.X., Baldwin, K.M. (2000). In vivo regulation of the beta-myosin heavy chain gene in soleus muscle of suspended and weight-bearing rats. *American Journal of Physiology, 278,* C1153–C1161.)

Strength Changes with Aging

Studies of muscle strength in humans across a range of ages have demonstrated that strength loss occurs in a fairly similar fashion in different muscle groups studied. The small intrinsic muscles of the hand seem to get about as weak as muscles within the proximal and distal leg segments. Thus, to a first approximation, when discussing muscle aging, the muscle group studied does not need to be extremely specified. Primarily for practical reasons, the most studied muscle group in humans is the vastus lateralis. You have already seen this muscle studied extensively in trying to understand muscle adaptation to exercise. Many of the

---

Box 5-6. Why Is Older Muscle Weaker?

With aging, muscle becomes weaker for several reasons. First, muscle fiber size decreases which results in a muscle that has a smaller cross-sectional area. Second, the number of fast muscle fibers decreases which itself causes strength loss. In addition, there is evidence that ability to activate motor units decreases with age so that even the fibers that remain in the muscle are not used. The good news is that exercise, even performed by patients older than 90, is effective at reversing many of these changes.

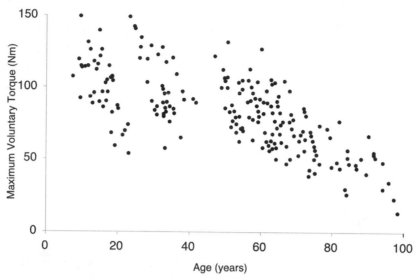

FIGURE 5-29. Maximum quadriceps extension torque measured in 111 healthy subjects ranging from 20 to 100 years old. Note that maximum strength declines near the sixth decade of life. (Data from: Vandervoort, A.A., McComas, A.J. (1986). Contractile changes in opposing muscles of the human ankle joint with aging. *Journal of Applied Physiology, 61,* 361–367.)

tools developed to study quadriceps in general and the vastus lateralis in particular have now been applied to studies of the aged individual.

Review of the quadriceps strength data available suggests that pronounced declines in strength do not occur until well into the sixth decade of life. At this point, across many studies and using a variety of methods, strength begins to decrease precipitously (Fig. 5-29). Of course, the underlying question is, "Why?" "Strength" is a very complex phenomenon that has underlying muscular, tendinous, nervous, and skeletal components. One of the first questions to be addressed is, "Is the strength loss associated with aging primarily muscular or neural in nature?" This is important if rational therapeutic measures are to be developed to combat the aging process and to understand the effects of age on each system independently. In much the same way as individuals study muscle fatigue to try to identify the "site" of fatigue (Chapter 2, pages 102–105) similar tools are applied to the study of neural drive in aged muscle. An individual is asked to maximally ac-

tivate their muscle and an electrically generated muscle "twitch" is superimposed upon the voluntarily contracting muscle. Although there are some technical limitations to this so-called "twitch interpolation method" (Enoka & Fuglevand, 1993), there are several reliable reports demonstrating that neural drive does not limit strength in aging (Vandervoort & McComas, 1986). Of course, the tasks measured were very simple and this does not imply that aging might be accompanied by more subtle neurological changes (see below).

Muscle Fiber Size and Number Changes with Aging

If strength is due to muscular changes, what types of changes have been measured? What do you think would be the most definitive demonstration that muscle changes cause muscle weakness? As you might expect, many studies report the fiber type and fiber size distribution within a relatively small, but hopefully representative, vastus lateralis muscle biopsy (Essen-Gustavsson & Borges, 1986; Larsson,

Sjodin, & Karlsson, 1978; Lexell, Taylor, & Sjöström, 1988). These authors generally agree that aging results in an increase in the relative percentage of type 1 muscle fibers and that the fiber atrophy observed is most pronounced for type 2 fibers. The magnitude of such changes ranges from about 5% to 15%, certainly not enough to explain the dramatic strength losses. Even so, how can the change in fiber type percentage be explained? The most obvious explanation invokes a type 2 to type 1 fiber type transformation secondary to chronic increased use. While this is attractive, it is a difficult proposition to test. It would require serial testing of muscle at very long time intervals. It has not yet been presented in this text, but another obvious explanation for an increase in the percentage of type 1 muscle fibers would be a selective loss of type 2 muscle fibers—type 2 muscle fiber death due to aging. Again, such a hypothesis would be extremely difficult to test. However, a series of excellent studies by the Swedish neurologist Dr. Jan Lexell and his colleagues have provided such a test. Lexell et al. developed a novel method for freezing, sectioning, staining, and sampling the *entire* vastus lateralis muscle from humans who had suffered a sudden accidental death (Lexell, Downham, & Sjöström, 1984). Muscles were obtained within 3 days post mortem and the histochemical methods described in Chapter 2 were used to create an entire profile of fiber type and fiber size across the muscle. This was performed in relatively young, healthy men as well as an aged population ranging from 19 to 84 years old (Lexell & Downham, 1992; Lexell, Henrikkson-Larsen, Winblad, Sjöström, 1983). These authors confirmed the increase in type 1 fiber type percentage from about 50% in the "20 year olds" to about 60% in the "70+ year olds" (Fig. 5-30A). However, this effect was weak and not statistically significant. What was more dramatic was the large atrophy in type 2-fiber area (almost 50%, Fig. 5-30B) and, unexpectedly, the large decrease in type 2 fiber number. Using these two parameters, they calculated the relative area of the muscle occupied by type 2 fibers and found that it decreased from

about 55% of the muscle in the younger age groups to only about 30% of the muscle in the older age groups (Fig. 5-30C). This then provided the explanation for the dramatic loss in strength and the relatively modest increase in the percentage of type 1 muscle fibers. More recently, the detailed properties of aged human muscle fibers have been studied with high-resolution mechanical and biochemical experimentation on single fibers obtained from human muscle and even myosin molecules obtained from single fibers of human muscle (Degens, Yu, Li, & Larsson, 1998; Hook, Li, Sleep, Hughes, & Larsson, 1999).

Motor Unit Changes with Aging

If muscle fiber number decreases with age, what happens to the number of muscle fibers within each motor unit? If motor neurons and muscle fibers are lost at the same relative rate, innervation ratio will stay constant. If relatively more muscle fibers than neurons are lost, innervation ratio will decrease whereas if relatively more neurons than fibers are lost, innervation ratio will increase. Using the spike-triggered averaging method presented in Chapter 2 (page 99), it has been demonstrated that the number of motor units decreases and the average motor unit innervation ratio increases after about age 60 (Brown, Strong, & Snow, 1988; McComas, 1995; Stalberg & Fawcett, 1982). In other words, there are more muscle fibers per motor unit and there are even electrophysiological and some morphological manifestations of denervation and reinnervation (giant electrical potentials and fiber type grouping). These observations suggest that, neurons may be lost and denervated muscle fibers remaining are reinnervated by nearby sprouting axons from existing motor units. There is evidence of a loss in alpha motor neurons within the spinal cord with subsequent degeneration of their axons (Kawamura, Okazaki, O'Brien, & Dych, 1977a,b). It is no wonder that many of the current "anti-aging" therapies focus on strategies to increase the quality and quantity of nervous tissue avail-

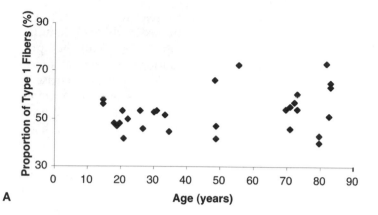

A

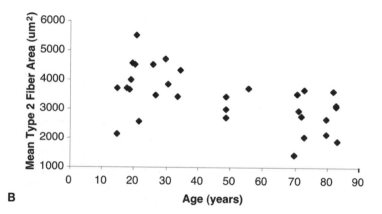

B

FIGURE 5-30. Muscle fiber characteristics change with age. **(A)** Proportion of slow (type 1) fibers, **(B)** Mean fast fiber area, and **(C)** Relative type 2 fiber area. The relative area of fast fibers across the muscle appears to decrease with age due to their decreased size. (Data from: Lexell, J., Henriksson-Larsen, K., Winblad, B., Sjöström, M. (1983). Distribution of different fiber types in human skeletal muscles: Effects of aging studied in whole muscle cross sections. *Muscle Nerve, 6,* 588–595.)

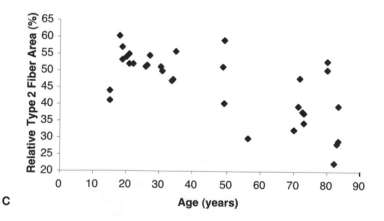

C

able. It is exciting to see such studies. Stay "tuned in" to the fantastic studies currently underway in this field throughout the world.

A final word about treating the aged muscle—there is conclusive evidence that even very old muscle (from individuals older than 90 years) can be strengthened using exercise therapy (Fiatarone et al., 1990; Hagberg et al., 1989; Pyka, Lindenberger, Charette, & Marcus, 1994). It was once thought that exercise in the elderly, which involved high exertion levels might be dangerous from the point of view of excessive blood pressure that could lead to stroke. However, several individuals have shown that this is not the case and, in fact, there are tremendous physical and psychological benefits to strength training in the elderly.

Mechanisms of Cellular Aging

THE OXIDATIVE STRESS HYPOTHESIS

Currently, there is not complete agreement on what defines aging at the cellular level. However, one idea that has been gaining momentum and for which a good deal of experimental support exists is the idea that free radicals generate by the normal oxidative processes might initiate damage and lead to degenerative changes (Sohal & Weindruch, 1996). Free radical scavengers naturally exist in nature and their quantity decreases with age. Thus, the free radicals produced by, for example, oxidative phosphorylation may cause damage to cellular components, most importantly nuclear DNA that could alter the lifespan of the cell. A fascinating experiment was performed by the gerontologists, Drs. Raj Sohal, Rick Weindruch, and colleagues in which the lifespan of insects was altered simply by adjusting the level of free radicals within their tissues. The experimental animal of choice was the fruit fly because it has such a short lifespan (~50 days) and literally hundreds of generations can be studied within a relatively short period of time. In an early ex-

periment, these authors created a genetically altered line of flies that overexpressed the free radical scavenger molecules superoxide dismutase (SOD) and catalase (Orr & Sohal, 1994; Sohal & Weindruch, 1996). Both of these molecules "absorb" free radicals that are generated by the tissue, presumably eliminating the damage that they would cause. Amazingly, transgenic flies overexpressing SOD and catalase had a lifespan that was nearly one-third longer than their nontransgenic controls and biochemical evidence of either protein damage or DNA damage was much attenuated (Fig. 5-31A). The flies with the longer life span (open circles, Fig. 5-31A) also had a lower fraction of oxidized proteins in the tissue. These flies also walked faster and consumed more oxygen over their lifespan (per unit body weight). Subsequently, the authors demonstrated that the ability of mice to swim through a maze was correlated with oxidative damage to the cerebral cortex (the portion of the brain that controls movement) and coordination during movement was correlated with oxidative damage to the cerebellum (the portion of the brain that controls coordination) (Forster et al., 1996). It thus appears that oxidative damage to tissue may be a general phenomenon not limited to muscle. Perhaps it even relates to differences in longevity among different populations around the world (Trichopoulou & Vasilopoulou, 2000).

CALORIC RESTRICTION AND AGING

A second method that these investigators used to minimize cellular oxidative stress was to limit the caloric intake of experimental animals. Obviously, food must be provided at some minimal level to maintain life itself, but there is conclusive evidence in laboratory rodents and supportive evidence in primates that food consumption above an optimal level progressively shortens lifespan. The authors have suggested that the "excess" calories (*i.e.*, those in excess of basic metabolic requirements) serve as fuel for the production of free radicals. This affect of caloric intact on life span was clearly seen in mice that were permitted to eat ad libidum, which weighed about 50 grams and

---

Therapist's Comments

Regarding the exercise studies for the elderly, I think it is important to remind therapists that the investigators were using a protocol that started with fairly light weights and progressed to a typical 3 sets of 8–12 repetitions with heavier weights. Specific sets and reps from these studies are difficult to come across but have been published elsewhere.

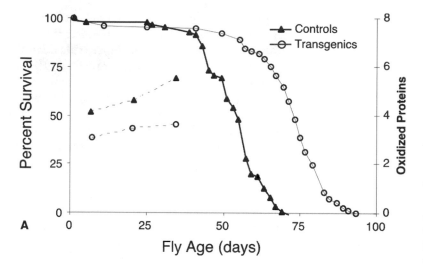

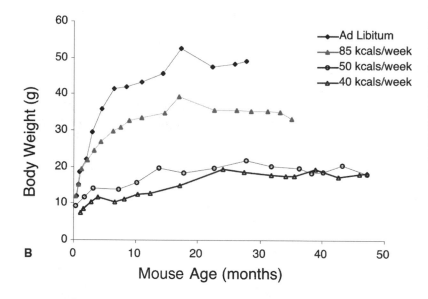

FIGURE 5-31. (A) Left symbols: Amount of DNA demonstrating "injury" in normal (filled symbols) and genetically altered fruit flies (open symbols) as indicated by the relative frequency of oxidized proteins. Right symbols: Difference in lifespan in fruit flies that overexpress a free-radical scavenger compared to normal fruit flies. Expression of a free radical scavenger decreases DNA damage and increases lifespan. **(B)** Body weight of mice permitted to eat different amounts of food ranging from 40 kcals/week to unlimited amounts (Ad libitum) (Data from: Sohal, R.S., Weindruch, R. (1996). Oxidative stress, caloric restriction, and aging. *Science, 215,* 1415–1418.)

which lived about 30 months (Fig. 5-31B). In contrast, mice that had their caloric intake restricted to about 40 kcal/week (less than half of the calories eaten by the other mice) only weighed about 20 grams and lived almost 50 months! These are clearly effects that are dramatic and deserve serious consideration for future aging studies. The data provide support for the consumption of enough calories to maintain normal physiological processes, but not so many that they serve as a source of free radicals that can themselves cause tissue damage.

A more recent caloric restriction study was performed by these same investigators using the modern molecular method of "gene array screening." This is a powerful method that is able to measure the expression levels of literally thousands of genes within an animal after a particular treatment and express those changes relative to some control animal (Lockhart et al., 1996; Marshall, 1999). The power of this method is that it provides a global indication of the large "players" in any treatment whether it be aging, exercise, disease, or surgery. This ap-

---

Box 5-7. Can You Really Eat Less and Live Longer?

It seems so. Fairly conclusive evidence in insect and rodent models demonstrate that caloric restriction results in greatly increased life spans. Increased life span also results from experimental treatments in which free-radical scavengers such as Vitamin E and superoxide dismutase (SOD) are given to the animals. Caloric restriction and antioxidants, at the molecular level, seem to prevent change in about 85% of the genes that normally change with age.

---

proach is more general in that the investigator, who may have a bias toward a particular gene or protein, can still obtain a "novel" result from a less familiar gene or protein. In addition, by investigating thousands of genes, it is possible to understand global changes to entire "classes" of genes (*e.g.*, genes encoding contractile proteins, metabolic enzymes, DNA repair enzymes, etc.). There is no doubt that you will see an increasing number of these types of studies.

Weindruch and colleagues compared 6,347 genes between adult (aged 5 months) and old (aged 30 months) mice (representing 5–10% of the mouse genome) (Fig. 5-32) (Lee, Klopp, Weindruch, & Prolla, 1999). Initially, you might think that the aged mice would simply show that all genes would merely "slow down" with time. In fact, this was clearly not the case. Specifically, only about 0.9% of the genes displayed a greater than 2-fold increase in expression while only about 0.9% displayed a greater than 2-fold decrease with age. Clearly aging was not synonymous with "running down." Most of the genes that increased with age (16% of those that changed) were mediators of the stress response such as proteins that "chaperone" other injured proteins for destruction or repair, DNA repair proteins, or other proteases (solid bars, Fig. 5-32). Consistent with changes that have already been discussed in aging—the inability for motor nerves to reinnervate muscle fibers, 9% of the upregulated genes were involved in neuronal growth. Of the genes that showed decreased expression with age, most (13%) were involved with energy metabolism

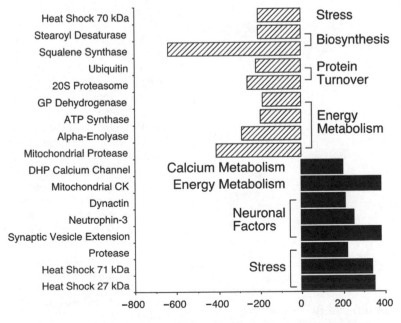

FIGURE 5-32. Summary of genes that are upregulated and downregulated with aging as determined by gene array screening. Filled bars represent upregulated genes while hatched bars represent downregulated genes. In spite of the large number of genes listed here, less than 1% of all the genes studied were affected. (Data from: Lee, C.K., Klopp, R.G., Weindruch, R., Prolla, T.A. (1999). Gene expression profile of aging and its retardation by caloric restriction. *Science, 285,* 1390–1393.)

Percent Change in Gene Expression

including glycolysis, ATP synthesis, and glycogen metabolism (hatched bars, Fig. 5-32). Other enzymes involved in protein and fatty acid synthesis decreased as well. The authors then used the same experimental approach applied to old mice who also had experienced a 24% caloric restriction similar to that described above and compared those results to aging alone (in this latter experiment, the aged mice became the "control" group). Recall that caloric restriction in fruit flies and in mice increased their life span significantly (Lee et al., 1999; Sohal & Weindruch, 1996). What was the molecular basis for such an effect? The authors found that caloric restriction completely or partially prevented the age-related changes in 84% of the genes that had shown significant changes with aging. Additionally, caloric restriction caused upregulation of other metabolic genes and synthetic genes with downregulation of DNA repair and stress genes. This implies an overall ability of the calorically restricted animals to resist the oxidative stress and decreased necessity to repair damaged cellular components—all good news.

AGED MUSCLE SUSCEPTIBILITY TO ECCENTRIC INJURY

The next chapter will provide a comprehensive discussion of mechanical injury to muscle that is forced to lengthen while activated (so-called "eccentric" contractions). For now, suffice it to say that forcing a muscle to lengthen while it is activated can cause injury and the greater the stretch, the greater the injury. To investigate the susceptibility of aged muscle to resist injury, Drs. Susan Brooks and John Faulkner compared the magnitude of force deficit after a single eccentric contraction between adult mice (aged 9–12 months) and aged mice (aged 27–34 months). They found that eccentric contractions caused injury in both adult and aged muscles. However, the magnitude of the force deficit was much greater in the aged muscles compared with the adult muscles (Fig. 5-33) (Brooks & Faulkner, 1990). This differential injury and limited recovery of aged muscles subjected to chronic eccentric exercise was even suggested as the explanation for the mechanism of loss in muscle force production in response to age that was shown above

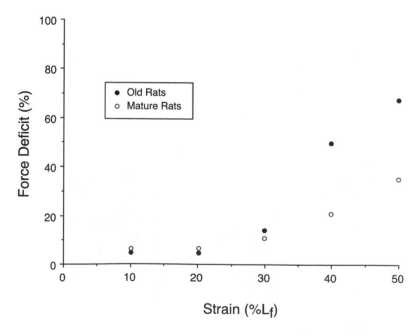

FIGURE 5-33. Relationship between muscle fiber strain (%L_f) and force deficit (percentage decline from initial force level) for adult (open circles) and aged (filled circles) extensor digitorum longus muscles. Force deficit increases with increasing strain and to a greater extent in the aged muscles. Aged muscles appear to be more sensitive to fiber strain compared with adult muscles. (Data from: Brooks, S.V., Faulkner, J.A. (1990). Contraction-induced injury: Recovery of skeletal muscles in young and old mice. *American Journal of Physiology, 258,* C436–C442.)

(Faulkner, Brooks, & Zerba, 1995). Whether injured aged muscles lose force-producing capability and are less able to mount the hypertrophic response has never been tested. This is, of course, a critical gap in our knowledge because if aged muscle is more easily injured and unable to adapt, then such injury should be judiciously avoided. If, however, injured aged muscle produces a vigorous strengthening response, the eccentric contractions would be expected to provide a potent strengthening stimulus to aged muscle. Again, future studies must resolve these unknown issues.

Adaptation to Tenotomy

Yet another model of decreased use is created when the insertion site of a tendon is surgically released or traumatically ruptures. This is known as tenotomy. In the early days of muscle research, this was used as a model to "create disuse atrophy" of the muscle. However, in the same way that a muscle without its associated motor nerve is neither normal nor "happy," a muscle under no load is also not "happy." As with denervation (see below) there are vast clinical implications of the changes that occur both in muscles and tendons after tenotomy because its occurrence is so common. There are numerous examples of tendon injuries that lead to severe debilitation. These include rotator cuff rupture, Achilles tendon injury, flexor and extensor tendon laceration in the hand, and patellar tendon rupture. Surgeons also intentionally cut tendons in corrective surgery. For example, surgical tenotomy is used in ophthalmology for realignment of the optic axis (Saunders, Bluestein, Wilson, & Berland, 1994). Tenotomy is commonly performed in foot and ankle surgery for treatment of hallux valgus, in hand surgery for tendon transfers and treatment of Mallet finger (Brzezienski & Schneider, 1995), in sports medicine for treatment of tendinitis (Leadbetter, Mooar, Lane, & Lee, 1992), in the treatment of rheumatologic diseases such as hamstring tenotomy for hemo-

philiac arthropathy of the knee, in pediatric orthopaedics for correction of deformities in cerebral palsy (Simon & Ryan, 1992), and in orthopedic traumatology for in the management of compartment syndrome contractures (Hargens et al., 1989). Thus, it is important to understand the effects of tenotomy on skeletal muscle both in the short term, immediately after surgery, as well as in the long term, after the muscle has had the chance to adapt to its new environment.

The immediate effects of tenotomy or tendon rupture on muscle are straightforward. Because most normal muscles are under resting tension, there is an immediate decrease in the tension across the muscle as well as muscle shortening after the muscle loses one of its attachments. Additionally, the specialized neural sensors are affected with respect to the length and tension information that they receive (see below).

Tenotomy Decreases Muscle Mass and Force-Generation Capacity

Tenotomy, studied across a wide range of species, results in decreased muscle mass. The specific effect of tenotomy depends both on the species and on the muscle studied. For example, in the rat soleus muscle, 12 days after tenotomy, muscle mass decreases by approximately 50% compared to a normal muscle (Buller & Lewis, 1965; Jakubiec-Puka, Catani & Carraro; 1992). As with the other models that have been presented, the antigravity muscles (composed primarily of slow fibers) atrophy to a greater extent than their antagonists (composed primarily of fast fibers). In many animal models, unintended reformation of a distal attachment of the muscle to either the tendon stump or surrounding connective tissue with subsequent application of tension may be a confounding factor in decreasing the true level of muscle atrophy after tenotomy. Since you have seen many examples in which muscle forces play a large role in causing the particular adaptive response, it is important to characterize the mechanical response to tenotomy to permit accurate interpretation.

Tenotomy, with intact innervation, leads to several changes in muscle contractile function. The eminent neurophysiologists Buller and Lewis performed pioneering studies in the 1960s (Buller & Lewis, 1965). They completely tenotomized all muscles around the rabbit ankle and showed significantly decreased twitch tensions in the tenotomized group to approximately 50% of the control values within only 3 weeks. Additionally, they noted an increase in the speed of muscle contraction, which may have indicated conversion of slow fibers to fast fibers, as occurs with other decreased use models. Of course, fiber type was not explicitly determined because, at that time, routine histochemistry was not available.

Tenotomy Causes Alterations in Sarcomeres and Supporting Structures

Tenotomy in general leads to an increase in the muscle connective tissue and microcirculation (Józsa et al., 1990). Within 1 week of tenotomy in the rat soleus and gastrocnemius muscles, there was a qualitative increase in both the epimysial and perimysial connective tissue layers. By 3 weeks after tenotomy, the volume density of connective tissue had increased by a factor of ten, with a greater increase in the soleus compared to the gastrocnemius. In parallel with the increase in connective tissue, there was a loss in the number of capillaries. By 3 weeks post-tenotomy, only 47% of the soleus capillaries remained. The capillary effect was more profound in the soleus compared to the gastrocnemius.

Tenotomy also plays a role in the organization of sarcomeres in series within a muscle. It was demonstrated that tenotomy of the proximal and distal tendons of rat soleus muscle not only lead to muscle belly shortening as one would expect, but that this shortening was distributed to the sarcomeres in such a way that they shortened proportionally from an average length of 2.6 μm to 1.8 μm (Baker & Hall-Craggs, 1978). These authors showed that over

the course of the following 4 weeks the sarcomere length returns to normal by reducing the sarcomere number, suggesting that the reduction of sarcomeres in series was made to optimize the contractile function of each sarcomere. If this were true, it would be similar to studies of immobilization in which sarcomere length returns to optimal by changing sarcomere number that was presented in Chapter 4. However, it should be noted that, as in the sarcomere number changes described in Chapter 4, tenotomy itself is not a model that isolates a single variable for study.

Relationship Between Tenotomy and Innervation

The effect of tenotomy on neural function is complex, involving both the efferent and afferent pathways. Tenotomy has been used as a method for simulating immobilization of muscle (Herbison, Jaweed, & Ditunno, 1979) but, this is probably not a clean treatment since the magnitude and the duration of muscle unloading are not explicitly known. EMG activity has been reported to be decreased or absent in animal tenotomy models (Vrbova, 1963) which is analogous to that observed with hindlimb unloading (Alford et al., 1987) and may represent an inability for the muscle to be reflexively activated or may truly represent decreased neural drive to the muscle itself.

Differential Response to Tenotomy of an Activated Compared to a Relaxed Muscle

In light of the strong influence on muscle mechanical properties on muscle plasticity, we were interested in comparing the response of skeletal muscle to what we termed "active" and "passive" tenotomy. Since tenotomy during muscle activation is a violent event, associated with rapid muscle shortening and even perforation of the Z-disk by myosin filaments, (Ramsey & Street, 1940) it was reasoned that it would be much more injurious to muscle compared with tenotomy of a muscle that was in a relaxed state. When relaxed muscle tendons are cut, there is a relatively modest retraction of the tendon. Distinguishing between the effects of these tenotomy types is clinically important because, as mentioned above, tenotomy occurs under both types of conditions and their treatments may not be identical.

To make this comparison, the effects of "active" tenotomy were compared with the effects of passive tenotomy, over the 3-week period after the tenotomy was performed (Abrams, Tsai, Watson, Jamali, & Lieber, 2000). It was discovered that after 1 week the active tenotomy group produced lower maximum tetanic tensions than the passive tenotomy, which was interpreted as indicating greater damage to the contractile elements (Fig. 5-34). By 21 days, however, the active tenotomy group had recovered to a significantly greater degree than the passive tenotomy group. One possible explanation of these findings was that the active tenotomy initially caused a greater muscle injury leading to a greater regenerative response, allowing more complete restoration of the contractile function. However, a number of important structural features of the muscle were measured to obtain support for this idea, but none was obtained. Surprisingly, differences between group P_o values were not explainable based upon careful quantitative analysis of

muscle architecture, muscle fiber size, or magnitude of regeneration as indicated by positive immunostaining with antibodies against developmental myosin (Table 5-1 and 5-2).

Based on the inability to explain contractile changes in terms of alterations in the contractile apparatus, it was hypothesized that the force changes resulted from disruption of the excitation-contraction (EC) coupling system within the muscle. As described in Chapter 2, the EC-coupling system includes the electrical and subcellular events such as muscle fiber action potential conduction, transverse tubule conduction, "activation" of the dihydropyridine (DHP) receptors and calcium release in the vicinity of the myofilaments (Ebashi, 1976). Precedent for selective disruption of EC-coupling after muscle injury already existed in the literature as will be discussed in Chapter 6 dealing with muscle injury (Warren et al., 1993). Perhaps tenotomy could lead to a similar effect. It was further hypothesized that, should EC-coupling be affected by tenotomy, upregulation of proteins associated with the EC-coupling apparatus could be observed such as the postsynaptic acetylcholine receptor or neural cell adhesion molecule (NCAM). During development, NCAM is expressed, presumably to attract motor nerves to innervate

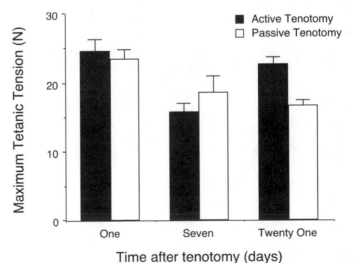

FIGURE 5-34. Maximum isometric tension generated by EDL muscles after active tenotomy (filled bars) or passive tenotomy (open bars). Active tenotomy represents tenotomy during muscle contraction while passive tenotomy represents tenotomy with the muscle at rest. (Data from: Abrams, R.A., Tsai, A.M., Watson, B., Jamali, A., Lieber, R.L. (2000). Skeletal muscle recovery after tenotomy and 7-day delayed muscle length restoration. *Muscle Nerve, 23,* 707–714.)

muscles. In adult muscle, NCAM is expressed after denervation (see page 273), presumably to "re-attract" a motor nerve to reinnervate the muscle and restore function.

NCAM Expression After Tenotomy

As a positive control for NCAM expression, Bupivicaine, which was markedly toxic to muscle fibers, led to disruption of muscle fibers and infiltration of leukocytes as well as a subsequent regenerative response characterized by formation of myotubes and immature myofibers observed on hematoxylin and eosin staining. Bupivicaine-injected muscles also demon-

strated pronounced expression of embryonic myosin in the regions of maximum myofiber disruption and, in many of those same fibers, positive staining for NCAM. Interestingly, NCAM was also expressed in a surrounding population of morphologically normal muscle fibers that did not express embryonic myosin. This indicates that regeneration is not required for NCAM expression.

Control micrographs of normal muscles did not express NCAM (Fig. 5-35A). NCAM was then expressed in tenotomized rabbit EDL muscle at levels significantly above (Józsa et al., 1990). Qualitatively, NCAM levels in-

TABLE 5-1   EDL Architectural Properties*

Experimental Group	Muscle Mass (g)	Muscle PCSA (cm²)	Serial Sarcomere Number
Active Tenotomy (n=9–12/group)			
1 day	3.68+/–0.24	2.54+/–0.26	6233+/–302
7 days	3.32+/–0.24	2.05+/–0.14	6193+/–190
21 days	3.89+/–0.13	2.23+/–0.50	5323+/–287
Passive Tenotomy (n=9–11/group)			
1 day	2.96+/–0.06	1.84+/–0.05	6170+/–159
7 days	3.40+/–0.31	2.44+/–0.28	5939+/–217
21 days	2.85+/–0.07	1.92+/–0.12	5844+/–185
Control Muscles (n=6)**			
	3.56+/–0.21	1.92+/–0.20	5844+/–185

Abbreviation: PCSA, physiological cross-sectional area

*Data are from Abrams, R.A., Tsai, A.M., Watson, B., Jamali, A., Lieber, R.L. (2000). Skeletal muscle recovery after tenotomy and 7-day delayed muscle length restoration. *Muscle Nerve, 23*, 707–714.

**Control data from: Lieber R.L., Blevins, F.T. (1989). Skeletal muscle architecture of the rabbit hindlimb. Functional implications of muscle design. *Journal of Morphology, 199*, 93–101.

TABLE 5-2   EDP Morphometric Properties*

Experimental Group	Fast Fiber Area (um²)	Number of Fast Fibers	Slow Fiber Area (um²)	Number of Slow Fibers
Active Tenotomy (n=9–12/group)				
1 day	2715+/–62	499	1598+/–58	95
7 days	2520+/–90	222	1429+/–30	66
21 days	2215+/–60	271	1451+/–31	65
Passive Tenotomy (n=9–11/group)				
1 day	2444+/–60	378	1506+/–36	117
7 days	2971+/–62	159	1544+/–41	53
21 days	2384+/–53	495	1393+/–31	134

*Data from Abrams, R.A., Tsai, A.M., Watson, B., Jamali, A., Lieber, R.L. (2000). Skeletal muscle recovery after tenotomy and 7-day delayed muscle length restoration. *Muscle Nerve, 23*, 707–714.

FIGURE 5-35. Representative micrographs of rabbit EDL muscles immunoassayed for NCAM. Quantitative results from stereological analysis shown in Table 5-2, page 268. **(A)** Control EDL muscle that received no treatment. **(B)** Tenotomized muscle, 1 day after tenotomy, **(C)** Tenotomized muscle, 7 days after tenotomy, and **(D)** Tenotomized muscle, 21 days after tenotomy. Darkly stained fibers are positive for the NCAM protein although the range in staining intensity varies among fibers. Arrows point to selected fibers expressing NCAM. (Used by permission from: Jamali, A., Afshar, P., Abrams, R., Lieber, R.L. (2002). Expression of neural cell adhesion molecule (NCAM) in tenotomized skeletal muscle. *Journal of Orthopaedic Research*, 20, 364–369.)

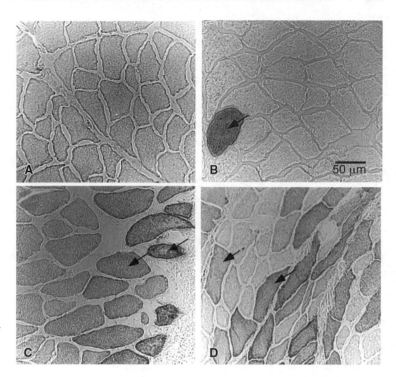

creased from barely detectable levels 1 day after tenotomy (Fig. 5-35B) to relatively high levels 7 and 21 days after tenotomy (Figs. 5-35C and 5-35D). Quantitatively, NCAM labeled from 2–5% of fibers 1 day after tenotomy. These data demonstrate a time-dependent effect of tenotomy type, reminiscent of, but certainly not proving, cause for the observed functional data (Fig. 5-34).

Probably the key question here is, what was the muscle "thinking" after tenotomy? Why would it be advantageous to interrupt neuromuscular communication? Clearly the answers to these questions are speculative at this point, but one possibility is that the muscle, somehow, "sensed" the loss of load and "turned off" the neuromuscular junction to prevent muscle activation and subsequent injury. This would represent a type of "circuit breaker" to protect the muscle from activation while unloaded. A second possibility is that there is a load sensing mechanism within the muscle that is related to its interpretation of the state of innervation. Perhaps when the muscle senses no load, it "thinks" that there is no motor nerve innervat-

ing it and expresses NCAM to "re-attract" the motor nerve. Many future studies are clearly required to understand both the muscle's response to tenotomy as well as methods to restore function after tenotomy. It should be noted that, in the study above, after a 7-day delay period, in a separate group of animal subjects, the distal tendons were reattached to the retinaculum to simulate a repair and the muscle properties recovered fully (Abrams et al., 2000).

Adaptation to Denervation

Now consider a "completely different" type of decreased-use model—denervation (Fig. 5-36). Denervation was used in early muscle plasticity studies as a model of disuse, because it was easy to perform and was viewed as a way to instantly and permanently decrease the use placed upon the muscle. However, as has been seen repeatedly, a denervated muscle is a "different" kind of muscle. For example, the denervated soleus muscle responded much differently to electri-

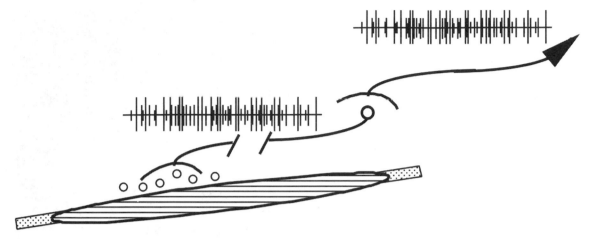

FIGURE 5-36. Schematic diagram of denervation model. Lower motor neuron is transected.

cal stimulation patterns than did a normally innervated muscle. As such, consider denervation, not so much as a typical model of decreased use, rather as a model that illustrates the intimate relationship between muscles and nerves. The unique aspects of denervation that have significant clinical implications will also be considered. Certainly, denervation is a relevant plasticity model and represents an important clinical treatment problem. How does one "treat" a denervated muscle? Are the adaptive responses to tension and stretch similar? How do denervated muscle fibers become reinnervated? Can muscle properties return to normal following reinnervation?

Muscle Strength Changes After Denervation

The most obvious muscular change that occurs after denervation is muscle "atrophy." This atrophy affects both fast and slow muscle fibers and results in decreased fiber diameter and decreased muscle force. Analogous to previously mentioned decreased use models, denervated muscles increase their contractile speed due to fiber type conversion in the slow-to-fast direction. In spite of this conversion, the muscles still generate much lower forces than normal.

Muscle Fiber Atrophy After Denervation

While the mechanism of muscle fiber atrophy is not fully understood in any experimental model, recent experiments have implicated some intramuscular proteolytic enzymes in the atrophic process. An interesting denervation/reinnervation experiment was performed by Dr. Marie Badalmente, who applied the protease inhibitor leupeptin to primate thenar muscles after median nerve denervation and surgical repair (Badalmente, Hurst, & Stracher, 1989). Muscle fibers normally contain enzymes within them that are capable of digesting the cell constituents. This is another way in which the muscle can alter properties in response to a change in environment (these enzymes will be discussed in more detail in Chapter 6 during the discussion of muscle injury and muscular dystrophy). Muscle fibers thus have the capability to "self-destruct" if these proteolytic enzymes are activated. One family of enzymes is activated automatically when the intracellular calcium levels rise too high for a prolonged period of time (the calcium activated neutral proteases, Calpain) (Croall & Demartino, 1991). Since intracellular calcium levels are not normally high for a long time, increased free calcium within a muscle fiber signifies that muscle fiber integrity has been lost (the cell membrane has been broken) and subsequent regeneration should occur. (see a further discussion of this mechanism in Chapter 6.) Badalmente and her colleagues injected monkeys with the Calpain inhibitor, leupeptin, in order to attenuate Calpain's effect. They confirmed that Calpain was suppressed by leupeptin and they then showed that the fiber diameter of leupeptin-treated abductor pollicis and opponens pollicis muscles were greater than the non-treated denervated muscles, suggesting less "atrophy" (Fig. 5-37). Additionally, a greater number of axons survived when muscles were treated with leupeptin. These data may suggest that maintenance of muscle properties following denervation may have a beneficial effect on the reinnervating nerve. Alternatively, Calpain may have a direct axon-sparing role. Again, here is a situation in which a muscle change may affect, in a retrograde fashion, changes within the nerve.

Muscle Fiber Changes After Denervation

Perhaps the most interesting muscle responses to denervation are the subtle changes around the fiber that "signal" to the outside world that the nerve and muscle are no longer in communication. This may not be surprising since there is not really anything more important to a muscle than maintaining an intact neural connection. For example, recall in muscle development, that the myotube was literally covered with acetylcholine receptors (AChR) until the nerve "arrived." After innervation, the density and number of extrajunctional AChRs de-creased dramatically and the only remaining receptors were those at the neuromuscular junction (NMJ, see Chapter 1, page 11). After denervation, a reversal of the developmental process is observed in that a proliferation of extrajunctional AChR occurs (Fig. 5-38). Some view this response as a sort of "signal" that causes nerves to sprout new axons and prepare to form a new neuromuscular junction. The fact that denervation mimics part of the development of the neuromuscular junction is one reason why developmental biologists use denervation as an experimental model to study the process of nerve-muscle connection. (see experiments described in Chapter 1).

What other signals are available to guide the incoming nerves? As mentioned above, the extracellular matrix molecule, NCAM, is implicated in the denervation-reinnervation process. Recall that during development, NCAM was expressed on the surface of the primitive myotubes to perhaps "guide" incoming nerves to the muscle fiber. In denervation, NCAM is again expressed by the muscle fiber (Fig. 5-39). In fact, the NCAM molecule appears to be expressed any time that the muscle fiber is "receptive" to incoming nervous innervation. Following are some of the experimental demonstrations of muscle fiber innervation by foreign nerves.

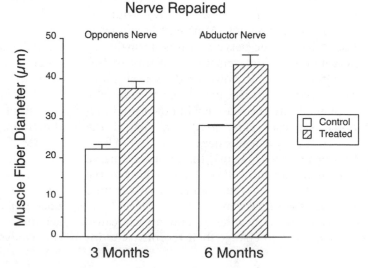

FIGURE 5-37. Muscle fiber diameter of primate muscles after application of leupeptin to muscles whose nerves were transected and then repaired. Treated muscles received application of leupeptin, the calcium protease inhibitor (hatched bars). Control muscles were simply denervated (open bars). (Data from: Badalmente, M.A., Hurst, L.C., Stracher, A. (1989). Neuromuscular recovery using calcium protease inhibition after median nerve repair in primates. *Proceedings of the National Academy of Sciences of the United States of America, 86*, 5983–5987.)

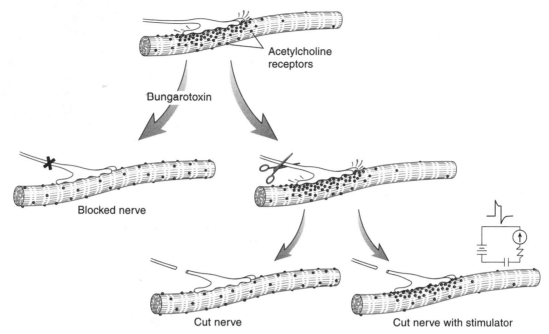

FIGURE 5-38. Relationship between the distribution of ACh receptors and the presence or absence of the nerve. If the nerve is blocked with bungarotoxin, ACh receptors are expressed along the fiber length similar to denervation (left path). However, if the nerve is cut and then stimulation is superimposed on denervation (right path), ACh receptor expression is suppressed.

Denervated Muscle Fibers Increase "Receptivity" to Nerves

A nerve can be surgically implanted into a normal skeletal muscle and will often continue to grow (Fig. 5-40). It will continue to grow and sprout small neuronal processes, but these processes will not form new synapses with the muscle fiber. Why not? Apparently, the muscle fiber "signals" the nerve that it is normally innervated and thus, remains refractory to further innervation. If, however, the muscle's normal nerve is cut, the nerve that is surgically implanted into the muscle will now form functional synapses (Fig. 5-40). In fact, if the muscle is only partially denervated (only a fraction of the nerve is cut), the implanted nerve will innervate only those fibers whose nerve branches were cut. Quite an effective signaling method is working here.

Experimentally, other treatments can cause muscle fibers to change their receptivity to in-nervation by foreign nerves. As you might predict, these are treatments that change the activity level of the muscle fibers. For example, a muscle can be paralyzed with botulinum toxin (a toxin that enters the presynaptic nerve terminal and inhibits ACh release) and the fibers will become receptive to innervation. Conversely, if a denervated muscle is electrically activated, it will not permit innervation by the incoming nerve in spite of the fact that it has no normal nerve of its own (Fig. 5-40). Why not?

Dr. Joshua Sanes and his colleagues showed that all of these conditions are consistent with the timing of a muscle fiber's expression of NCAM (Fig. 5-39). Thus, under conditions of high activity (normally innervated muscle or electrically stimulated, denervated muscle), NCAM is not expressed and synapse formation does not occur. However, when muscle fiber activity is low (in denervation, pharmacological paralysis, or development), NCAM is ex-

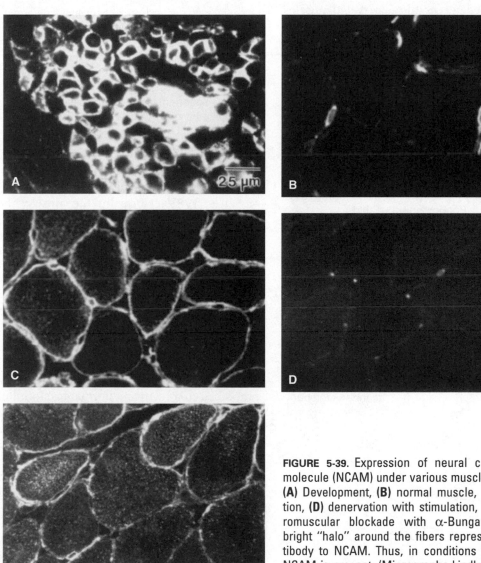

FIGURE 5-39. Expression of neural cell adhesion molecule (NCAM) under various muscle conditions. **(A)** Development, **(B)** normal muscle, **(C)** denervation, **(D)** denervation with stimulation, and **(E)** neuromuscular blockade with α-Bungarotoxin. The bright "halo" around the fibers represents the antibody to NCAM. Thus, in conditions A, C, and E, NCAM is present. (Micrographs kindly provided by Dr. John Covault, University of Connecticut.)

pressed and nerves synapse with the fiber (Sanes & Covault, 1985).

Formation of New Muscle Synapses

Sanes and his colleagues, as well as others, have implanted nerves into denervated muscles to determine where along the fiber length the synapse is formed. If nerves are implanted close to the original neuromuscular junction (NMJ), the synapse forms at exactly the original location. If, however, a site remote from the original NMJ is chosen, a new, ectopic synapse will form. In an effort to determine what was special about the NMJ, Glicksman and Sanes experimentally "killed" muscle fibers

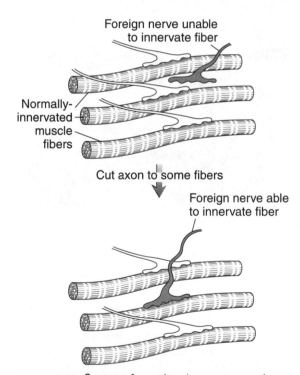

FIGURE 5-40. Synapse formation does not occur in an already-innervated muscle fiber (upper panel). Note that a foreign nerve (thick wiggly line) growing in a muscle composed of innervated fibers does not form an additional synapse. However, if the motor nerve to a muscle fiber is cut (lower panel), a new synapse will form.

> **Box 5-8. Why Is Reinnervated Muscle Weak?**
>
> The main cause for weakness after reinnervation is a decrease in the number of functional neurons that actually grow back into the correct muscle. These nerve fibers must grow from the site of the lesion back into the correct muscle. Even if they grow back, if they synapse with the wrong muscle, they will be dysfunctional. Thus, nerve injuries that occur very close to a muscle have a better prognosis of functional recovery compared with nerve injuries that occur far away from the muscle.

by mechanically crushing them (Glicksman & Sanes, 1983). Normally, the muscle fibers would regenerate (Chapter 6) to form a new muscle. However, these investigators prevented muscle regeneration by repeated exposure to intense X-rays leaving only the muscle-free ghosts—essentially only the basal lamina filled with muscle fiber debris. Recall that the basal lamina is the structure that ensheathes muscle fibers during development (pages 9–10). It is outside of the sarcolemma and is thus an extracellular structure. Interestingly, reinnervation of these muscle-free ghosts proceeded in a relatively normal fashion. Relatively normal NMJs were formed in precisely the location of the original NMJ and the nerve presynaptic terminals were "loaded" with normal-appearing ACh vesicles. These data provide strong evidence that, at least in the early stages of synapse formation, the basal lamina provides a sufficient molecular signal to the nerve for synaptogenesis. But what about the expression of NCAM? Didn't that cause the reinnervation? No. This experiment reinforces an important lesson: just because one event is associated with another event does not mean that it causes it. Clearly, NCAM expression was associated with reinnervation, but it alone did not cause it.

Muscle Fiber Specificity to Reinnervation

The conditions surrounding reinnervation of a muscle fiber were discussed, but take this one step further: How does a nerve select which muscle fiber type to innervate? This is a "hot" research area and definitive answers are not yet available. The reason it is so important is that in Chapter 2, muscle fiber recruitment proceeds in an orderly fashion according to the size principle (pages 98 to 100). This is one of the important bases for motor control and coordination. If that sophisticated relationship between nerve and muscles is lost during reinnervation, it will have profound functional consequences. Therefore, there is great interest in understanding the factors that control reinnervation in an effort to improve the functional results after reinnervation. A number of clever experiments have been devised to study this problem. You can imagine that determining experimentally, which muscle fiber is attached to which axon, would be technically difficult. However, in spite of these difficulties, several experiments have provided clues that lead us to believe that nerves generally innervate the nearest receptive fiber, regardless of type. But the story is not that simple.

Motor Unit Properties Following Cross-Reinnervation

To study the specificity of reinnervation, a nerve that normally innervates slow fibers is given the opportunity innervate slow or fast fibers (or vice versa). This can be done by surgically cross-reinnervating the triceps surae muscles with the antagonistic motor axons from the common peroneal nerve. In this case flexor neurons are forced to innervate extensor muscles. Such an experiment was performed by Drs. Tessa Gordon, Richard Stein, and their colleagues using the cat hindlimb model (Fig. 5-41). After performing the surgical reanasto-

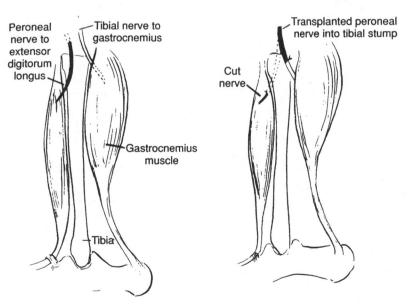

FIGURE 5-41. Schematic diagram of the cross-reinnervation experiment. Peroneal nerve, which normally innervates the anterior compartment muscles, is surgically reattached to the distal stump of the tibial nerve, which normally innervates the plantarflexors.

mosis (micro-reconnection) of the proximal flexor nerve with the distal extensor nerve stump (and vice versa), they waited 1–2 years, and again measured motor unit properties (as discussed in Chapter 2, pages 92 to 94) (Gordon, Thomas, Stein, & Erdebil, 1988).

Motor Unit Tension After Reinnervation

These investigators had already documented the relationship between motor unit tension and axon size as a function of unit type (Fig. 5-42A). As expected, a wide range of normal MG motor unit tensions were observed, ranging from only 10–20 mN to over 1000 mN (1 mN equals 1.0×10^{-3} N or 9.8 grams). Also, as

expected based on the size principle, the normal MG units that generated the smallest tensions had the smallest axon action potentials and therefore, the smallest axon size. Units that developed the highest tensions had the largest axon sizes. Finally, low-tension units were identified as S units, the intermediate tension units as FR units and the high-tension units as FF units. This was all consistent with the idea of the "size principle" previously presented (Henneman, Somjen, & Carpenter, 1965).

After reinnervation was induced by cutting the nerve and then surgically repairing it to the antagonistic nerve, a number of changes occurred. Before you read the results, try to pre-

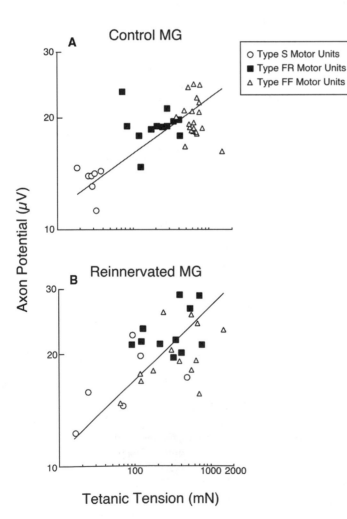

FIGURE 5-42. Relationship between motor unit tension and action potential amplitude for **(A)** normal and **(B)** cross-reinnervated cat medial gastrocnemius. Each symbol represents a different motor unit type. Normally, S units are associated with the smallest axons, represented by low axon potentials with FR and FF units having increasing tension and axon potential amplitude. However, after reinnervation, this relationship is dramatically altered. (Data from: Gordon, T., Thomas, C.K., Stein, R.B., Erdebil, S. (1988). Comparison of physiological and histochemical properties of motor units after cross-reinnervation of antagonistic muscles in the cat hindlimb. *Journal of Neurophysiology, 60,* 365–378.)

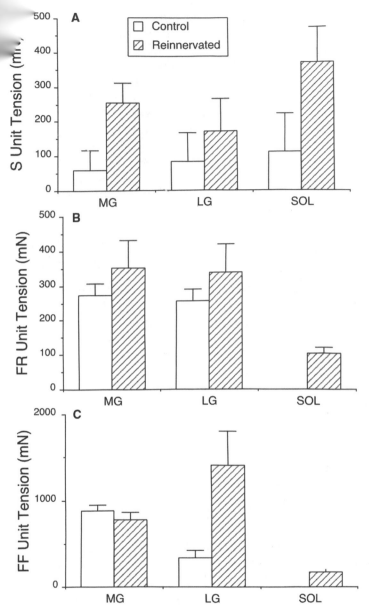

FIGURE 5-43. Graph of t different motor units fro bars) or cross-reinnerva bars) cat skeletal muscles the normal motor units gener according to the size princip ever, following reinnervation, th tionship no longer holds. (Data Gordon, T., Thomas, C.K., Stein, Erdebil, S. (1988). Comparison of ph ological and histochemical properties motor units after cross-reinnervation o antagonistic muscles in the cat hind-limb. *Journal of Neurophysiology, 60,* 365–378.)

reasons than the S units. This is a good exercise to see if you understand the contributing factors to motor unit tension). Since the MG motor unit specific tensions were "correct" after reinnervation (in the sense that they were ordered correctly although their absolute values were different) but innervation ratio and fiber

area were not, the conclusion was that specific tension was the only parameter which was uniquely determined by the innervating axon. The main limitation of this interpretation is that calculation of innervation ratios and specific tensions using this model are very indirect. Specific tension is always the term that is "left over" to balance the motor unit tension equation. Future experiments are required to clarify these issues.

To summarize, denervated muscle represents a "different beast" since loss of neuromuscular communication leads to dramatic alterations in muscle structure, function, and adaptive ability. In this exciting research area, you are beginning to understand the factors that regulate nerve-muscle interaction. It is critical to make advances in this area in order to improve muscle function after traumatic nerve injury.

Evidence for Specificity of Reinnervation

The previous denervation-reinnervation might lead one to the conclusion that reinnervation is completely random. However, this is far from the truth. Many studies have demonstrated that many axons, which grow out from a denervated stump are able to "navigate" to the correct distal stump and reinnervate the appropriate muscle. This was shown in a most dramatic earlier this century by Cajál, who cut the motor nerve to a fast muscle and then constructed a Y-chamber to give this reinnervating nerve a choice of

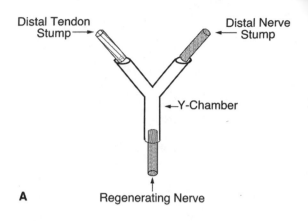

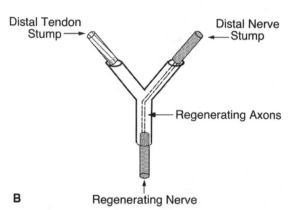

FIGURE 5-45. (A) Representation of the experiment in which a severed nerve was given the option of growing through a Y-tube into either the original nerve or a tendon. **(B)** In all cases, the nerve selectively chose to grow toward the distal nerve stump. This experiment suggests some type of attraction of nerve for incoming axons. (Figure redrawn after: Lundborg, G. (1988). *Nerve injury and repair* (page 18). New York: Churchill Livingstone.)

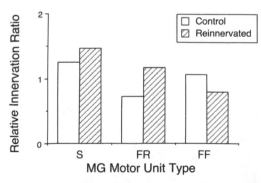

FIGURE 5-44. Innervation ratios calculated for normal (open bars) or cross-reinnervated (hatched bars) cat skeletal muscles. (Data from: Gordon, T., Thomas, C.K., Stein, R.B., Erdebil, S. (1988). Comparison of physiological and histochemical properties of motor units after cross-reinnervation of antagonistic muscles in the cat hindlimb. *Journal of Neurophysiology, 60*, 365–378.)

either the original fast muscle, or a different slow muscle (Fig. 5-45). If reinnervation were completely random, an equal number of axons would have chosen each "branch" of the Y (Cajal, 1928). However, almost 80% of the reinnervating axons "chose" to innervate the correct distal stump, providing evidence that some type of signal permitted specific reinnervation. More recent experiments have implicated vari-

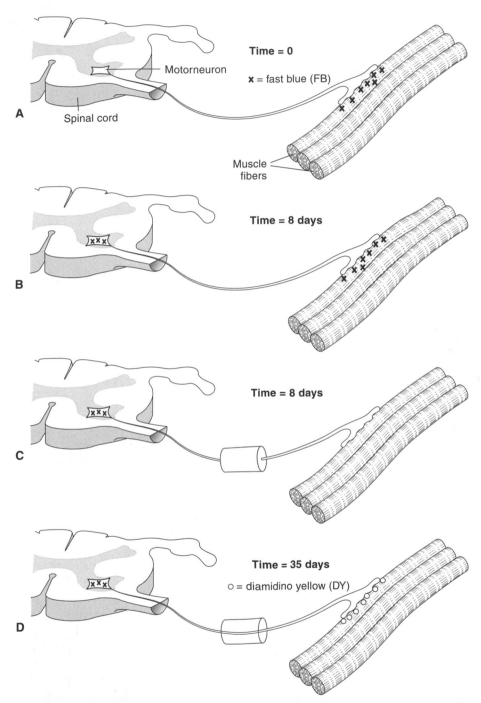

FIGURE 5-46. Schematic representation of the double tracer method used to identify specificity of connections between motoneurons in the spinal cord and peripheral muscle targets. **(A)** Original connections between nerves innervating tibialis anterior labeled using fast blue (FB). **(B)** After 8 days, FB is transported retrograde to cell bodies in spinal cord. **(C)** Nerve cut and allowed to grow back through a 10-mm gap in a plastic tube. **(D)** After TA reinnervation, connections between TA and spinal cord labeled using diamidine yellow (DY).

ous chemicals such as growth factors and specific extracellular proteins as the chemical signals for providing navigational aid to incoming axons.

A more recent demonstration of reinnervation specificity was provided by Rende et al. who used the "double labeling" technique to trace the connections between axons and motoneuron cell bodies in the spinal cord (Fig. 5-46) (Rende, Granato, Monaco, Zelano, & Toesca, 1991). The experimental model was the rat tibialis anterior (TA). Most of the motoneuron cell bodies to the TA are located at spinal cord level L3. Rende et al. used two separate tracer dies to follow the connections between the TA and spinal cord motoneurons before and after denervation-reinnervation. They started by injecting the blue tracer known as "fast blue" into the TA muscle. Fast blue (FB) is taken up at the neuromuscular junction and moved via axonal transport into the motoneuron cell bodies (Fig. 5-46A). After 8 days (enough time for the axons to transport FB to the motoneuron cell bodies) they cut the sciatic nerve (which contains the motor nerves to the TA, other dorsiflexors, and plantarflexors, as well as many sensory nerves) and placed both cut ends of the nerve in a small plastic tube, leaving a long 10 mm gap between ends (Figs. 5-46B and 5-46C). This configuration allowed the outgrowing axons to make a choice between several nerve fascicles—some correct, some incorrect. After 30–35 days (enough time for many outgrowing axons to arrive at the muscles), they re-injected the TA muscles with a different tracer known as "diamidino yellow dihydrochloride" or, more simply, DY (Fig. 5-46D). The DY acts similarly to the FB in that it is transported back to the motoneurons where it can be observed microscopically. Before reading on, try to predict the appearance of motoneuron cell bodies, which were correctly innervated. Which tracers would be present? How would motoneurons appear which had originally projected to the TA but were not correctly innervated?

The results, shown schematically in Figure 5-47, provided convincing evidence that 30% of the reinnervating axons found the TA muscle. Motoneurons that showed both the FB and DY tracers were those that had originally been labeled with FB and then subsequently labeled with DY after correct reinnervation. However, many other motoneurons at the L3 level showed only FB which suggested either that they were originally labeled and failed to reinnervate anything, or that they were originally labeled and reinnervated the wrong muscle (Fig. 5-47). Current research in this area will use this type of model to investigate the signals (chemical, mechanical, hormonal) that control specificity of reinnervation. Ultimately, improved reinnervation specificity will improve functional recovery of patients following nerve injury. It looks like the main hope is not so much in expert microsurgical technique (note 30% specific reinnervation when no surgery was performed) but rather in identifying the appropriate biological signals (Lundborg, 1988). In fact, one of the pioneers in this area, the Swedish hand surgeon Dr. Göran Lundborg has performed a long-term follow-up study to his original study that compared the effects of direct microsurgical nerve repair to nerve repair in which the axons were allowed to "grow across" a small tube place between the severed ends. Lundborg and colleagues had already shown that axons would grow across the gap and there was evidence that the specificity was better in the presence of the tube (Lundborg 1988). Much to their credit, they published an excellent report stating that the long-term function of these patient groups were identical (Lundborg, 2000).

■ Chapter Summary

Skeletal muscle response to decreased used is characterized by muscle fiber atrophy, decreased muscle force generating capacity, and a slow-to-fast muscle fiber type conversion if the disuse is extreme enough. Generally, muscle oxidative capacity and endurance do not change. This essentially represents a reversal of

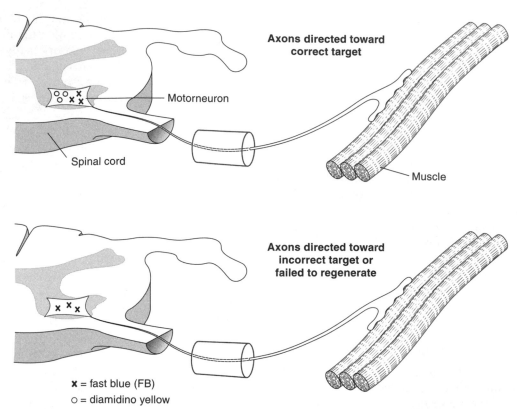

Axons directed toward
correct target

Motorneuron

Spinal cord

Muscle

Axons directed toward
incorrect target or
failed to regenerate

x = fast blue (FB)
o = diamidino yellow

FIGURE 5-47. Schematic representation of innervation specificity following denervation of the rat sciatic nerve and permitting regrowth across a 10-mm gap within a plastic tube. Symbols refer to the tracers described in Figure 5-46. Note that if the reinnervating axon is directed toward one of the originally innervated fibers, both tracers are in the cell body. However, if axons are directed toward the wrong target (where no diamidine yellow was applied) or if the axon failed to regenerate, only fast blue is found in the cell body.

the increased use response. Glycolytic response seems to match the fiber type: increased percentage of fast fibers is accompanied by increased glycolytic capacity. The magnitude of the atrophic and adaptive response is related to the change in use experienced by the muscle. Thus, the often-used antigravity muscles atrophy to a greater extent than their less-often used antagonists. Regulation of muscle mass represents the balance between protein synthesis and degradation. In the hindlimb unloading model, muscle loss was initiated at the transnational level. Pretranslational and posttranslational regulation have been observed in unloading and other models of decreased use.

When the nerve to a muscle is cut, the muscle fiber becomes a qualitatively different entity. A reversal of some of the developmental processes, which serve as signals to nerves for reinnervation to occur, is observed. The reinnervation process itself does not appear to be fiber type specific although some signals are conveyed between the reinnervating stump and its target. At this point, muscle adaptation to the relatively "normal" perturbations has been discussed. However, in some cases the level of use is so intense or extreme that the muscle itself becomes injured or even killed. In still other cases muscle malformation during development imparts specific properties to the muscle.

In the next chapter, these muscle responses to exercise-induced injury, surgical trauma, and muscle disease will be considered.

REFERENCES

(2000). Genetic epidemiologic studies on age-specified traits. NIA Aging and Genetic Epidemiology Working Group. *American Journal of Epidemiology, 152*, 1003–1008.

Abrams, R.A., Tsai, A.M., Watson, B., Jamali, A., Lieber, R.L. (2000). Skeletal muscle recovery after tenotomy and 7-day delayed muscle length restoration. *Muscle Nerve, 23*, 707–714.

Akeson, W.H., Amiel, D., Abel, M.F., Garfin, S.R., Woo, S.L. (1987). Effects of immobilization on joints. *Clinical Orthopaedics, 219* 28–37.

Alford, E.K., Roy, R.R., Hodgson, J.A., Edgerton, V.A. (1987). Electromyography of rat soleus, medial gastrocnemius, and tibialis anterior during hindlimb suspension. *Experimental Neurology, 96*, 635–649.

Andersen, J.L., Mohr, T., Biering-Sorensen, F., Galbo, H., Kjaer, M. (1996). Myosin heavy chain isoform transformation in single fibres from m. vastus lateralis in spinal cord injured individuals: effects of long-term functional electrical stimulation (FES). *Pflugers Arch, 431*, 513–518.

Armstrong, R.B., Saubert, C.I., Seeherman, H.J., Taylor, C.R. (1982). Distribution of fiber types in locomotory muscles of dogs. *American Journal of Anatomy, 153*, 87–98.

Babij, P., Booth, F.W. (1988a). Actin and cytochrome c mRNAs in atrophied adult rat skeletal muscle. *American Journal of Physiology, 254*, C651–C656.

Babij, P., Booth, F.W. (1988b). Clenbuterol prevents or inhibits loss of specific mRNAs in atrophying rat skeletal muscle. *American Journal of Physiology, 254*, C657–C660.

Badalmente, M.A., Hurst, L.C., Stracher, A. (1989). Neuromuscular recovery using calcium protease inhibition after median nerve repair in primates. *Proceedings of the National Academy of Science of the United States of America, 86*, 5983–5987.

Baker, J.H., Hall-Craggs, E.C. (1978). Changes in length of sarcomeres following tenotomy of the rat soleus muscle. *Anatomy Record, 192*, 55–58.

Baldi, J.C., Reiser, P.J. (1995). Intermediate filament proteins increase during chronic stimulation of skeletal muscle. *Journal of Muscle Research and Cell Motility, 16*, 587–594.

Booth, F.W., Thomason, D.B. (1991). Molecular and cellular adaptation of muscle in response to exercise: perspectives of various models. *Physiology Review, 71*, 541–585.

Brooks, S.V., Faulkner, J.A. (1990). Contraction-induced injury: Recovery of skeletal muscles in young and old mice. *American Journal of Physiology, 258*, C436–C442.

Brown, W.F., Strong, M.J., Snow, R. (1988). Methods for estimating numbers of motor units in biceps-brachialis muscles and losses of motor units with aging. *Muscle Nerve, 11*, 423–432.

Brzezienski, M.A., Schneider, L.H. (1995). Extensor tendon injuries at the distal interphalangeal joint. *Hand Clinics of North America, 11*, 373–386.

Buller, A.J., Lewis, D.M. (1965). Some observations on the effects of tenotomy in the rabbit. *Journal of Physiology (London), 178*, 326–342.

Burke, R.E., Levine, D.N., Tsairis, P., Zajac, F.E. (1973). Physiological types and histochemical profiles in motor units of the cat gastrocnemius. *Journal of Physiology (London), 234*, 723–748.

Cajal, R. (1928). *Degeneration and regeneration of the nervous system.* London: Oxford University Press.

Chilibeck, P.D., Jeon, J., Weiss, C., Bell, G., Burnham, R. (1999). Histochemical changes in muscle of individuals with spinal cord injury following functional electrical stimulated exercise training. *Spinal Cord, 37*, 264–268.

Croall, D.E., Demartino, G.N. (1991). Calcium-activated neutral protease (calpain) system: structure, function, and regulation. *Physiology Review, 71*, 813–847.

De Leon, R.D., Hodgson, J.A., Roy, R.R., Edgerton, V.R. (1998). Locomotor capacity attributable to step training versus spontaneous recovery after spinalization in adult cats. *Journal of Neurophysiology, 79*, 1329–1340.

De Leon, R.D., Hodgson, J.A., Roy, R.R., Edgerton, V.R. (1999). Retention of hindlimb stepping ability in adult spinal cats after the cessation of step training. *Journal of Neurophysiology, 81*, 85–94.

Degens, H., Yu, F., Li, X., Larsson, L. (1998). Effects of age and gender on shortening velocity and myosin isoforms in single rat muscle fibres. *Acta Physiologica Scandinavica, 163*, 33–40.

Ebashi, S. (1976). Excitation-contraction coupling. *Annual Review of Physiology, 38*, 293–313.

Edgerton, V.R., Barnard, R.J., Peter, J.B., Maier, A.,

Simpson, D.R. (1975). Properties of immobilized hind-limb muscles of the galago senegalensis. *Experimental Neurology, 46*, 115–131.

Edgerton, V.R., Roy, R.R. (2000). Invited review: Gravitational biology of the neuromotor systems: A perspective to the next era. *Journal of Applied Physiology, 89*, 1224–1231.

Enoka, R.M., Fuglevand, A.J. (1993). Neuromuscular basis of the maximum voluntary force capacity of muscle. In M.D. Grabiner (Ed.), *Current Issues in Biomechanics* (215–235). Champaign, IL: Human Kinetics.

Essen-Gustavsson, B., Borges, O. (1986). Histochemical and metabolic characteristics of human skeletal muscle in relation to age. *Acta Physiologica Scandanavica, 126*, 107–114.

Faulkner, J.A., Brooks, S.V., Zerba, E. (1995). Muscle atrophy and weakness with aging: contraction-induced injury as an underlying mechanism. *Journal of Gerontology, 50A*, 124–129.

Fiatarone, M.A., Marks, E.C., Ryan, N.D., Meredith, C.N., Lipsitz, L.A., Evans, W.J. (1990). High-intensity strength training in nonagenarians. Effects on skeletal muscle. *Journal of the American Medical Association, 263*, 3029–3034.

Forster, M.J., Dubey, A., Dawson, K.M., Stutts, W.A., Lal, H., Sohal, R.S. (1996). Age-related losses of cognitive function and motor skills in mice are associated with oxidative protein damage in the brain. *Proceedings of the National Academy of Science of the Unites States of America, 93*, 4765–4769.

Fournier, M., Roy, R.R., Perham, H., Simard, C.P., Edgerton, V.R. (1983). Is limb immobilization a model of muscle disuse? *Experimental Neurology, 80*, 147–156.

Giger, J.M., Haddad, F., Qin, A.X., Baldwin, K.M. (2000). In vivo regulation of the beta-myosin heavy chain gene in soleus muscle of suspended and weight-bearing rats. *American Journal of Physiology, 278*, C1153–C1161.

Glicksman, M.A., Sanes, J.R. (1983). Differentiation of motor nerve terminals formed in the absence of muscle fibres. *Journal of Neurocytology, 12*, 661–671.

Gordon, T., Thomas, C.K., Stein, R.B., Erdebil, S. (1988). Comparison of physiological and histochemical properties of motor units after cross-reinnervation of antagonistic muscles in the cat hindlimb. *Journal of Neurophysiology, 60*, 365–378.

Grimby, G., Broberg, C., Krotkiewska, I., Krotkiewski, M. (1976). Muscle fiber composition in patients with traumatic cord lesion. *Scandinavian Journal of Rehabilitation Medicine, 8*, 37–42.

Hagberg, J.M., Graves, J.E., Limacher, M., Woods, D.R., Leggett, S.H., Cononie, C., Gruber, J.J., Pollock, M.L. (1989). Cardiovascular responses of 70 to 79 year-old men and women to exercise training. *Journal of Applied Physiology, 66*, 2589–2594.

Haggmark, T., Eriksson, E. (1979). Cylinder or mobile cast brace after knee ligament surgery. *American Journal of Sports Medicine, 7*, 48–56.

Hargens, A.R., Akeson, W.H., Mubarak, S.J., Owen. C.A., Gershuni, D.H., Garfin, S.R., Lieber, R.L., Danzig, L.A., Botte, M.J., Gelberman, R.H. (1989). Kappa Delta Award paper. Tissue fluid pressures: From basic research tools to clinical applications. *Journal of Orthopaedic Research, 7*, 902–909.

Harkema, S.J., Hurley, S.L., Patel, U.K., Requejo, P.S., Dobkin, B.H., Edgerton, V.R. (1997). Human lumbosacral spinal cord interprets loading during stepping. *Journal of Neurophysiology, 77*, 797–811.

Hauschka, E., Roy, R., Edgerton, R. (1987). Size and metabolic properties of single muscle fibers in rat soleus after hindlimb suspension. *Journal of Applied Physiology, 62*, 2338–2347.

Henneman, E., Somjen, G., Carpenter, D.O. (1965). Functional significance of cell size in spinal motorneurons. *Journal of Neurophysiology, 28*, 560–580.

Herbison, G.J., Jaweed, M.M., Ditunno, J.F. (1979). Muscle atrophy in rats following denervation, casting, inflammation, and tenotomy. *Archives of Physical Medicine and Rehabilitation, 60*, 401–404.

Hook, P., Li, X., Sleep, J., Hughes, S., Larsson, L. (1999). The effect of age on in vitro motility speed of slow myosin extracted from single rat soleus fibres. *Acta Rhematologica Scandanavica, 167*, 325–326.

Jakubiec-Puka, A., Catani, C., Carraro, U. (1992). Myosin heavy-chain composition in striated muscle after tenotomy. *Biochemical Journal, 282*, 237–242.

Jamali, A., Afshar, P., Abrams, R., Lieber, R.L. (2002). Expression of neural cell adhesion molecule (NCAM) in tenotomized skeletal muscle. *Journal of Orthopaedic Research, 20*, 364–369.

Józsa, L., Kannus, P., Thöring, J., Reffy, A., Järvinen, M., Kvist, M. (1990). The effect of tenotomy and immobilisation on intramuscular connective tissue. A morphometric and microscopic study in rat calf muscles. *Journal of Bone and Joint Surgery, British Volume, 72*, 293–297.

Kawamura, Y., O'Brien, P., Okazaki, H., Dyck, P.J. (1977a). Lumbar motoneurons of man II: the number and diameter distribution of large- and intermediate-diameter cytons in "motoneuron columns" of spinal cord of man. *Journal of Neuropathology and Experimental Neurology, 36,* 861–870.

Kawamura, Y., Okazaki, H., O'Brien, P.C., Dych, P.J. (1977b). Lumbar motoneurons of man I: Number and diameter histogram of alpha and gamma axons of ventral root. *Journal of Neuropathology and Experimental Neurology,36,* 853–860.

Larsson, L., Sjodin, B., Karlsson, J. (1978). Histochemical and biochemical changes in human skeletal muscle with age in sedentary males, age 22–65 years. *Acta Physiologica Scandinavica, 103,* 31–39.

Leadbetter, W.B., Mooar, P.A., Lane, G.J., Lee, S.J. (1992). The surgical treatment of tendinitis. Clinical rationale and biologic basis. In *Clinics in sports medicine.* Vol. 11 (pp. 679–712). Chicago, IL: American Academy of Orthopaedic Surgeons.

Lee, C.K., Klopp, R.G., Weindruch, R., Prolla, T.A. (1999). Gene expression profile of aging and its retardation by caloric restriction. *Science, 285,* 1390–1393.

Lexell J, Downham D. What is the effect of ageing on type 2 muscle fibres? [letter]. *Journal of Neurological Science, 107,* 250–251.

Lexell, J., Downham, D., Sjöström, M. (1984). Distribution of different fiber types in human skeletal muscles. A statistical and computational study of the fiber type arrangement in m. vastus lateralis of young, healthy males. *Journal of Neurological Science, 65,* 353–365.

Lexell, J., Henriksson-Larsen, K., Winblad, B., Sjöström, M. (1983). Distribution of different fiber types in human skeletal muscles: effects of aging studied in whole muscle cross sections. *Muscle Nerve, 6,* 588–595.

Lexell, J., Taylor, C.C., Sjöström, M. (1988). What is the cause of the ageing atrophy? Total number, size and proportion of different fiber types studied in whole vastus lateralis muscle from 15- to 83-year-old men. *Journal of Neurological Science, 84,* 275–294.

Lieber, R.L., Blevins, F.T. (1989). Skeletal muscle architecture of the rabbit hindlimb. Functional implications of muscle design. *Journal of Morphology, 199,* 93–101.

Lieber, R.L., Fridén, J.O., Hargens, A.R., Danzig, L.A., Gershuni, D.H. (1988). Differential response of the dog quadriceps muscle to external skeletal fixation of the knee. *Muscle Nerve, 11,* 193–201.

Lieber, R.L., Fridén, J.O., Hargens, A.R., Feringa, E.R. (1986b). Long-term effects of spinal cord transection of fast and slow rat skeletal muscle. II. Morphometric properties. *Experimental Neurology, 91,* 435–448.

Lieber, R.L., Jacks, T.M., Mohler, R.L., Schleim, K., Haven, M., Cuizon, D., Gershuni, D.H., Lopez, M.A., Hora, D., Nargund, R., Feeney, W., G.J. H. (1997). Growth hormone secretagogue increases muscle strength during remobilization after canine hindlimb immobilization. *Journal of Orthopaedic Research, 15,* 519–527.

Lieber, R.L., Johansson, C.B., Vahlsing, H.L., Hargens, A.R., Feringa, E.R. (1986a). Long-term effects of spinal cord transection on fast and slow rat skeletal muscle I. Contractile properties. *Experimental Neurology, 91,* 423–434.

Lieber, R.L., McKee-Woodburn, T., Fridén, J., Gershuni, D.H. (1989). Recovery of the dog quadriceps after ten weeks of immobilization followed by four weeks of remobilization. *Journal of Orthopaedic Research, 7,* 408–412.

Lockhart, D.J., Dong, H., Byrne, M.C., Follettie, M.T., Gallo, M.V., Chee, M.S., Mittmann, M., Wang, C., Kobayashi, M., Horton, H., Brown, E.L. (1996). Expression monitoring by hybridization to high-density oligonucleotide arrays. *Nature Biotechnology 14,* 1675–1680.

Lundborg, G. (1988). *Nerve injury and repair.* New York: Churchill Livingstone.

Lundborg, G. (2000). A 25-year perspective of peripheral nerve surgery: Evolving neuroscientific concepts and clinical significance. *Journal of Hand Surgery, 25,* 391–414.

Marshall, E. (1999). Do-it-yourself gene watching. *Science, 286,* 444–447.

McComas, A.J. (1995). Motor unit estimation: Anxieties and achievements. *Muscle Nerve, 18,* 369–379.

McDonald, K.S., Blaser, C.A., Fitts, R.H. (1994). Force-velocity and power characteristics of rat soleus muscle fibers after hindlimb suspension. *Journal of Applied Physiology, 77,* 1609–1616.

Miller, J.B., Stockdale, F.E. (1987). What muscle cells know that nerves don't tell them. *Trends in Neurosciences, 10,* 10–14.

Morey, E.R., Sabelman, E.E., Turner, R.T., Baylink, D.J. (1979). A new rat model simulating some aspects of space flight. *Physiologist, 22,* S23–S24.

Orr, W.C., Sohal, R.S. (1994). Extension of life-span by overexpression of superoxide dismutase and catalase in *Drosophila melanogaster. Science, 263,* 1128–1130.

Pyka, G., Lindenberger, E., Charette, S., Marcus, R. (1994). Muscle strength and fiber adaptations to a year-long resistance training program in elderly men and women. *Journal of Gerontology, 49,* M22–M27.

Ramsey, R.W., Street, S.F. (1940). The isometric length-tension diagram of isolated skeletal muscle fibers of the frog. *Journal of Cell and Comparative Physiology, 15,*11–34.

Rende, M., Granato, A., Monaco, M.L., Zelano, G., Toesca, A. (1991). Accuracy of reinnervation by peripheral nerve axons regenerating across a 10-mm gap within an impermeable chamber. *Experimental Neurology, 111,* 332–339.

Roy, R., Bello, M., Bouissou, P., Edgerton, R. (1987). Size and metabolic properties of fibers in rat fast-twitch muscles after hindlimb suspension. *Journal of Applied Physiology, 62,* 2348–2357.

Roy, R.R., Talmadge, R.J., Hodgson, J.A., Oishi, Y., Baldwin, K.M., Edgerton, V.R. (1999). Differential response of fast hindlimb extensor and flexor muscles to exercise in adult spinalized cats. *Muscle Nerve, 22,* 230–241.

Roy, R.R., Talmadge, R.J., Hodgson, J.A., Zhong, H., Baldwin, K.M., Edgerton, V.R. (1998). Training effects on soleus of cats spinal cord transected (T12-13) as adults. *Muscle Nerve, 21,* 63–71.

Safran, M.R., Zachazewski, J.E., Benedetti, R.S., Bartolozzi, A.R., 3rd, Mandelbaum, R. (1999). Lateral ankle sprains: a comprehensive review part 2: treatment and rehabilitation with an emphasis on the athlete. *Medicine and Science in Sports and Exercise, 31,* S438–S447.

Sanes, J.R., Covault, J. (1985). Axon guidance during reinnervation of skeletal muscle. *Trends in Neurosciences, 8,* 523–528.

Saunders, R.A., Bluestein, E.C., Wilson, M.E., Berland, J.E. (1994). Anterior segment ischemia after strabismus surgery. *Survey of Ophthalmology, 38,* 456–466.

Shields, R.K., Chang, Y.J., Ross, M. (1998). Neuromuscular propagation after fatiguing contractions of the paralyzed soleus muscle in humans. *Muscle Nerve, 21,* 776–787.

Shields, R.K., Law, L.F., Reiling, B., Sass, K., Wilwert, J. (1997). Effects of electrically induced fatigue on the twitch and tetanus of paralyzed soleus muscle in humans. *Journal of Applied Physiology, 82,* 1499–1507.

Simard, C.P., Spector, S.A., Edgerton, V.R. (1982). Contractile properties of rat hindlimb muscles immobilized at different lengths. *Experimental Neurology, 77,* 467–482.

Simon SR, Ryan AW. *Biomechanical/neurophysiologic factors, related to surgical correction of equinus deformity.* In M.D. Sussman, (Ed), *The diplegic child* (pp. 365–381). Rosemont, IL: American Academy of Orthopaedic Surgeons.

Sohal, R.S., Weindruch, R. (1996). Oxidative stress, caloric restriction and aging. *Science, 215,* 1415–1418.

Spector, S.A., Simard, C.P., Fournier, M., Sternlicht, E., Edgerton, V.R. (1982). Architectural alterations of rat hindlimbs skeletal muscles immobilized at different lengths. *Experimental Neurology, 76,* 94–110.

Stalberg, E., Fawcett, P.R. (1982). Macro EMG in healthy subjects of different ages. *Journal of Neurology, Neurosurgery, and Psychiatry, 45,* 870–878.

Thomason, D.B., Biggs, R.B., Booth, F.W. (1989). Protein metabolism and B-myosin heavy-chain mRNA in unweighted soleus muscle. *American Journal of Physiology, 257,* R300–R305.

Thomason, D.B., Herrick, R.E., Surdyka, D., Baldwin, K.M. (1987). Time course of soleus muscle myosin expression during hindlimb suspension and recovery. *Journal of Applied Physiology, 63,* 130–137.

Trichopoulou, A., Vasilopoulou, E. (2000). Mediterranean diet and longevity. *British Journal of Nutrition, 84,* S205–S2059.

Vandervoort, A.A., McComas, A.J. (1986). Contractile changes in opposing muscles of the human ankle joint with aging. *Journal of Applied Physiology, 61,* 361–367.

Vrbova, G. (1963). Changes in the motor reflexes produced by tenotomy. *Journal of Physiology (London), 166,* 241–250.

Warre, G.L., Lowe, D.A., Hayes, D.A., Karwoski, C.J., Prior, B.M., Armstrong. R.B. (1993). Excitation failure in eccentric contraction-induced injury of mouse soleus muscle. *Journal of Physiology (London), 468,* 487–499.

Weibel, E.R. (1979). *Point counting methods: Practical methods for biological morphometry* (pp. 101–161). London: Academic Press.

Weibel, E.R. (1980). Practical methods for biological morphometry. In *Stereological methods.* New York, NY: Academic Press.

CHAPTER 6

Skeletal Muscle Response to Injury

Chapter Overview

Numerous examples in the world of sports, therapy, surgery, and trauma support the idea that skeletal muscle is one of the most adaptable tissues in the body. Whether the level of use increases or decreases, muscle responds accordingly. As you have seen, muscles are always "trying" to tailor their structural and functional properties to the level of use they experience. However, at times the level of use, metabolic load, or the level of stress on a muscle fiber is so great that the fiber actually suffers damage— the fiber breaks. When the fiber breaks, all or part of the muscle cell degenerates and it is replaced with new muscle tissue. The replacement process is termed regeneration. Skeletal muscle mounts a vigorous regenerative response following injury. Such a response has important implications for both the normal developmental process and the potential use of regenerating muscle in the treatment of diseased muscle. The processes of injury, degeneration and regeneration are the subjects of this final chapter. In this chapter, a number of the lessons previously learned will be applied to understanding muscle adaptation to injury.

Educational Objectives

● To be able to describe the anatomical location and developmental origin of the muscle satellite cell.
● To be able to describe the basic morphological events in the muscle cell degeneration-regeneration process.
● To be able to describe the eccentric injury model in terms of muscle physiology and human performance.
● To be able to discuss proposed mechanisms of eccentric injury along with their clinical relevance.

Introduction

In addition to skeletal muscle's ability to adapt, it also possesses a great ability to regenerate. For years, skeletal muscle's capacity for regeneration was doubted. Some believe that this was because of the distinguished Oxford anatomist Dr. Wilfred E. Le Gros Clark who performed studies of gunshot wound healing around World War II and claimed that, while muscle repaired itself following injury, regeneration of new muscle cells was not possible. There are still some histology and physiology textbooks today that state patently that muscle cells do not regenerate. However, muscle cells certainly do regenerate.

Causes of Muscle Regeneration

Numerous experimental and pathological conditions induce muscle cell degeneration and regeneration. Experimentally, muscles can be crushed, minced, transplanted, exercised, or grafted to initiate this process. Clinically, muscles experience degeneration after blunt trauma, surgical manipulation, ischaemia, and in direct response to the myotoxic effect of local anesthetics. All of these "treatments" have as a common theme, the complete or partial disruption of the muscle cell. After having read through the first chapters of this book, you can probably make a fairly accurate guess at the cellular events associated with the process of degeneration and regeneration. In fact, many events involved in the regenerative process recapitulate the developmental processes outlined in Chapter 1. As a result, it is not uncommon to study regenerating muscle as a model for development. The cellular basis of the muscle regenerative response will be discussed by first describing the "typical" degeneration-regeneration cycle followed by a discussion of various experimental models that have provided insights into the mechanism of muscle regeneration.

Morphology of the Degeneration-Regeneration Cycle

The regeneration sequence conceptually resembles the process of repairing a damaged car: the existing damaged components are removed, replacement components are made, and then they are inserted into their final location. This cycle in muscle, described in detail by Dr. Bruce Carlson, proceeds in much the same way: damaged cellular components are digested, satellite cells proliferate to form new muscle fiber building material, and satellite cells fuse to form new myotubes and muscle fibers, thus recovering cellular function (Carlson, 1973).

Digestion of Damaged Cellular Components

After physical damage to the muscle cell, the degeneration process begins with digestion of damaged cellular components by endogenous protease enzymes released from muscle cell lysosomes and by exogenous proteases released from infiltrating mononuclear macrophages. These macrophages serve as scavengers that "pick up" or phagocytose the cellular debris (Fig. 6-1). The source of these infiltrating cells is the microcirculation surrounding the fibers so that if circulation is absent for any reason (e.g., the cellular necrosis is due to ischaemia or the circulation has been traumatized), the repair process is delayed or aborted. In mammalian muscle, cellular infiltration begins within hours of the initial injury and is well-developed within a few days.

During this digestion phase of degeneration, most cellular components are affected. A beautiful chronicle of cellular responses to degeneration has been published by Carpenter and Karpati (Carpenter & Karpati, 1984). Myofibrils lose their regularity and begin to appear disorganized in the region of the Z-disk. Mitochondria appear more rounded and lose their regular distribution within the cell. Actin and myosin filaments begin to lose their regularity and may even intertwine with the cytoplasmic processes of the macrophage. Glycogen particles, which are plentiful in normal (especially fast) muscle fibers, disappear and the cell no longer stains positively with the PAS stain or for the enzymes used in glycogenolysis (e.g., phosphorylase). Later, the muscle cytoplasm appears as a jumbled mesh of poorly-staining filaments. Degeneration therefore represents the "dismantling phase" of the damaged cell.

Proliferation of Satellite Cells

The next stage in the regeneration cycle is the proliferation of skeletal muscle satellite cells (Fig. 6-1). Recall from Chapter 1, that satellite cells arrange themselves peripherally between the basal lamina and sarcolemma during development during the time period when primary and secondary myotubes are being formed. Satellite cells have not been discussed in detail so far in this text, but now they occupy center stage. Satellite cells are present along the periphery of muscle fibers at less frequent intervals than myonuclei. They resemble myonuclei in many ways but have a more-developed cytoplasm and as such can be identified to represent from 1% to 10% of the total number of nuclei in

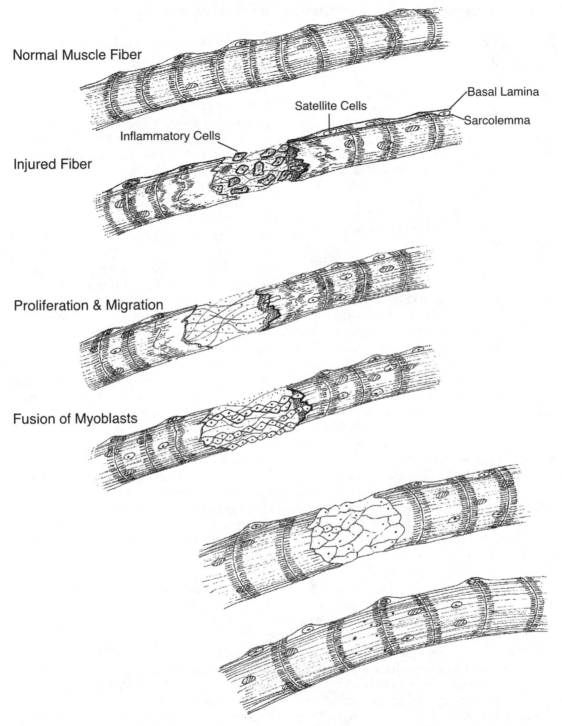

Normal Muscle Fiber

Basal Lamina

Sarcolemma

Satellite Cells

Inflammatory Cells

Injured Fiber

Proliferation & Migration

Fusion of Myoblasts

FIGURE 6-1. Schematic diagram of the degeneration-regeneration process. After a normal muscle fiber is injured, the following events occur (top to bottom): cellular infiltration and inflammation to digest damaged cellular components; proliferation of satellite cells; fusion of satellite cells into myotubes to form new myofibrils; synthesis of myofibrillar proteins to "fill" new fiber.

Box 6-1 Isn't It True That Muscles Do Not Regenerate?

Absolutely not. Unlike other tissues, such as nerves, internal organs, or heart muscle, muscles contain satellite cells—muscle stem cells that serve as muscle cell precursors. These satellite cells are typically quiescent but, upon injury to the fiber, satellite cells begin rapidly dividing and replacing the injured muscle tissue. As a result of the presence of satellite cells, muscles are one of the best tissues in the body at regenerating and are a prime target for gene therapy.

---

the fiber periphery. Because there are relatively few satellite cells, it is not always easy to observe them. In fact, the discovery of the satellite cell was relatively recent and was received by the scientific community with some skepticism (Mauro, 1961). However, it is now known that these satellite cells represent precursor cells to myoblasts that associated with myotubes during development but did not fuse with them. As such, many prefer the terms "presumptive myoblast," or "myogenic precursor cell" to satellite cell in order to specifically refer to their origin and function. There is growing evidence that satellite cells actually represent a muscle population of stem cells that can differentiate into muscle and other tissue types (Hawke & Garry, 2001). In spite of the then lack of understanding of satellite cell activity by the scientific community, it was well known that when a muscle fiber was injured, cellular proliferation occurred within the cell. The question was, "What is the origin of the cells?" In the late 1960s, one school of thought claimed that the source of the proliferating cells was the nuclei within the damaged muscle fiber. They believed that, after injury, the mature muscle fiber fragmented (along with a nucleus) into mononuclear myoblast-like cells, which then recapitulated the developmental process. Others claimed that the satellite cell itself entered a dramatic mitotic phase and began to proliferate in response to some unknown stimulus (see description of this controversy in Mauro, 1970.)

The answer to this dilemma was provided in 1976 by Dr. Mike Snow in radioactive tracer experiments (Snow, 1976). Snow performed two series of experiments: In the first series, he caused developing muscle nuclei to take up radioactive thymidine (a component of DNA). The thymidine base was rendered radioactive by replacing one of the normal (^2H) hydrogen atoms with radioactive hydrogen, known as tritium (^3H). Pregnant rats were injected with ^3H-thymidine at several intervals during their pregnancy (Fig. 6-2). The offspring were allowed to mature for 5–7 weeks. During growth, myonuclei became radioactively labeled whereas any label present in satellite cells was diluted past the point of detection. Then their muscles were minced and forced to degenerate and then regenerate. Snow then measured the radioactivity of the cells involved in the regeneration process. What do you predict would happen? Virtually none of the regenerating cells were radioactive, implying that the nuclei of the regenerated fibers came from something other than normal myonuclei. To investigate this phenomenon further, Snow selectively labeled satellite cells and again, forced these muscles to degenerate and regenerate and found that the regenerating nuclei were indeed radioactive. These experiments established that the cellular source of myonuclei during regeneration was the satellite cells. In fact, satellite cell proliferation represents one of the most impressive biological examples of high synthetic activity.

Signals for Satellite Cell Proliferation

What causes this impressive induction of satellite cell mitotic activity? What is the signal that induces satellite cell proliferation? Dr. Richard Bischoff has performed a series of interesting experiments that have identified some signals that control the behavior of satellite cells (Bischoff, 1986). In one experiment, Bischoff developed a method for "growing" isolated

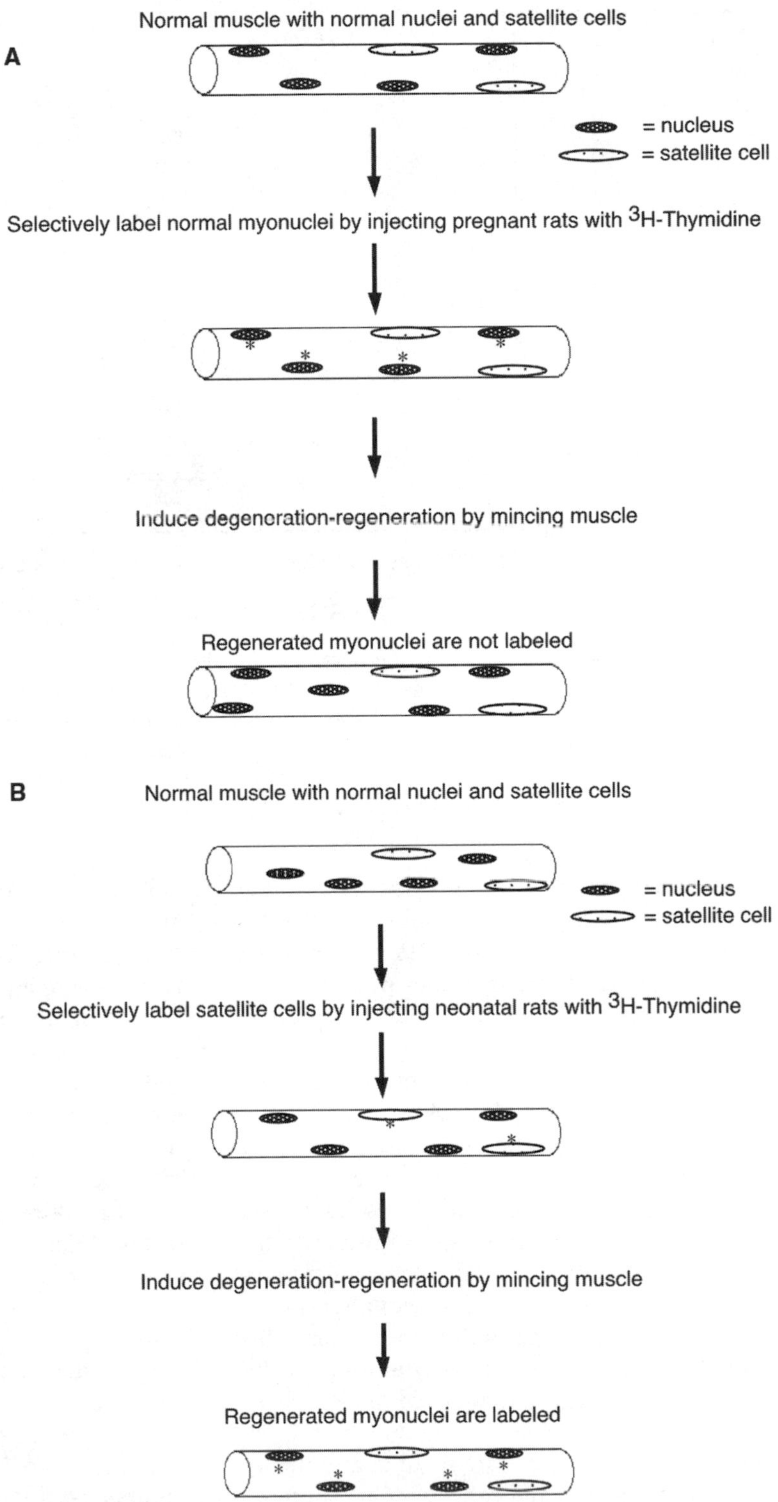

FIGURE 6-2. Experimental demonstration of the source of regenerating myonuclei. **(A)** normal myonuclei were radioactively labeled. Then, upon regeneration, cells in the new fiber were measured for radioactivity. Regenerated myonuclei were not labeled. **(B)** Satellite cells were first radioactively labeled. Then, upon inducing regeneration, cells in the new fiber were measured for radioactivity. Regenerated myonuclei were labeled. These experiments showed that satellite cells were the source of myonuclei in regenerating fibers. (Figure redrawn based on data in: Snow, M.H. (1976). Myogenic cell formation in regenerating rat skeletal muscle injured by mincing. *Anatomical Record, 188,* 201–217.)

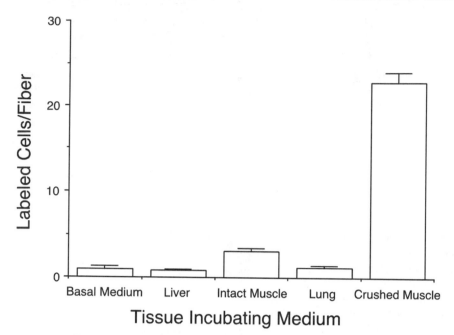

FIGURE 6-3. Experimental determination that a crushed muscle extract causes satellite cell proliferation. Muscle fibers with their associated satellite cells were incubated with various tissue extracts. Only with the extract from crushed muscle, did satellite cells proliferate. This experiment demonstrates that normal muscle contains a mitogen. (Data from: Bischoff, R. (1986). A satellite cell mitogen from crushed adult muscle. *Developmental Biology, 115,* 140–147.)

muscle fibers in culture—outside of the animal, to test various "factors" that might cause satellite cell proliferation. If muscles were crushed and the crushed muscle extract was placed on the cultured muscle fiber, satellite cells proliferated (Fig. 6-3). However, neither "intact muscle extract" (extract from normal muscle) nor extract from other crushed tissues caused satellite cell proliferation. Bischoff concluded that satellite cells were under "positive control." That is, some factor(s) from crushed muscles caused satellite cells to proliferate when normally, they would remain quiescent. This experiment suggested the appealing scenario that after a muscle fiber was damaged and released this mitogenic "factor," satellite cell proliferation would be induced, resulting in muscle repair.

Since the satellite cell is "sandwiched" in between the muscle fiber sarcolemma and the basal lamina, Bischoff and colleagues attempted to determine the relative influence of sarcolemma and basal lamina on the satellite cell proliferative response (Bischoff, 1990). The experimental system again involved isolation of single rat muscle fibers and their associated satellite cells. These cells were placed in a specially-designed cell culture apparatus and allowed to proliferate under a variety of conditions. In the first condition, muscle fibers were killed by application of the local anesthetic Marcaine (Fig. 6-4). This left satellite cells along with their basal lamina to proliferate. In another treatment, the fibers were again killed with Marcaine, but the satellite cells were removed from the basal lamina by spinning them off using a centrifuge. Finally, control fibers with both the intact muscle sarcolemma and the fiber basal lamina were allowed to proliferate.

Satellite cell proliferation was induced by incubating the culture systems in "muscle extract," the soluble portion obtained when muscle fibers were minced. Muscle extract induced cell proliferation (as seen above), but the magnitude of the proliferation was greater if the satellite cells were not in contact with the sarcolemma. Bischoff and colleagues concluded that the sarcolemma exerted a negative control on

> **Box 6-2 What Signals a Satellite Cell to Begin Dividing Within an Injured Muscle?**
>
> The molecular details are not fully known but it almost certainly involves some type of self-activation of the satellite cell by growth factors. In any case, satellite cell activation occurs when the normal inhibitions imposed by the muscle membrane and cell's basal lamina are removed due to injury to either of these tissues. Common events that activate satellite cells include muscle trauma, exercise-induced injury, chronic stretch, significant muscle fiber hypertrophy and injection of local anesthetics.

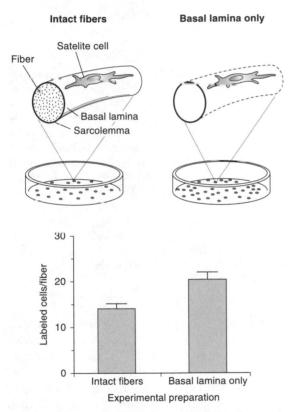

FIGURE 6-4. Schematic representation of experiments used to determine the effect of basal lamina and sarcolemma on satellite cell proliferation. Two experimental conditions were studied: the intact fiber with satellite cells in contact with both the sarcolemma and basal lamina (top left), and satellite cells dissociated from both the sarcolemma and basal lamina (top right). Satellite cells proliferated to a greater extent when the muscle fiber was removed (lower panel). (Data from: Bischoff, R. (1990). Interaction between satellite cells and skeletal muscle fibers. *Development, 109*, 943–952.)

satellite cells to prevent proliferation. In this way it was possible to explain why one portion of a damaged fiber might mount a large regenerative response (since its sarcolemma was damaged and thus not in contact with the satellite cell) while another portion might remain quiescent (since the satellite cell was still in contact with the sarcolemma).

Thus, satellite cells are under both positive and negative control: positive control by some mitogenic factor within the muscle and negative control because of sarcolemmal contact. The molecular details of each of these control processes remain to be elucidated.

Growth Factor Effects on Satellite Cells

It is known that skeletal muscle fibers have various growth factors beneath the basal lamina in some type of bound form that can be released upon fiber breakage. But just which growth factor is involved in satellite cell proliferation such as is seen when muscle extract is placed on satellite cells in culture and causes them to divide (such as that shown in Fig. 6-3)? There is evidence that a specific growth factor, the hepatocyte growth factor (HGF), is able to activate satellite cells powerfully and specifically (Johnson & Allen, 1993; 1995). HGF was originally discovered in liver (hence the name) and caused proliferation and "scattering" of hepatocytes in culture. Subsequently, it was shown to have mitogenic activity even for satellite cells (Allen, Sheehan, Taylor, Kendall, & Rice, 1995; Jennische, Ekberg, & Matejka, 1993). But was it present in muscle and would it activate satellite cells in vivo? This question was definitively answered in the affirmative by Dr. Ron Allen and colleagues (Tatsumi, Anderson, Nevoret, Halery, & Allen, 1998). They first showed that HGF was present in the extracellular matrix, surrounding the muscle fibers in uninjured muscle. They then showed that HGF was present in "crushed muscle extract" and that when muscle was injured, both HGF and its cellular receptor were located in the same region of regenerative muscle. Incubation of the crushed muscle extract with an antibody to HGF (which would bind it and render it biologically inactive) rendered the extract ineffective. Finally, when HGF was directly injected into rat tibialis anterior muscles, satellite cell proliferation was clearly observed based on uptake of a synthetic nucleotide used during DNA replication (Fig. 6-5). These experiments provide fairly conclusive evidence of the autocrine nature of growth factors, specifically HGF, in causing satellite cell proliferation.

Fusion of Satellite Cells into Myotubes

After only a few days after injury, proliferation of satellite cells is noticeable and, within 3–4 days, their presence is unmistakable (Fig. 6-1). Now, the regeneration process resembles, in many ways, the normal developmental process. Satellite cells begin to express the myogenic regulatory factors *myoD* and *myf-5*, which was shown in development, and resulted in the commitment of stem cells to the myogenic lineage (Megeney, Kablar, Garrett, Anderson, & Rudnicki, 1996). Satellite cells begin to align themselves along the basal lamina and fuse into myotubes (Fig. 6-1). The presence of the basal lamina has been considered to be of critical importance as a substrate for satellite cell proliferation and fusion. For example, it is known that satellite cells when placed in cell culture proliferate and fuse better on a collagen substrate (the primary component of the basal lamina) compared with a plastic substrate. It is known

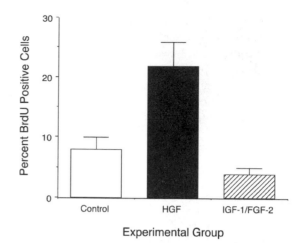

FIGURE 6-5. Proliferation of satellite cells under different conditions indicated by the appearance of BrdU positive cells in tissue. BrdU positive cells are those that are involved in cellular replication such as proliferating satellite cells. Treatments of satellite cells represent saline control (open bar), hepatocyte growth factor, HGF (filled bar), and a combination of insulin-like growth factor-1 (IGF-1) and fibroblast growth factor-2 (FGF-2). Only HGF shows the activation with the muscle in the in vivo condition. (Data from: Tatsumi, R., Anderson, J.E., Nevoret, C.J., Halevy, O., Allen, R.E. (1998). HGF/SF is present in normal adult skeletal muscle and is capable of activating satellite cells. *Developmental Biology, 194,* 114–128.)

that the basal lamina is not a completely passive structure during regeneration in that it expresses various extracellular matrix components along a certain time course. Thus, its characteristics change continually throughout the regeneration process and it is unlikely that it maintains a central controlling influence (Gulati, Reddi, & Zalewski, 1983). In fact, a recent report demonstrated satellite cell proliferation and fusion under conditions where the basal lamina was actually absent. It may be, therefore, that other factors are actually responsible for the alignment of myoblasts as they fuse into myotubes. For example, a novel myoblast cell culture system was developed by Dr. Herman Vandenburgh (Vandenburgh, 1982; Vandenburgh, Hatefaludy, Karlisch, & Shansky, 1991). He showed that myoblasts grown in a simple, nonmoving culture system proliferated with random orientation and remain relatively immature (Fig. 6-6). However, if the cells were cyclically lengthened and shortened, the cells became well-aligned, took up greater amounts of amino acids, and synthesized more proteins (Shansky, Del Tatto, Chromiak, & Vandenburgh, 1997). These data suggested that, in addition to certain chemical factors, mechanical stress, or at least strain, had a pronounced effect on the myoblastic maturation process (Vandenburgh, et al., 1996; Vandenburgh, Swasdison, & Karlisch, 1991). This type of experiment may also be relevant in the tissue engineering approach to creating artificial skeletal muscle, which is an exciting new area of biotechnology (Huard & Fu, 2000; Niklason 1999; Niklason et al., 1999).

Synthesis of Contractile Proteins

As satellite cells proliferate and regeneration continues, myotubes mature, continue to differentiate, and synthesize new myofibrillar proteins. As in development, new myoblasts are deposited in the outer subsarcolemmal region of the regenerating fiber. Thus, regenerating fibers, like developing fibers, when stained for myofibrillar proteins, appear as doughnuts with light central cores (Fig. 6-1). As fibers continue to fill with contractile protein, muscle nuclei are usually pushed to the periphery and the fiber takes on the appearance of a mature skeletal muscle fiber. Sometimes regenerated fibers fail to move the nucleus to the periphery and a central nucleus remains. This central nucleus serves as a pathological statement that the fiber has undergone degeneration and regeneration. Often, the number or percentage of central nuclei within a muscle is used to express the level of regeneration of muscle tissue. The entire regeneration process requires about 6 months in most higher mammals although regeneration in rat muscle is quite a bit faster, requiring only about 2 months. It should be obvious from this discussion, that the control and coordination of muscle events is not fully understood during regeneration. Many of these questions are also relevant to the muscle developmental process and are being actively pursued.

Muscle Properties After Regeneration

After regeneration occurs, do muscle properties return to their original values? Do all properties recover to the same extent? You have seen dramatic demonstrations of muscle plasticity under various conditions. How "plastic" is regenerating muscle? Answers to these questions have important clinical implications in which performance is affected after injury or trauma.

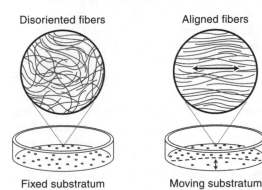

Disoriented fibers   Aligned fibers

Fixed substratum   Moving substratum

FIGURE 6-6. Effect of strain on avian myoblasts in culture. When the substratum on which these myoblasts are grown remains fixed, myofibers grown in a disoriented fashion (left) whereas cultured myoblasts align themselves and mature faster when mechanically strained in vitro (arrow represents strain direction on right). (Figure drawn based on observations in: Vandenburgh, H.H. (1982). Dynamic mechanical orientation of skeletal myofibers in vitro. *Developmental Biology, 93*, 438–443.)

Recovery of Muscle Contractile Properties in Cat Muscle

To address the question of muscle recovery following regeneration, Dr. John Faulkner and his colleague (Faulkner, Niemeyer, Maxwell, & White, 1980) induced cat extensor digitorum longus muscle regeneration by surgically removing the muscle, transecting the nerve and neurovascular supply and replanting the entire muscle (Fig. 6-7). Muscles were allowed to re-

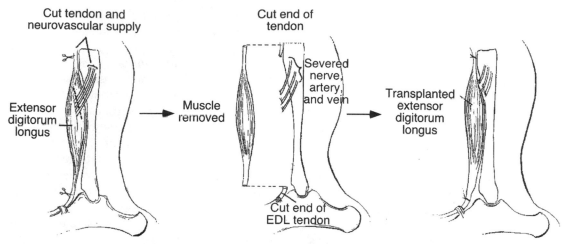

FIGURE 6-7. Experimental method for transplantation of the cat extensor digitorum longus (EDL). The EDL was removed and the neurovascular supply severed. It was then replaced in the original site where reinnervation and regeneration could occur. (Figure based on method in: Faulkner, J.A., Niemeyer, J.H., Maxwell, C., White, T.P. (1980). Contractile properties of transplanted extensor digitorum longus muscles of cats. *American Journal of Physiology, 238,* C120–C126.)

cover from 40 to 400 days, and contractile properties measured at specific intervals. After a few weeks, muscles developed measurable tension and maximum tetanic tension continued to increase for about 8 months at which point it stabilized to about 50% of the level reached in control muscles (Fig. 6-8). This relative recovery was increased if the nerve was left intact. In contrast to P_o, these investigators found that many properties demonstrated complete recovery after graft stabilization (stabilization was defined as the time when fibers in the central muscle core were the same size as fibers in the periphery). For example, time-to-peak tension (Fig. 2-2), half-relaxation time (Fig. 2-2), V_{max} (Fig. 2-7), fiber length, and individual fiber cross-sectional area returned to control levels after 6 months. Apparently, not all of the fibers regenerated since, although fiber area and length were normal, muscle mass and P_o decreased significantly, implying a decrease in fiber number. Alternately, perhaps the force generated per fiber decreased. This is a difficult question to resolve since direct mea-surement of muscle fiber number is difficult and controversial.

Metabolically, regenerated muscle demonstrated a decrease in endurance after transplantation. Capillary density and succinate dehydrogenase activity recovered to only about 50% of control levels rendering the muscle dramatically more fatigable. Fortunately, since you have learned that muscle endurance is very plastic in response to increased muscle use (Chapter 4), it is possible that training of these muscles might significantly improve fatigability. This is an area of ongoing investigation and early experimental results are promising. Incidentally, muscle endurance in regenerated rat muscle is much greater than that observed in cat muscle so there is apparently a species difference that may make the results a bit difficult to apply to the human situation.

Plasticity of Regenerating Muscle Fibers

Faulkner and his colleague (Donovan & Faulkner, 1987) also investigated a regenerating muscle's adaptive capacity by comparing surgical transplantation (in which the muscle was removed without its neurovascular supply and placed in a new site) to surgical transposition (in which the muscle was removed with its vascular supply intact and moved to a new site and innervated by the new nerve; Fig. 6-9). In transplantation, the muscle fibers degenerated due to ischaemia and, in addition, the investigators injected the local anesthetic Bupivacaine to obtain a uniform regenerating population of fibers. In surgical transposition, the fact that the vascular supply was left intact insured muscle fiber survival. Implantation of the new motor nerve would thus be similar to a cross-reinnervation experiment.

Donovan and Faulkner compared the adaptation of rat soleus and extensor digitorum longus (EDL) muscles following either transposition or transplantation. In all cases, transposition resulted in muscle fibers, which recovered the greatest strength (Fig. 6-10A). For example, the transposed EDL P_o was 830 mN compared with the transplanted EDL P_o of only 590 mN. Similarly, the transposed soleus P_o was 710 mN compared with the transplanted soleus P_o of 660 mN. However, what was perhaps more interesting was the change in contractile speed and fiber type distribution following the treatments. In all cases, the transplanted muscle became more like the muscle, which had been in the recipient site. Thus, the transplanted soleus time-to-peak twitch tension (TPT) was 29 ms, very close to the control EDL TPT of 24 and very different from either the transposed SOL TPT of 67 ms or the control SOL TPT of 83 ms (Fig. 6-10B). In the same way, the transplanted EDL contained only 33% fast fibers, closer to the control soleus fast fiber percentage of 15% than either the transposed EDL percentage (86%) or the control EDL percentage (97%; Figure 6-10C). Thus, in all cases, the transplanted

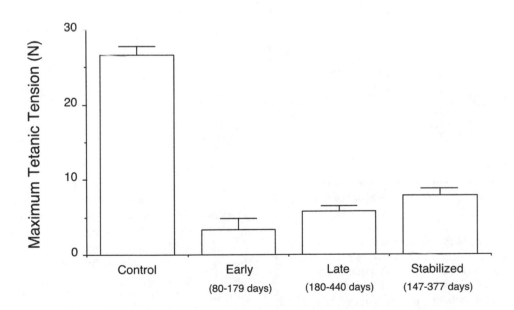

Graft Measurement Interval

FIGURE 6-8. Time course of tetanic tension in the cat EDL after induced degeneration and regeneration. (Data from: Faulkner, J.A., Niemeyer, J.H., Maxwell, C., White, T.P. (1980). Contractile properties of transplanted extensor digitorum longus muscles of cats. *American Journal of Physiology*, *238*, C120–C126.)

Rat Hindlimb

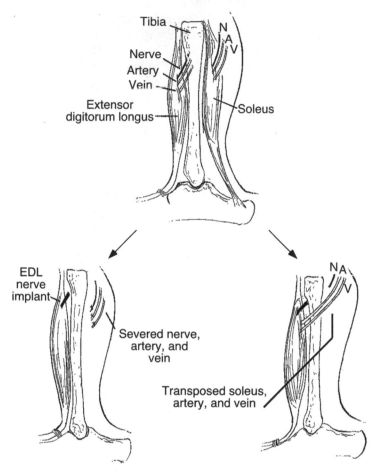

FIGURE 6-9. Schematic diagram comparing muscle transplantation (left panel) with muscle transposition (right panel) in rat soleus and EDL muscles. After transplantation, the muscle degenerates and then regenerates whereas after transposition, the muscle does not degenerate due to the intact neurovascular supply, but adapts to the new motor nerve. (Figure based on methods in: Donovan, C.M., Faulkner, J. (1987). Plasticity of skeletal muscle: regenerating fibers adapt more rapidly than surviving fibers. *Journal of Applied Physiology, 62,* 2507–2511.)

muscles, consisting of regenerating fibers, were the most adaptable fibers present.

These experiments raised the intriguing possibility that, since regenerating fibers were highly adaptable, that a specific strategy to enable muscle fiber adaptation might be to enter the regeneration cycle. While this is certainly not the typical mechanism of muscle adaptation, the possibility exists that a greater degree of adaptation might occur in muscle after traumatic laceration of skeletal muscle, free muscle graft (transplantation) or muscle fiber adaptation to intense exercise which is accompanied by fiber breakage (see page 304).

Box 6-3 Why Can Muscle Regeneration Be Good?

There is evidence that, as a muscle regenerates, it takes on the characteristics of its new environment. Thus, if the goal is to transplant a muscle into a new area, the regenerative response of muscle that occurs, places it in a much more "plastic" state—readily able to adapt to the new neural input and level of use. Currently, the tremendous regenerative capacity of muscle is not exploited very often clinically.

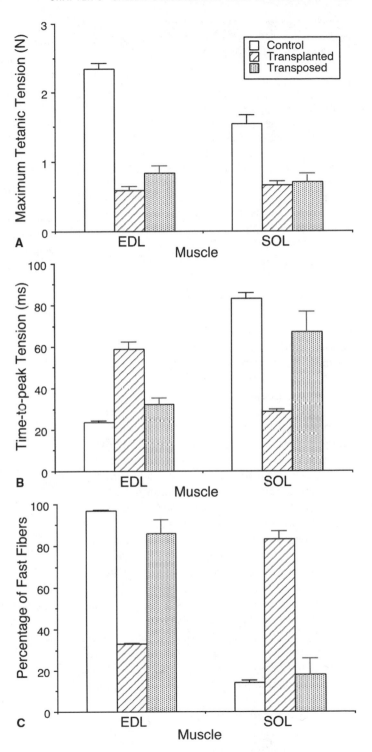

FIGURE 6-10. Muscle properties after transplantation (hatched bars) compared with transposition (stippled bars). **(A)** Maximum tetanic tension of muscles following transplantation and transposition. **(B)** Time-to-peak tension of muscles following transplantation and translocation. **(C)** Fast fiber percentage of muscles following transplantation and translocation. (Data from: Donovan, C.M., Faulkner, J. (1987). Plasticity of skeletal muscle: regenerating fibers adapt more rapidly than surviving fibers. *Journal of Applied Physiology, 62*, 2507–2511.)

Box 6-4 Does Young Muscle Regenerate Better Than Old Muscle?

Interestingly, transplantation experiments have shown that "old" muscle doesn't regenerate as well as "young" muscle. However, the caveat is that, in almost all experiments, "old" muscles were transplanted back into "old" animals. It turns out, that the problem with the "old muscle" experiments was the older *animal*, not the older *muscle*. There was no difference in the older muscle's intrinsic regenerative ability. This fact was demonstrated clearly, for when old muscles were transplanted into young animals, they regenerated perfectly!

Regeneration of Aged Muscle

Chapter 5 showed that aged muscle demonstrates a variety of changes that could in theory, render it more or less capable of regeneration. In fact, the regeneration experiments do not produce as successful a result in old compared to young animals. The regenerative response is less vigorous and the muscles regain a smaller proportion of their pre-degeneration properties. Why should this be the case? Dr. Bruce Carlson pursued this question by transplanting young muscle into aged rats and aged muscle into young rats (Carlson & Faulkner, 1989). His hypothesis was that there was a difference between the old and young muscles themselves that caused the differential regenerative response. Of course, he also performed the control experiments of transplanting young muscles into young rats and old muscles into old rats. The results were, to say the least, surprising (Fig. 6-11). Carlson and colleagues demonstrated that the level of regeneration depended on the age of the recipient animal much more than the age of the donor tissue. Thus, old muscle transplanted into young rats regenerated almost as well as young muscle transplanted into young rats (Fig. 6-11, hatched bars). Similarly, young muscle transplanted into old rats did not regenerate well at all, despite the presumed high quality of the young tissue (Fig. 6-11, open bars). These data demonstrate that, with ageing, there is not necessarily any loss in muscle's ability to regenerate, but rather, that the muscle tissue milieu has a profound influence on regenerative capacity. As you might expect, the hormonal and other cellular factors that affect regeneration are active areas of current research. Carlson and colleagues have since showed that one of the major factors that limit a muscle's ability to regenerate effectively has to do with the quality of the reinnervation response. They showed that one of the main problems with regeneration of either young or old muscle in the older animals was the "impaired" ability of old motor nerves to reinnervate muscles (Carlson & Faulkner, 1989). This is reminiscent of the other aging experiments in which motor neuron number decreased with aging. These types of results point to the nervous system as a major factor causing reduced muscle function and plasticity observed with age.

Clinical Application to Muscular Dystrophy

An improved understanding of skeletal muscle regeneration promises to provide improved functional recovery after surgical repair and grafting. However, nowhere is the promise of muscle regeneration so bright as in the application of modern biological techniques to the "repair" of diseased muscle tissue.

Duchenne Muscular Dystrophy

The most common type of genetic dystrophy that affects children is known as Duchenne muscular dystrophy (DMD), named for its original descriptor. DMD is a devastating myopathy, which is sex-linked, striking young boys (about 1 in 3,500) early in the first years of life. By the age of about 13 most DMD patients must use a wheelchair for mobility and weakness of the intercostal muscles often leads to death by age 20. Upon histological examina-

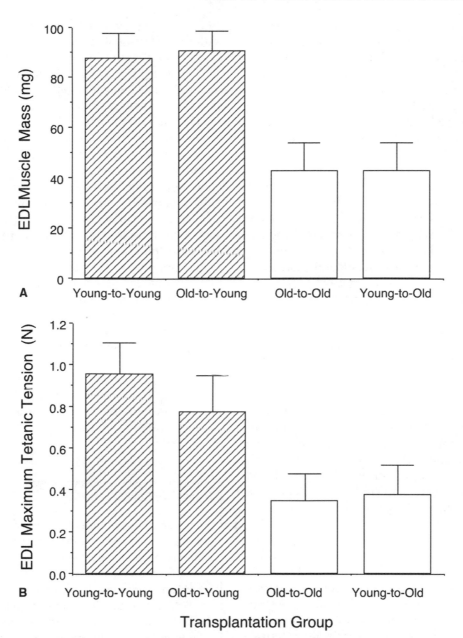

FIGURE 6-11. Maximum tetanic tension generated by regenerated muscle as a function of muscle age and host age. **(A)** EDL mass of young and old muscles transplanted into young animals (hatched bars) or old animals (open bars). **(B)** EDL maximum tetanic tension of young and old muscles transplanted into young animals (hatched bars) or old animals (open bars). Data demonstrate that the quality of muscle recovery after transplantation is determined by the age of the host. (Data from: Carlson, B.M., Faulkner, J.A. (1989). Muscle transplantation between young and old rats: age of host determines recovery. *American Journal of Physiology, 256,* C1262–C1266.)

tion, the muscle reveals tremendous variation in fiber size and central nuclei, suggesting repeated cycles of degeneration and regeneration. However, the regeneration does not compensate for the degeneration, leading to a progressive loss of muscle fibers. In parallel with the muscle fiber changes is a proliferation of connective tissue and fat cells within the tissue such that the muscle ultimately becomes nonfunctional.

The actual "cause" of Duchenne muscular dystrophy was not known until 1987. Prior to that, numerous morphological observations of dystrophic muscles had led to several hypotheses for this cyclic dysfunctional process including ischemia, neural degeneration, and leaky membranes (Brown & Lucy, 1997). Certainly, these hypotheses were consistent with many of the observations that had been made.

It was found that dystrophic muscle lacked a specific protein product that came to be known as "dystrophin" in deference to its absence in dystrophic tissue (Hoffman, Brown, & Kunkle, 1987a). Dystrophin was found to be associated with the sarcolemma (Ohlendieck, Ervasti, Snook, & Campbell, 1991) as a long filamentous network. The DNA sequence of the protein suggested that it was structurally similar to spectrin, a protein that allows red blood cells to have their characteristic biconcave disk shape and also that it was able to bind actin, much like α-actinin within the sarcomere. Taken together, these observations suggested a polymerized filament network, lying below the sarcolemma that was believed to stabilize the muscle membrane during contraction (Petrof, Shrager, Stedman, Kelly, & Sweeney, 1993). In the absence of dystrophin, the muscle membrane would not be able to tolerate repetitive contraction leading to loss of membrane integrity and the morphological appearance described above. An animal model of DMD was also discovered that mimicked some (but, importantly, not all) of the morphological affects of DMD. The so-called *mdx* mouse muscles show segmental clusters of necrotic fibers at the age of 10–12 days. The muscles then degener-

ate and regenerate over the next few months with regenerating fibers achieving near-normal diameters but with centrally-placed nuclei (see above, page 295). The centrally-placed nuclei thus provide a morphological label for degenerated and regenerated fibers.

The subsarcolemmal dystrophin protein forms a network that integrates the myofibrillar force generating components with the surface membrane. Importantly, a collection of transmembrane proteins is associated with dystrophin in much the same way that the intermediate filaments are associated with the costameres across the muscle fiber. Thus, the dystrophin and dystrophin-associated proteins (DAP) are critical not only to the maintenance of cellular integrity but also perhaps to the cell's ability to respond appropriately to stress. In fact, the loss of even one of the components of the DAP complex can give rise to one of many muscle myopathies. Using modern molecular methods, these myopathies are now being classified in terms of the specific missing protein (Campbell, 1995; Dalakas et al., 2000), which provides insights into the normal functions of these components (Table 6-1).

Therapist's Comments

Because of the potential for muscle injury in the muscles of children with Duchenne muscular dystrophy, the child must be protected from overuse early in the disease process. I recommend the use of lightweight bracing and judicious early use of powered wheelchairs to protect the muscles from injury. However, some exercise is needed and is beneficial.

Low impact exercise, such as swimming, lessens the chance of muscle injury (since the muscle action is primarily concentric), and it emphasizes aerobic conditioning which is particularly helpful for the child.

TABLE 6-1	Localization of Proteins Involved in Different Muscular Dystrophies	
Cellular Localization	Protein Involved	Type of Muscular Dystrophy
Nucleus	Emerin	x-linked Emery-Dreifuss muscular dystrophy
	Lamin	Autosomal dominant Emery-Dreifus muscular dystrophy
Cytoplasm	Calpain	Limb girdle muscular dystrophy (2A)
Cytoskeleton	Dystrophin	Duchenne/Becker muscular dystrophy
	Telethonin	Limb girdle muscular dystrophy (2G)
Sarcolemma	Sarcoglycans	Limb girdle muscular dystrophy (2C-F)
	Caveolin	Limb girdle muscular dystrophy (1C)
	$\alpha 7$ Integrin	Congenital myopathy
Extracellular Matrix	Laminin	Congenital muscular dystrophy
	Collagen	Bethlem myopathy

Therapeutic Implantation of Myoblast Cells in mdx Mice

A potentially thrilling set of experiments has suggested that it might be possible to "fix" affected muscle from mdx mice by implanting normal myoblasts into the DMD muscle during early development. This work has been performed in different laboratories around the world. One set of illustrative experiments was performed by the muscle pathologists Drs. George Karpati, Sterling Carpenter and colleagues in which nondystrophic myogenic cells which had been labeled with ^{3}H-thymidine (as described earlier) were implanted into the quadriceps of young (3–15 day old mdx mice [Karpati, Pouliot, Stirling, & Holland, 1989]; Fig. 6-12). At this young age, mdx mice have not yet begun to shown muscle necrosis. The mdx mice were allowed to grow and the developed quadriceps muscles were screened for the presence of radioactive myonuclei. Karpati

et al. found heavily labeled myonuclei in the host fibers implying that implanted "normal" nuclei had fused with the mdx myoblasts and formed what are called "mosaic" or "chimeric" muscle fibers—fibers with nuclei of different

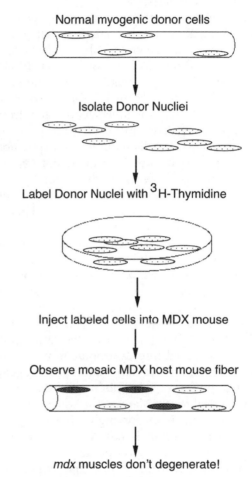

FIGURE 6-12. Experimental manipulation of mouse mdx cells by fusion with normal satellite cells. Incorporation of normal myogenic donor cells into mdx cells results in expression of dystrophin and normal cellular morphology. (Figure based on experimental methods in: Karpati, G., Pouliot, Y., Stirling, C., Holland, P. (1989). Implantation of nondystrophic allogenic myoblasts into dystrophic muscles of mdx mice produces "mosaic" fibers of normal microscopic phenotype. In L.H. Kedes and F.E. Stockdale (Eds.), Cellular and Molecular Biology of Muscle Development. (pp. 973–985). New York: Alan R Liss, New York.)

origin. Subsequent work from this and other laboratories have also demonstrated that, after formation of mosaic fibers, many of the normal degenerative features of dystrophic muscle are not seen—the fibers are "fixed" by the addition of normal myoblasts.

A similar experiment was performed by Partridge et al. in which chimeric muscle fibers were formed as described above (Partridge, Morgan, Coulton, Hoffman, & Kunkel, 1989). Importantly, using a relatively low ratio of normal donor to *mdx* nuclei, these investigators showed that the fibers converted from dystrophin-negative to dystrophin-positive. Thus, the normal cells induced the expression of the dystrophin protein. Subsequent experimentation has shown that dystrophin is expressed even in muscle fiber regions in which the original *mdx* nuclei are present (Huard, Lebrecque, Dansereau, 1991).

Obviously, the therapeutic potential of these treatments is immense. As a result of these basic science experiments, clinical application of this work to patients with muscular dystrophy has been attempted (Blau & Springer, 1995; Gussoni, Blau, & Kunkel, 1997; Rando & Blau, 1994). At this point, it is clear that dystrophin genes introduced into dystrophic muscles can allow the muscle to re-express this missing gene product but, as yet, it has not produced a significant clinical result. Many of the issues relate to developing methods for high efficiency gene transfer into human muscles and forcing muscles to make the appropriate gene products (Huard & Fu, 2000). This, of course, is an exciting and promising area of research.

Muscle Response to Exercise-Induced Injury

It has been repeated that skeletal muscle actions associated with lengthening (eccentric) contractions are also associated with high muscle forces. Numerous investigators have demonstrated that when eccentric exercise is performed, muscle damage and muscle soreness result. The term eccentric "contraction" does not, therefore, imply muscle shortening and is the term most often used to describe the active stretch of an activated muscle. Eccentric contractions are interesting to study not only to understand how muscle is injured during intense exercise, but because there is evidence that these types of contractions produce very high strengthening effects. This is sort of a two-edged sword: eccentric contractions can produce strengthening, but also injure the muscle. Thus, the question is should they be used in therapy? Such a question can only be answered after both the mechanisms of injury and strengthening are understood. In this section, this will be addressed.

Mechanics of Eccentric Contractions

Our first evidence that something is "strange" regarding eccentric contractions, is based on the observation that muscle behaves mechanically different when shortening compared with lengthening. This shows up as a dramatic discontinuity of the force-velocity relationship for shortening compared with lengthening. Chapter 2 showed, for example, that when a muscle shortens at about 1% V_{max} that maximum tetanic tension drops to about 95% P_o (Fig. 2-7). However, when a muscle is forced to lengthen at the same slow velocity, 1% V_{max}, tension rises precipitously to over 125% P_o (Fig. 6-13)! In Chapter 2, this behavior was explained based on the asymmetrical mechanical properties of the cross-bridge. However, it is becoming increasingly clear that the classic cross-bridge theory is really not able to explain a number of mechanical phenomena that are known to occur with muscle lengthening (Harry, Ward, Heglund, Morgan, & McMahon, 1990; Morgan, 1990). The exact details of these phenomena are beyond the scope of this textbook, even though they do make for some fascinating reading. This fact is raised to point out that, despite eccentric contractions being a normal part of the gait cycle (Chapter 3) and experienced by most muscles in the body, relatively little is known of the physiology of eccentric

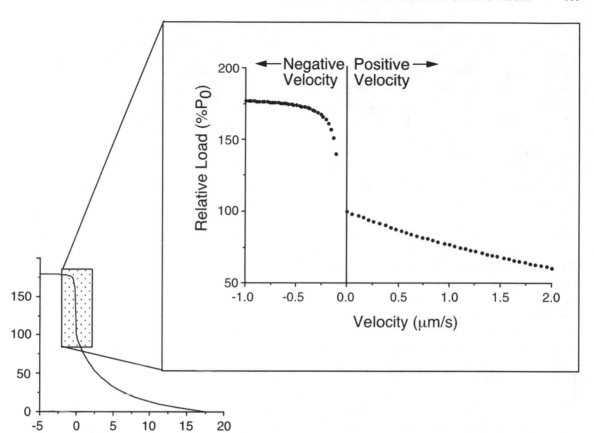

FIGURE 6-13. Enlargement of the positive and negative force–velocity relationship in the region very near the zero velocity point (isometric contraction). Note the force increase per unit negative velocity is over six times the force decrease per unit positive velocity. Thus, muscles are very "stiff" in resisting active stretch.

contractions. Many investigators agree that eccentric contractions, if performed at a high intensity, can cause injury, but as the physiologist Dr. Herman deVree pointed out, ". . . it is difficult to image why a structure would be injured when performing the very act for which it was designed!" In fact, you have seen that most physiological experiments have been performed with maximal activation under steady state conditions (isometric or isotonic contractions) when, in reality, these conditions are rarely achieved. "Eccentric contraction physiology" is an exciting area of research that promises new vistas in therapeutic and exercise treatment.

Box 6-5 Why Should Active Muscle Lengthening Make A Muscle Stronger?

Lengthening of an activated muscle is known as an eccentric contraction, and results in very high muscle force, muscle soreness, and tissue injury. Some or all of these factors provide a powerful strengthening stimulus to the muscle. As a result, eccentric contractions, practically known as "negatives" and "plyometrics" are commonly used by individuals who want to gain muscle strength.

A common eccentric contraction experienced during the gait cycle is the active lengthening of the quadriceps musculature as the foot strikes the ground (Fig. 6-14A). As foot strike occurs and the momentum of the body carries it forward and down, the quadriceps lengthen and the knee flexes. This is especially pronounced if deceleration is required such as in downhill running or walking down steps. How many people have felt sore quadriceps after a long downhill hike? Indeed downhill running in animals and humans remains a favorite physiological model to induce muscle injury and soreness.

Human Models of Eccentric Contraction

One finding on which many agree is that, after an intense bout of eccentric exercise, muscle soreness is not immediately experienced, but is maximum about 24–48 hours later. This phenomenon has been termed delayed onset muscle soreness (DOMS). There is no question that DOMS is uniquely related to the eccentric contraction and not to exercise itself. This is easily demonstrated by comparing subjective impressions of soreness between individuals who have performed exercise involving eccentric contractions to those who have performed exercise involving isometric contractions. Unfortunately, it is difficult to quantify soreness and therefore investigators have searched for other more objective parameters to study eccentric exercise. One such parameter that is measurable in both animals and humans is the circulating level of creatine kinase.

In Chapter 2, we noted that creatine kinase (CK) is an enzyme found in striated muscle, and which catalyzes the conversion of ADP to ATP according to the reaction:

$$\text{Creatine Phosphate} + \text{ADP} \rightarrow \text{Creatine} + \text{ATP} \quad \text{(Eq. 2-18)}$$

(In fact, ATP is so rapidly regenerated from ADP by CK that ATP levels remain almost unchanged during muscle contraction, even during very intense anaerobic exercise.) CK is located inside muscle fibers and, under normal conditions, remains there. However, when exercise is extremely intense and a cell is injured, CK is released into the bloodstream where it can be detected. (In fact different isozymes of CK exist in heart and skeletal muscles so that serum cardiac CK levels can be used to diagnose myocardial infarction.) CK therefore serves as an indirect measure of myofiber integrity and injury.

Serum CK Levels After Eccentric Contraction

Dr. Bill Evans and colleagues measured serum CK levels after intense eccentric exercise in young college students (Evans et al., 1986). Subjects performed an eccentric exercise bout consisting of a single 45 minute bout of high intensity exercise. He presented two major experimental findings: First, he showed that CK levels did not immediately increase after eccentric exercise, but were elevated a few days after the exercise bout, peaked 5 days after the exercise bout and remained elevated for several days thereafter (Fig. 6-15). Think about what this infers regarding muscle fiber breakdown. Clearly, the data suggest that muscle fibers do not simply "break" in response to exercise and release their contents like a popped water balloon. The CK data suggest that the muscle fibers experienced some type of injury that then initiated a cascade of events that included loss of intracellular muscle components. The cascade may involve events that continue for several days as illustrated by the protracted elevated CK levels shown in Figure 6-15.

Evans et al. also importantly demonstrated that if subjects had been trained by performing the same eccentric exercise training protocol before an eccentric exercise bout, that the magnitude and duration of the elevated CK levels were greatly attenuated (Fig. 6-15). These trained subjects also had elevated CK levels before the experimental exercise bout, suggesting that they were experiencing greater muscle fiber turnover, probably due to the eccentric training. The study therefore presents two important results on which most investigators

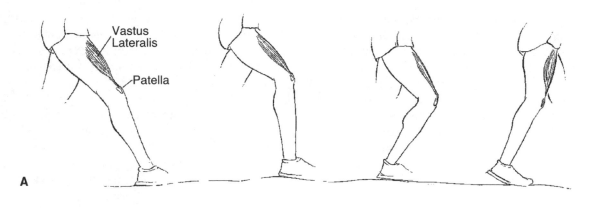

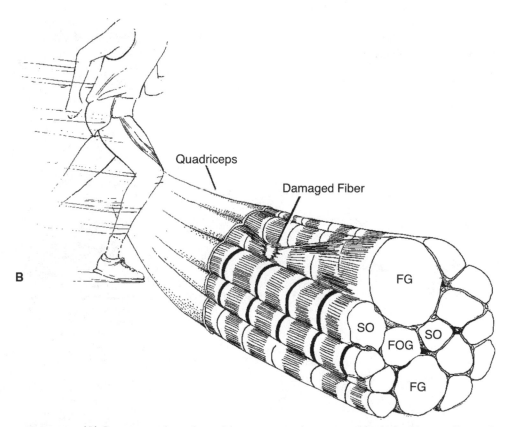

FIGURE 6-14. **(A)** Representation of quadriceps eccentric contraction during foot strike and subsequent toe-off. As the momentum of the body forces knee flexion, vastus lateralis is forced to actively lengthen. **(B)** Schematic illustration of damage to specific muscle fibers following eccentric contraction (Compare with Figs. 6-24 and 6-40A)

agree: (1) muscle damage and soreness due to eccentric contraction is delayed and prolonged and (2) prior eccentric training provides a "protective" effect on further muscle damage.

Studies of serum CK levels have provided information regarding the types of exercise that cause injury (those that are biased toward eccentric contractions) and the protective effects of prior eccentric training (as seen above). A very dramatic demonstration of the muscle adaptations that occur with repeated exercise bouts was provided by Dr. Diane Newham and her colleagues. They studied the effects of eccentric exercise of elbow flexor muscles performed three different times separated by 2 weeks (Newham, Jones, & Clarkson, 1987). After the first bout, as expected, maximum strength dropped precipitously (Fig. 6-16A) and creatine kinase levels began to rise dramat-

ically (Fig. 6-16B). However, 2 and 4 weeks later, a different result was observed. A significant drop in maximum strength again occurred (arrows, Fig. 6-16A), but there was no accompanying change in serum CK levels (Fig. 6-16B). These data indicated some type of a "remodeling" of the muscle that occurred due to the initial eccentric contraction and that persisted even 2 weeks later. This striking result made the muscle physiology community think long and hard about both the nature of muscle adaptation and the stimuli that cause the adaptations to occur. More will be said about this below.

Serum CK is Not a Good Predictor of the Magnitude of Muscle Injury

Using serum CK measurements such as those provided above, investigators have made ad-

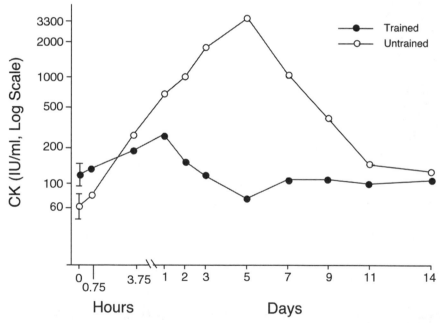

FIGURE 6-15. Time course of serum creatine kinase (CK) levels following eccentric exercise in untrained (open circles) and trained (filled circles) subjects. Note the delay between the exercise bout and subsequent peak serum enzyme levels. (Data from: Evans, W.J., Meredith, C.N., Cannon, J.G., Dinarello, C.A., Frontera, W.R., Hughes, V.A., Jones, B.H., Knuttgen, H.G. (1986). Metabolic changes following eccentric exercise in trained and untrained men. *Journal of Applied Physiology, 61,* 1864–1868.)

Therapist's Comments

In humans, as in animal models, strength decreases after eccentric exercise-induced muscle injury. This strength loss, measured as the maximum voluntary contraction, is quite severe, often reaching 25–50% loss of strength immediately after a single exercise bout. More importantly for the clinician, the loss of strength can easily last several weeks. This suggests that a patient who is beginning an exercise program that includes a significant amount of eccentric muscle actions may be significantly weaker for a few weeks after the initial bout. The clinician must account for the potential loss of strength by decreasing the exercise intensity to avoid possible further injury to the muscle. They must also educate the patient that this is the natural time-course of the injury-repair-strengthening process so that the strength loss is not viewed by the patient as unexpected or overly depressing.

vances in our understanding of eccentric exercise, demonstrating, for example, that creatine kinase levels are significantly elevated after eccentric exercise (Byrnes et al., 1985; Evans, et al., 1986), that the perception of soreness after eccentric exercise is out of phase with serum creatine kinase levels (Newham, 1988), and that a protective effect of previous training can be demonstrated by comparing creatine kinase levels to untrained control values (Evans et al., 1986). Unfortunately, it is also often assumed that the level of creatine kinase activity is somehow related to the magnitude of muscle injury, although this idea has not been explicitly tested (Kyrolainen, Takala, & Komi, 1998; McHugh et al., 1999). There is a great need in the muscle exercise community for some type of serum marker of muscle injury that provides an estimate of the magnitude of muscle injury, similar

to the serum assay for troponin I that provides a rough estimate of the amount of heart muscle involved in a myocardial infarction (Jaffe, 2001).

To measure the relationship (if any) between CK levels and muscle injury, serum CK levels were measured in New Zealand White rabbits subjected to noninvasive eccentric exercise of the ankle dorsiflexors by rotating the ankle 30° in dorsiflexion while directly stimulating the muscles via the peroneal nerve. This pattern was repeated every 2 seconds for 30 minutes resulting in 900 eccentric contractions of the dorsiflexors, simulating a single, but intense eccentric exercise bout (Lieber, Schmitz, Mishra, & Fridén, 1994). After 1, 2, 7, 14, or 28 days, maximum dorsiflexion torque was measured directly by activating the peroneal nerve transcutaneously and measuring dorsiflexion torque. In addition, a blood sample was collected and immediately centrifuged for measurement of serum CK activity.

The lack of association between dorsiflexion torque and serum CK revealed that serum creatine kinase levels provided poor predictive power in estimating skeletal muscle function (Fig. 6-17). No significant correlation was observed between creatine kinase activity and torque with the regression relationship calculated describing only ~8% of the experimental variability (Fridén & Lieber, 2001).

It may not be surprising that this relationship is relatively poor since a muscle fiber's permeability to intramuscular enzymes may or may not be correlated with cellular contractile function. For example, in a separate study, it was demonstrated that numerous muscle fibers subjected to eccentric exercise that retained their ability to exclude plasma fibronectin demonstrated significant structural abnormalities such as loss of intracellular desmin, myofibrillar disruption, and Z-disk disintegration (Lieber et al., 1994). These fibers would be considered injured but would not contribute to the total pool of serum creatine kinase. Thus, while serum creatine kinase levels may provide a gross indication that skeletal muscle injury

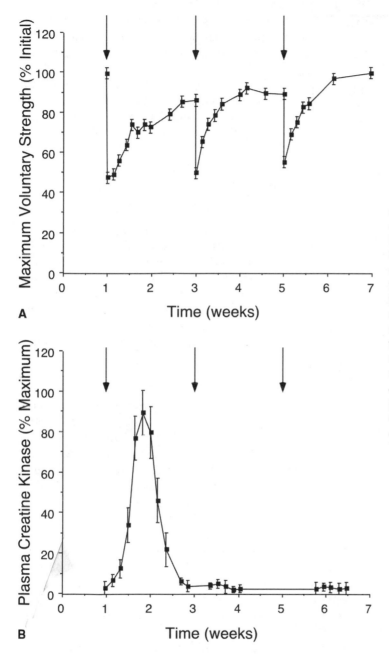

FIGURE 6-16. Changes in muscle strength and serum creatine kinase levels measured after three eccentric exercise bouts of human elbow flexors. **(A)** Maximum voluntary contraction level measured at times ranging from initially to 7 weeks after exercise. **(B)** Serum creatine kinase levels measured at times ranging from initially to 7 weeks after exercise. Vertical arrows represent separate exercise bouts. (Data from: Newham, D.J., Jones, D.A., Clarkson, P.M. (1987). Repeated high-force eccentric exercise: effects on muscle pain and damage. *Journal of Applied Physiology, 63,* 1381–1386.)

has occurred, the precise CK level does not provide an indicator of muscle injury magnitude. This is seen clearly in the data when creatine kinase levels and dorsiflexion torque measured 1 day after eccentric exercise are compared with those measured 7 days after exercise (Fig. 6-17). After 1 day, CK levels (3846 IU/L) were over 6 times those obtained for the samples obtained after 7 days (618 IU/L; Fig. 6-17, filled arrows) even though dorsiflexion torque for the 1 day samples (0.584 Nm) was only 10% less than torque measured 7 days after eccentric

Box 6-6 Is the Pain of Eccentric Exercise Due to Lactic Acid Buildup?

No. The pain resulting from eccentric exercise is apparently related more to the inflammatory response and tissue reaction to the injury rather than the buildup of any metabolic products. In fact, eccentric contractions are more energy efficient than, for instance, isometric contractions that produce much more lactic acid and which, as you probably know cause almost no soreness. The precise basis of muscle pain after eccentric exercise is not clear but there is evidence implicating the very small sensory nerve endings within the muscle and even the muscle spindles. Interestingly, there is evidence that if pain is suppressed with antiinflammatory medications, muscle function is compromised.

exercise (0.646 Nm; Fig. 6-17, open arrows). For these data, a significant difference between CK activities was accompanied by no significant difference between torque values. Therefore, investigators were encouraged to use caution when attempting to infer muscle functional properties based on serum enzyme levels.

Muscle Ultrastructure After Eccentric Contraction

What morphological changes occur in skeletal muscle after such intense eccentric contractions? Dr. Jan Fridén, working in Dr. Björn Ekblom's laboratory of exercise physiology quantified the extent and type of muscle injury that occurred in humans following "model" eccentric contractions (Fridén, Sjöström, and

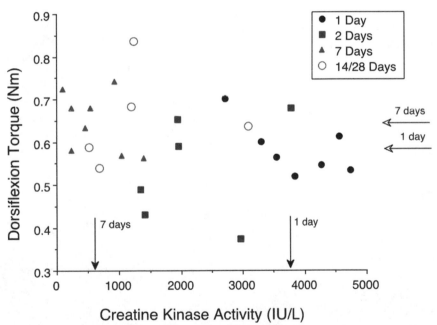

FIGURE 6-17. Relationship between serum creatine kinase (CK) and maximum dorsiflexion torque. Data are presented for torque measured 1, 2, 7, or 14/28 days after a single eccentric exercise bout. Note the ~6-fold variation in serum CK levels between measurements obtained 1 or 7 days after exercise (filled arrows) with a corresponding ~10% difference in maximum tetanic tension (open arrows). (Used with permission from: Fridén, J., Lieber, R.L. (2001). Serum creatine kinase level is a poor predictor of muscle function after injury. *Scandinavian Journal of Medicine and Science in Sports, 11*, 126–127.)

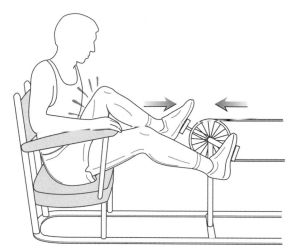

FIGURE 6-18. Experimental method for inducing eccentric muscle contractions in human quadriceps femoris muscles. The individual pushes against the pedal, which is being driven in the reverse direction by a torque motor. (Figure modified from: Fridén, J., Sjöström, M., Ekblom, B. (1983). Myofibrillar damage following intense eccentric exercise in man. *International Journal of Sports Medicine, 4*, 170–176.)

Ekblom, 1981; 1983). Subjects were asked to pedal against a motor-driven ergometer that was moving in the opposite direction to their applied force (Fig. 6-18). Subjects generated extremely high power levels for 30 minutes and

exercised at 80–100% of their VO_{2max}. This was intense exercise. Immediately and 3 and 6 days after the exercise bout, small biopsies were taken from their vastus lateralis muscles. The most consistent change observed in the experimental muscle biopsies was the disorganization of the myofibrillar material, especially at the Z-disk (Fig. 6-19B). The nature of the disruption was relatively focal, often extending only a few sarcomeres. This myofibrillar disruption was accompanied by breakage of the myofibrillar cytoskeleton as evidenced by significant redistribution of proteins associated with the cytoskeleton such as vimentin, laminin, and desmin. Fridén et al. demonstrated that the ultrastructural disruption was only observed after eccentric contraction and, again, the magnitude of the disruption was greatly attenuated if the subjects had been previously trained by performing the same eccentric exercise.

When isokinetic strength was measured from subjects after eccentric exercise, a small but significant decrease in isokinetic torque was observed at high angular velocities even 6 days following the exercise bout. These investigators cautiously interpreted their data as indicating that preferential damage to the fast muscle fibers had occurred due to the eccentric exercise.

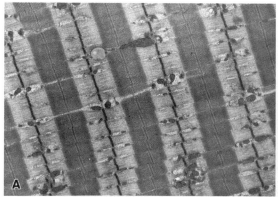
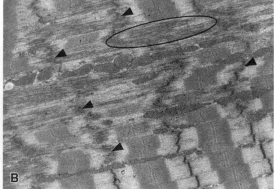

FIGURE 6-19. Ultrastructural changes in human muscle following eccentric contraction. **(A)** Normal muscle. **(B)** Muscle obtained 3 days after eccentric contraction. Note that the disruption is focal and primarily in the region of the Z-disk. (Unpublished micrograph courtesy of Dr. Jan Fridén, Professor of Hand Surgery, Salgrenska University Hospital, Göteborg, Sweden.)

Many questions regarding eccentric contraction-induced exercise remain. What are the cellular signals that initiate the damage process? What can be done to prevent the muscle damage? What can be done to facilitate recovery following muscle damage? How often should repeat exercise bouts be experienced to maximally strengthen the muscle but so as not to cause excessive damage?

As seen throughout this text, significant advances in understanding are only made using well-designed and carefully planned experiments. When mechanism questions are addressed, excellent animal models are required to provide unequivocal answers.

Recall that, in isolated skeletal muscle, a muscle that is eccentrically activated, generates more tension compared with a muscle that is isometrically activated (Fig. 6-20). A muscle can also generate relatively high tensions even if it is only passively stretched. These isolated contractile events can serve as models for eccentric contraction-induced injury studies and are usually performed in combination during experimental studies of eccentric contraction in animal models.

Eccentric Exercise of Isolated Muscles

Dr. John Faulkner and his colleagues were the first to report the results of eccentric contractions imposed directly in isolated animal muscles to investigate muscle function and the cellular response to injury (McCully & Faulkner, 1985). They attached the distal portion of the mouse extensor digitorum longus (EDL) muscle to a specially-designed motor that could forcibly lengthen the muscle by a controlled amount. Using this apparatus, they

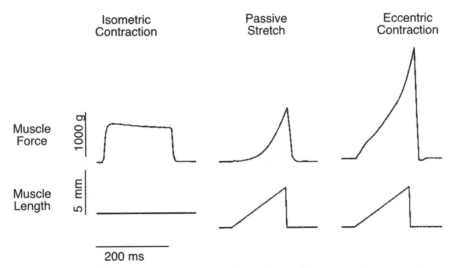

FIGURE 6-20. Tension comparison under different conditions for the rabbit tibialis anterior muscle. Contractile records from isometric contraction (left panel), passive stretch (middle panel), and eccentric contraction, (right panel). The upper trace depicts muscle force, the lower trace depicts muscle length (motor length control output). In the isometric contraction panel, muscle length was held constant while the muscle was stimulated for 400 ms at 40 Hz resulting in a tension equivalent to about 50% P_o. In panel passive stretch, the unstimulated muscle was stretched 25% of the muscle fiber length in 400 ms (corresponding to a strain rate of 63%/sec). In panel eccentric contraction, the stimulation pattern from isometric contraction and the length change from passive stretch were superimposed to yield the eccentric contraction shown. Note that tension was greatest for eccentric contraction followed by passive stretch and isometric contraction. Muscle stimulation coincided with lengthening.

exercised animals eccentrically, isometrically, and isotonically and compared the muscular response.

Force Changes After Eccentric Exercise

McCully and Faulkner found that, after a single 30 minute bout of "exercise," P_o decreased the most when the exercise was eccentric compared to isometric or isotonic (Fig. 6-21). The decrease in P_o after eccentric contraction was greatest 5 days after the exercise and recovered to control levels after about 30 days. During this time period, significant cellular infiltration was observed—again only in the eccentrically exercised muscles. Although all groups decreased in P_o, only the eccentric group showed such dramatic signs of inflammation.

We repeated the type of experiment per-

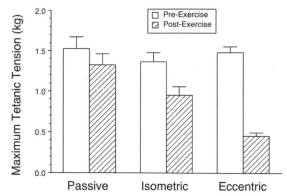

FIGURE 6-22. Maximum tetanic tension generated by TA muscles before (open bars) and after (hatched bars) one of the three experimental treatments. P_o decreased following all treatments. However, the magnitude of the decrease was greater for EC, followed by IC, followed by PS. (Data from: Lieber, R.L., McKee-Woodburn, T., Fridén, J. (1991). Muscle damage induced by eccentric contractions of 25% strain. *Journal of Applied Physiology, 70*, 2498–2507.)

formed by Faulkner's group in order to investigate the fiber type-specific effects of eccentric contraction (Lieber & Fridén, 1988). Again, three groups of experimental animals were used: eccentric contractions (EC), isometric contractions (IC), and passive stretch (PS; Fig. 6-20) to determine whether the stretch damaged the muscle. Muscles were "exercised" in one of the three modes for 30 minutes and muscle contractile properties were measured. Contractile and morphological results will be discussed serially to build the "case" for a putative damage mechanism.

As expected, we found that, after 30 minutes of EC, IC or PS exercise, P_o decreased to the greatest extent in the EC group compared with either the IC or PS group (Fig. 6-22). In addition, the tension decrease was accompanied by a muscle "slowing" as evidenced by a significant decrease in twitch and tetanic rate of rise of tension.

Time Course of Tension Change During Exercise

For all three treatments, peak tension decreased monotonically with time (Fig. 6-23). No abrupt drop in tension was observed for EC

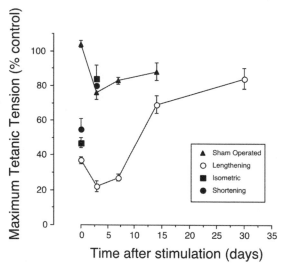

FIGURE 6-21. Time course of change in maximum tetanic tension following various experimental treatments such as eccentric contraction (open circles), isometric contraction (filled squares), concentric contractions (filled circles) or sham operation (filled triangles). Note that only the eccentrically exercised muscles demonstrate the large, prolonged force decline and that the experimental method itself resulted in ~20% decline in maximum tetanic tension. (Data from: McCully, K.K., Faulkner, J.A. (1985). Injury to skeletal muscle fibers of mice following lengthening contractions. *Journal of Applied Physiology, 59*, 119–126.)

treatment that would have suggested that the damage had occurred as a discrete, coordinated "event" or that a tear had occurred along the length and width of the muscle. Instead, the eccentric contraction time-course showed a very interesting phenomenon that was elicited based on an indirect calculation. The logic of this indirect calculation was that, in effect, an eccentric contraction could be viewed as a simultaneous isometric contraction and a passive stretch. If an eccentric contraction were no more than these two phenomena occurring at the same time and in parallel, then the eccentric contraction force would just be the sum of the passive stretch force plus the isometric force. Therefore, the "added" component of tension was defined due to EC (Fig. 6-23, open circles) as the difference between the peak EC tension level (P_{EC}) and the sum of the peak IC tension (P_{IC}) and peak PS tension (P_{PS}). That is, $P_{ADD} = P_{EC} -$

($P_{IC} + P_{PS}$). Notice that early in the treatment period, P_{ADD} exceeded 500 grams, but decayed relatively rapidly and became zero after about 7 minutes. Thus, early in the treatment period the muscle experienced 500 grams more tension than it would have experienced as the simple algebraic sum of IC and PS. The significance of this finding is addressed below as the damage mechanism is discussed. The important point to note about these data is that the "action" associated with eccentric contraction happens relatively rapidly and early in the exercise bout.

Muscle Morphological Changes Following Eccentric Exercise

In an effort to understand the basis for the contractile results, the morphology of the muscles was observed at both the light microscopic and electron microscopic levels. Although the morphology of samples from the PS and IC groups

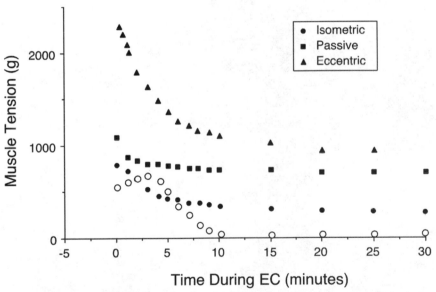

FIGURE 6-23. Time course of tension decline during the three experimental treatments. In each case, data were acquired on-line during 30 minutes of eccentric contractions (EC) (triangles), isometric contractions (IC) (squares), or passive stretch (PS) (circles). Note that EC resulted in the greatest tension. The open circles represent the parameter, P_{ADD}, the addition tension, which is calculated as the difference between the EC tension and the sum of IC and PS tensions. See text for explanation of the significance of P_{ADD}. (Data from: Lieber, R.L., McKee-Woodburn, T., Fridén, J. (1991). Muscle damage induced by eccentric contractions of 25% strain. *Journal of Applied Physiology, 70,* 2498–2507.)

appeared normal, the most obvious result was that the eccentrically exercised muscles exhibited increased portions of abnormal fibers when viewed in cross-section. These fibers appeared rounded, more lightly stained on H&E, and approximately four times the normal size (Fig. 6-24). Only fibers from muscles in the EC group demonstrated this abnormal appearance and they were always depleted of glycogen confirming that they had been activated.

What fiber type were these "enlarged" fibers? Fiber type was determined by staining serial sections as described in Chapter 2, for myofibrillar ATPase activity, succinate dehydrogenase (SDH) activity, and α-glycerophosphate dehydrogenase (αGP) activity. It was found that all enlarged fibers were exclusively of the FG fiber type (Figs. 6-24). What might this mean? Our impression was that it provided insights into the damage mechanism as described below.

While no ultrastructural abnormalities were observed in any of the muscles from the IC or PS groups, a significant portion of the fibers in the EC group displayed various degrees of disorganization of the sarcomeric band pattern such as Fridén et al. had observed after eccentric exercise in human subjects (Fridén, Sjöström, & Ekblom, 1983). Streaming and smearing of the Z-disk material, focal loss of

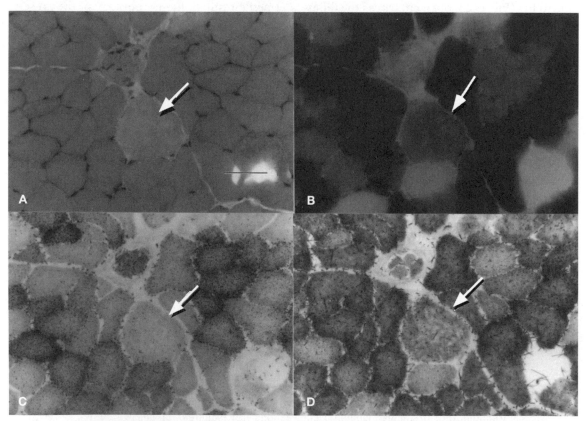

FIGURE 6-24. Cross-sectional light micrographs of rabbit TA under different staining conditions. Arrows point to enlarged fibers, which are of the FG fiber type. Calibration bar = 50 μm. **(A)** Hematoxylin & eosin **(B)** Myofibrillar ATPase following preincubation at pH = 9.4 **(C)** Succinate dehydrogenase **(D)** α-glycerophosphate dehydrogenase. (Micrograph from: Lieber, R.L., Fridén, J. (1988). Selective damage of fast glycolytic muscle fibers with eccentric contraction of the rabbit tibialis anterior. *Acta Physiologica Scandinavica, 133*, 587–588.)

Z-disks and extension of Z-disks into adjacent A-bands were commonly seen (Fig. 6-25). The Z-disk smearing was always located in specific locations within the same fiber and never extended across the whole fiber (and infrequently over more than three sarcomeres). In these areas, thick filaments were out of register, overlapping each other and/or the I-bands. Fine structural deviations appeared randomly distributed across and along the fibers.

Putative Mechanisms of Eccentric Contraction-Induced Damage

The fact that only FG fibers demonstrated histological abnormalities suggested that fiber oxidative capacity was important in determining the extent of fiber damage that occurs immediately following EC.

Based on the hypothesis that muscle fiber oxidative capacity was a determining factor in fiber damage, we hypothesized a damage scheme that predicted that muscle injury during eccentric contraction occurred as follows:

1. Early in the exercise period (i.e., within the first 10 minutes) FG fibers fatigue.
2. Based on their inability to regenerate ATP, they enter a rigor or high-stiffness state.
3. Subsequent stretch of stiff fibers mechanically disrupts the fibers, resulting in the observed cytoskeletal and myofibrillar damage.

This hypothesis was appealing for several reasons. First, it explained the well-known "protective" effect of endurance training on EC-induced damage, which was mentioned above. Endurance training is known to result in an increased muscle oxidative capacity, and therefore, FG to FOG fiber subtype conversion. Because FOG fibers do not fatigue and enter rigor as readily as the FG fibers, EC-induced damage would be expected to be lower following endurance training. An appeal of this hypothesis is that it made a testable prediction. (As you have seen, it is always preferable to perform an experiment that can clearly disprove a hypoth-

esis without ambiguity.) A second damage mechanism that could depend on fiber oxidative capacity relates to the other cellular processes that rely on oxidative metabolism. We could again hypothesize a damage scheme that occurs as follows:

1. Early in the exercise period FG fibers fatigue.
2. Based on their inability to regenerate ATP, mitochondria lose their calcium buffering capacity.
3. Increased intracellular calcium results in activation of the calcium-activated neutral proteases (which were active in denervation), lysosomal proteases, and other cellular processes that are calcium-mediated.

Test of Oxidative Capacity As a Causative Factor in Muscle Injury

As a test of the idea that low oxidative capacity predisposes a muscle to eccentric contraction-induced injury, we "artificially" increased muscle oxidative capacity using a chronic electrical stimulation protocol. Since FG fiber oxidative capacity is extremely low and since training can dramatically increase FG fiber oxidative capacity, actually converting it to the FOG fiber type (Chapter 4), we hypothesized that the protective effect of training was to increase fiber oxidative capacity. This hypothesis was directly tested by pre-treating rabbit anterior compartment muscles with electrical stimulation for 30 minutes/day × 5 days/week × 3 weeks. It was important to stimulate the muscles enough to cause the oxidative capacity change but not so much as to transform fiber type or cause dramatic muscle fiber size changes as are observed with chronic stimulation patterns (See Chapter 4, pages 174 to 179). This required careful "titration" of the stimulation dose to achieve the desired effect.

To document muscle changes due to electrical stimulation, muscle fiber oxidative enzyme activity (as indicated by the citrate synthase enzyme) and muscle capillary density and geometry were measured. As anticipated, we mea-

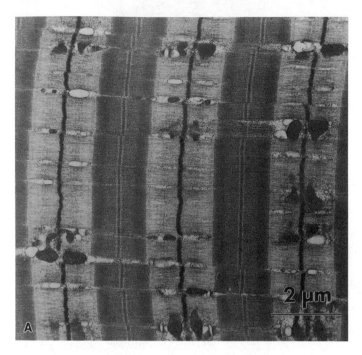

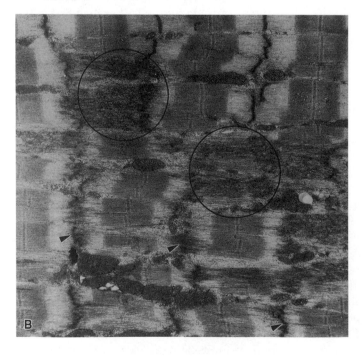

FIGURE 6-25. Longitudinal electron micrographs of rabbit TA. **(A)** Sample from isometric contraction group, which shows normal striation pattern and Z disks, which are perpendicular to the long myofibrillar axis. **(B)** Sample from eccentric contraction group, which demonstrates various disrupted regions. Note streaming and smearing of the Z-disk material (arrows) and extension of the Z-disks into adjacent A-bands (circled areas). (Micrograph from: Lieber, R.L., McKee-Woodburn, T., Fridén, J. (1991). Muscle damage induced by eccentric contractions of 25% strain. *Journal of Applied Physiology, 70*, 2498–2507.)

sured a significant increase in EDL oxidative activity and capillary density with smaller changes in the TA (Patel, Cuizon, Mathieu-Costello, Fridén, & Lieber, 1998). Note that the normal EDL and TA muscles have differing oxidative capacity (Fig. 6-26A) but, after 3 weeks of stimulation, their activities are nearly identical. This represents yet another illustration of the fact that a muscle will adapt to the new use conditions placed upon it. Before any stimulation, TA and EDL have different oxidative capacities but, after 3 weeks of stimulation, due to the "same" level of use, their oxidative capacities are nearly identical. In this case, a low level of stimulation applied for 30 minutes per day caused a large oxidative activity increase without concomitant changes in muscle injury level (Fig. 6-26). Yet, in spite of these well-documented increases in the muscle's ability to deliver oxygen and use it within the cell, there was no significant correlation between oxidative capacity and maximum tetanic tension for either the TA or EDL, and maximum tetanic tension not altered after injury preceded by electrical stimulation training (Fig.

Box 6-7 How Does "Getting into Shape" Prevent Further Eccentric Contraction-Induced Muscle Injury?

There is no question that, while the initial bout of eccentric exercise results in much pain, this pain level is greatly reduced after subsequent bouts. After a fair amount of eccentric training, an individual feels almost no pain even though they are performing the same exercise! At the muscle level, to prevent soreness and injury, the exercise being used to "get into shape" must involve eccentric contractions themselves, not simply increasing aerobic fitness or muscular oxidative capacity. The precise change that occurs within the muscle that protects it from further injury is not known, but there is evidence that muscles "remodel" by changing sarcomere number to keep sarcomeres operating at relatively short lengths.

6-26B). Therefore, low oxidative capacity did not provide the explanation for selective FG fiber damage.

Mechanical Factors Causing Muscle Injury

Numerous studies had established that muscle injury can occur relatively rapidly (c.f., P_{ADD} in Fig. 6-23) and several studies have since attempted to measure mechanical factors that cause injury. The fact that, as you have seen from the force-velocity relationship (Fig. 6-13), eccentric contractions are associated with high force and result in muscle damage has typically led to the presumption that the high muscle forces imposed upon the muscle caused the muscle injury. Although this was attractive in theory there was only anecdotal experimental evidence in support of such a claim. Therefore, we designed an experiment in which muscle stress and strain were systematically altered and muscle strength measured after cyclic eccentric contraction at different stresses and strains (Lieber & Fridén, 1993). Specifically, stimulation timing was altered relative to the muscle deformation to achieve altered stresses at identical strains (Fig. 6-27A) at two different strain magnitudes. Note that, mechanically, by delaying the muscle stretch and permitting the muscles to develop force prior to stretch, the force achieved during the stretch could be increased. Therefore we eccentrically exercised muscles at high strain (25% L_f) and low strain (12.5% L_f) and at high and low force at each of these strains. Maximum tetanic tension was the main parameter analyzed. When two "input" variables are changed (in this case, strain and force level) and one "output" variable is measured, the appropriate method for analysis of these data is to a stepwise regression model. In the case of our analysis, stepwise regression "partitioned" the effect stress and strain on the magnitude of decrease in tetanic tension. We found that the magnitude of injury was more closely related to the magnitude of the muscle strain as opposed to the stress imposed on the fibers (Fig. 6-27B). These data suggested that it is how far the muscle is stretched rather than the peak stress reached that causes injury. This result does not generally apply to other muscles. Interestingly, a recent report presented a different result for predominantly slow-contracting soleus muscles (Warren et al., 1993a) which may be due to the different muscles used or the different protocols designed to impose different stresses and strains upon the different muscles. Also, using multiple regression, they concluded that muscle stress was the primary mechanical factor that affected muscle injury magnitude. However, there were enough methodological differences between the studies to render neither completely conclusive.

The main problem with both studies described above was that both groups of investigators assumed that deformation was equally distributed along the muscle-tendon unit. Tendon compliance can result in mechanical situations in which the muscle length change is not the same as the change in the length of the

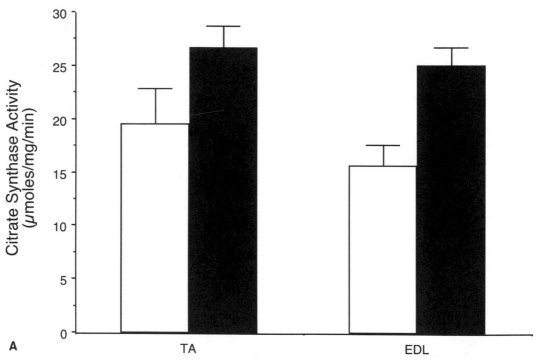

FIGURE 6-26. (A) Citrate synthase activity of rabbit tibialis anterior (TA) and extensor digitorum longus (EDL) muscles before (open bars) and after (filled bars) three weeks of low frequency stimulation. In both cases, citrate synthase activity significantly increased, but, for the EDL, the increase was more dramatic. **(B)** Maximum tetanic tension activity of rabbit tibialis anterior (TA) and extensor digitorum longus (EDL) muscles before (open bars) and after (filled bars) 3 weeks of low frequency stimulation. Horizontal hatched bars above graphs represent normal TA or EDL maximum tetanic tension (Experimental data from: Patel, T., Cuizon, D., Mathieu-Costello, O., Fridén, J., Lieber, R.L. (1998). Increased oxidative capacity does not protect skeletal muscle from eccentric contraction-induced muscle injury. *American Journal of Physiology, 274*, R1300–R1308. Comparative normal data in part (B) from: Lieber, R.L., Schmitz, M.C., Mishra, D.K., Fridén, J. (1994). Contractile and cellular remodeling in rabbit skeletal muscle after cyclic eccentric contractions. *Journal of Applied Physiology, 77*, 1926–1934.)

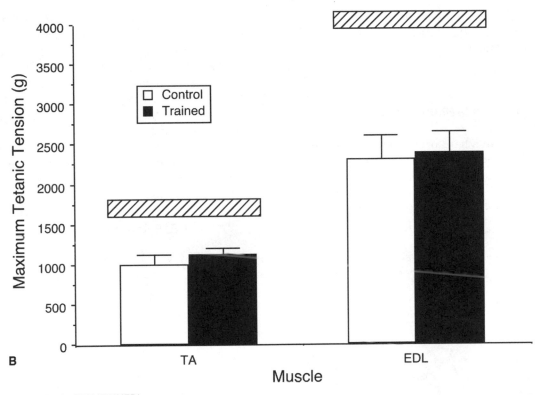

B

FIGURE 6-26. *(CONTINUED)*

muscle-tendon unit (see Fig. 3-4, page 121, for an example). Since both experiments described above were performed on intact muscle-tendon units, interpretation of these experiments was confounded by lack of precise strain measurements at the level of the sarcomere. Since sarcomeres may not lengthen proportionally to the deformation applied to the entire muscle-tendon unit, assumption of uniform deformation along the muscle-tendon unit under these experimental conditions is questionable. This limitation was overcome by directly measuring sarcomere strain in small bundles of muscle fibers during eccentric contraction treatment to explicitly determine the effect of fiber strain on injury (Patel, Fridén, Lutz, & Lieber, 2002). The data trace themselves illustrate a number of muscle mechanical properties and will be described in a bit of detail. During the eccentric contraction treatment, the muscle is first stimulated isometrically (Point #1 in Fig. 6-28B).

Note that force rapidly increases and, even though the muscle bundle is tightly held at the ends, sarcomere shortening occurs during this "isometric" contraction. The only thing isometric here is the overall length of the bundle (Fig. 6-28A). The sarcomeres are shortening considerably. At point #2 in Figure 6-28B the bundle of fibers is stretched and force rapidly increases. Note that the increase occurs in two phases—an early stiff phase and a later less stiff phase. This two-phased stiffness is characteristic of skeletal muscle (Rack & Westbury, 1974). At point #3, the bundle (and sarcomeres) is held a constant length and muscle force declines to a new resting level. Finally, muscle activation is halted, force returns to baseline, and the cycle is repeated. Using a protocol like this, muscle fiber bundles were eccentrically exercised to different strains and maximum tetanic tension measured. It was found that force decline was directly related to fiber strain, supporting muscle length change as a cause of injury (Fig. 6-29). Keep this idea in mind since another damage mechanism will be considered that is also related to fiber strain but in a unique manner.

SARCOMERE "POPPING" AS THE CAUSE OF INJURY

Several points have been made throughout this text that the mechanics of stretched muscle is very unique. This has been known for some time and yet the uniqueness of these mechanical events has been difficult to explain. In what must be considered an extremely creative and insightful probe into this question, the Australian electrical engineer Dr. David Morgan proposed a dramatic "phenomenon" to explain muscle injury with eccentric contraction. Instead of proposing muscle injury to individual sarcomeres, Morgan proposed that it is the interaction between sarcomeres that results in the injury (Morgan, 1990). Briefly, the theory pro-

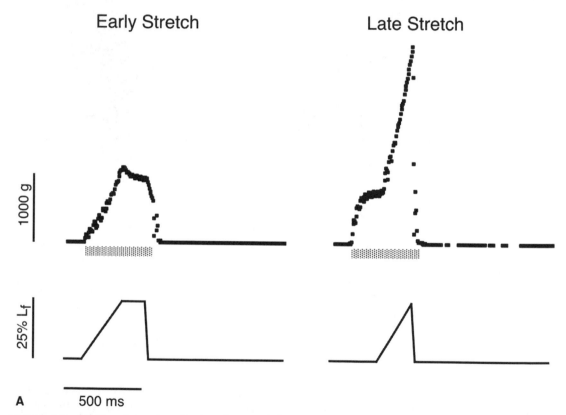

FIGURE 6-27. (A) Sample contractile data from early stretch (left panel) and late stretch (right panel) experimental groups. Note that both groups receive identical deformation patterns (lower records). However, due to the timing of the applied deformation, the late stretch group experiences much higher forces (upper records). Stippled area beneath force record represents stimulation duration. Abbreviation L_f: muscle fiber length. **(B)** Summary of maximum tetanic tension generated by the various treatment groups. No significant difference in maximum tension generated was observed between groups that experienced early stretch compared with late stretch at either 25% or 12.5% strain. However, a significant difference in tension generation was observed between groups strained 25% versus 12.5% of muscle fiber length. (Used with permission from: Lieber, R.L., Fridén, J. (1993). Muscle damage is not a function of muscle force but active muscle strain. *Journal of Applied Physiology, 74*, 520–526.)

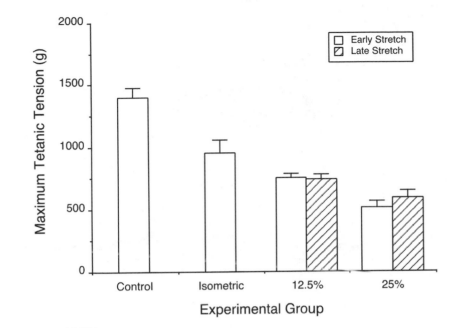

FIGURE 6-27. *(CONTINUED)*

poses that small strength differences along the length of the myofibril (due to small sarcomere length differences or even cross-sectional area variation) means that sarcomeres may be pulling against each other with slightly different forces during contraction. Sarcomere length differences could result in different sarcomere strengths because, at longer sarcomere lengths on the descending limb of the length-tension curve (Fig. 2-4), sarcomeres have less filament overlap and thus generate lower forces compared with their shorter counterparts in series (Fig. 6-30A). This difference in sarcomere strength can permit a differential length change of sarcomeres during stretch, whereby the longer sarcomeres are stretched more than the shorter ones and thus take up a disproportionate fraction of the length change (Fig. 6-30B). This differential length change continues during a stretch until finally, Morgan proposes, the lengthening sarcomeres get so long that the myofilaments no longer overlap and then "pop" to a very long length (Fig. 6-30C).

Although such a phenomenon sounds strange and definitely caught the muscle mechanics and muscle injury community by sur-

prise, the theory makes testable predictions. Time and again this text has shown that, a theory that makes testable predictions is useful to advance the field. Morgan's "popping sarcomere" hypothesis suggests that muscle adaptation after eccentric exercise will occur to keep sarcomeres from attaining the longer sarcomere lengths that render them vulnerable to the instability described above. Can you predict what this adaptation would be? How would you change the range of sarcomere lengths over which a muscle would operate during an eccentric contraction? The most obvious adaptation is for the muscle to increase serial sarcomere number and therefore decrease the magnitude of the stretch absorbed by each sarcomere population.

EXPERIMENTAL SUPPORT FOR THE "POPPING SARCOMERE" THEORY

The proposed adaptation mechanisms were tested in a number of ways. In one experiment, Morgan and colleagues trained rats by running downhill running, which induced eccentric contractions of the quadriceps, especially of the

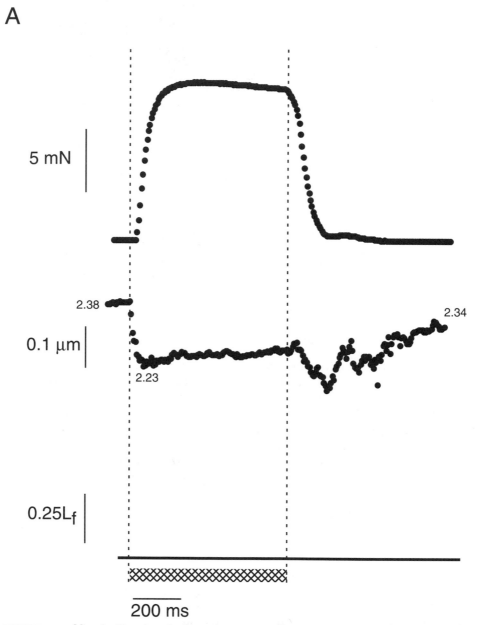

FIGURE 6-28. Muscle fiber bundle force (upper panel), sarcomere length (middle panel), and fiber bundle length (lower panel) associated with the contractile experiments performed. This panel demonstrates these parameters under conditions of **(A)** isometric contraction, **(B)** eccentric contraction of 25% strain. Hatched bar at the bottom of the figure indicates the period during which the muscle is electrically stimulated. Vertical lines denote corresponding time periods between force, sarcomere length, and fiber length records. Sarcomere length values on traces represent group means across all specimens. (From: Patel, T.J., Fridén, J., Lutz, G.J., Lieber, R.L. Active sarcomere strain causes injury to frog skeletal muscle fiber bundles. Submitted, 2002.)

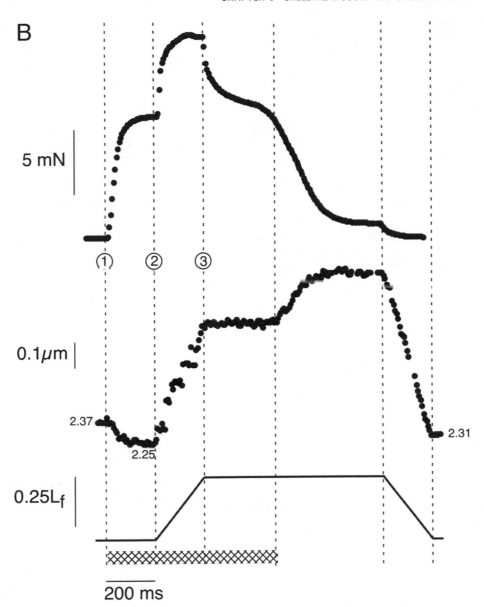

FIGURE 6-28. *(CONTINUED)*

vastus intermedius. The rats were exercised for 30 minutes per day × 5 days. Three days after the five day training period, the muscles were harvested and detailed architectural studies performed to determine serial sarcomere number within the fibers. The number of sarcomeres in series within the vastus intermedius fibers was shown to increase due to downhill running (Fig. 6-31A), which was amazing. Chapter 4 showed that the serial sarcomere number changes due to chronic length changes; however, this is the first time that serial sarcomere number changes associated with a particular mode of exercise has been seen. The investigators also tested whether run training alone could induce such a sarcomere number

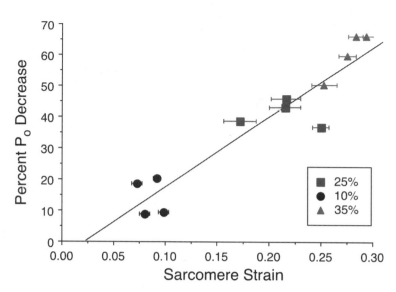

FIGURE 6-29. Relationship between average sarcomere strain measured during the eccentric exercise bout and the loss in maximum tetanic tension measured 30 minutes after the exercise bout for each experimental group. Data are presented for (●) 10% nominal strain, (■) 25% nominal strain, and (▲) 35% nominal strain. A highly significant relationship between sarcomere strain and percent loss in P_0 was observed. Standard error bars in strain direction represents variability measured among the 10 contractions for a given fiber bundle. (From: Patel, T.J., Fridén, J., Lutz, G.J., Lieber, R.L. Active sarcomere strain causes injury and differential cytoskeletal damage to frog skeletal muscle fiber bundles. Submitted, 2002.)

change, by training another group of rats to run uphill. The uphill-trained rats showed no sarcomere number increase and even a slight decrease providing support for increase in sarcomere number only due to eccentric training (Lynn & Morgan, 1994; Morgan & Allen, 1999). One appealing feature of this hypothesis is that it provides a mechanistic explanation for muscle adaptation observed after eccentric training—sarcomere number changes. Such changes have about the right time course to cause the protection and, as seen in Chapter 4, are readily accomplished by muscle.

A second test of the hypothesis was to rapidly chemically fix eccentrically contracting muscles and "look" for the popped sarcomeres (Talbot & Morgan, 1996). You might imagine that this is a difficult experiment. Morgan and colleagues used the appropriate random sampling methods that would avoid bias, as well as a reasonable statistical approach to analyzing their data, and provided evidence for the presence of popped sarcomeres (Fig. 6-31B). Again, the data are a bit controversial, but the results are extremely intriguing. Do muscles get injured by "popping sarcomeres?" At this point,

there is excellent theoretical support and some experimental evidence for the theory. The predictions made by the theory have generally been supported. The experiments being performed around the world will address this question in the next few years.

Therapist's Comments

As seen in Chapter 4, muscle-stretching exercises increase range of motion but do not appear to increase actual muscle fiber length. It has been suggested that if one of the muscle adaptations to eccentric exercise is to add sarcomeres in series, then eccentric exercise could be used to increase muscle length. This could, theoretically, increase range of motion. Although there are no definitive data currently available in this area, a recent experiment suggests that serial sarcomere addition may occur in humans after eccentric exercise. As Dr. Lieber has said before, "stay tuned."

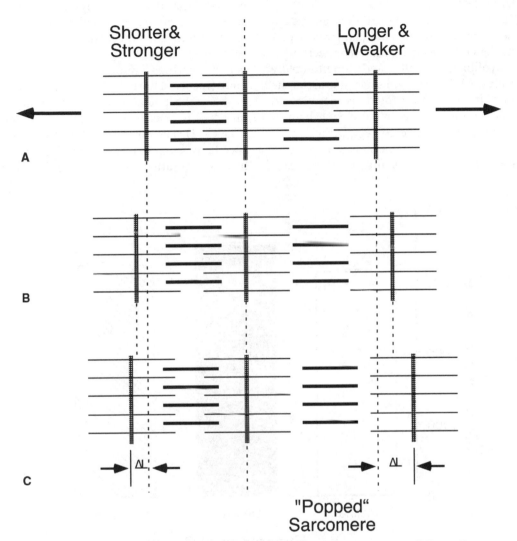

FIGURE 6-30. Schematic representation of the process of sarcomere "popping." Two adjacent sarcomeres are illustrated that are of slightly different strengths. **(A)** Sarcomeres are slightly different strengths due to differences in sarcomere length or due to intrinsic strength differences. **(B)** As the muscle is lengthened, the sarcomeres lengthen different amounts due to different strengths and one (on the right side) reaches the sarcomere length where no myofilament overlap occurs. **(C)** The sarcomere without myofilament overlap "pops" to a longer length where the tension is born by passive muscle elements (not shown). Notice that, overall, the length change in each sarcomere (ΔL) is not equal. This nonuniformity of sarcomere length is the fundamental idea behind the "popping sarcomere" hypothesis. (Based on ideas presented in: Morgan, D.L. (1990). New insights into the behavior of muscle during active lengthening. *Biophysical Journal, 57,* 209–221.)

RAPID CYTOSKELETAL DISRUPTION AFTER ECCENTRIC EXERCISE

In Chapter 2 it was shown that an extensive network of intermediate filaments is present in skeletal muscle that interconnects adjacent myofibrils radially and longitudinally (Lazarides, 1980, 1982). In skeletal muscle, the intermediate filament protein is desmin. In light of the rapid changes in muscle mechanical property that was observed (P_{ADD}, Fig. 6-23), tissue was stained at time periods ranging from 5 minutes to several days after eccentric exercise for desmin presence. Surprisingly, it was observed that there was a significant and widespread loss of the intermediate filament protein, desmin after eccentric exercise. In some cases, desmin loss was extremely rapid—it happened as early as 5 minutes into the EC exercise bout (Lieber, Thornell, & Fridén, 1996). This is the earliest documented structural change observed in muscle after eccentric contraction (Fig. 6-32). The rapidity of the effect points to a specific type of enzymatic hydrolysis as a likely mechanism rather than gene regulation would

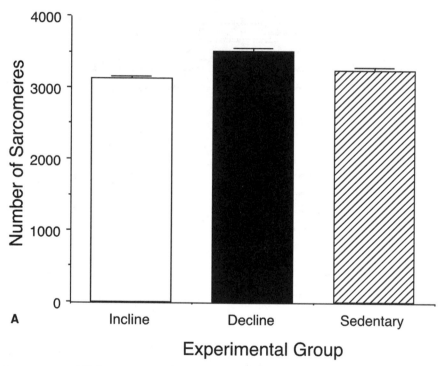

FIGURE 6-31. (A) Average number of sarcomeres in series for uphill running-trained (open bar), downhill running- (filled bar), and sedentary (hatched bar) rats. Note that the chronic eccentric contraction training (downhill running) caused an increase in serial sarcomere number, consistent with the predictions made by the "popping sarcomere" hypothesis. (Data from: Lynn, R., Morgan, D.L. (1994). Decline running produces more sarcomeres in rat vastus intermedius muscle fibers than does incline running. *Journal of Applied Physiology, 77*, 1439–1444.) **(B)** Sarcomere length distribution measured from a muscle after eccentric contraction. Notice the relatively gaussian distribution of shorter sarcomere lengths (open bars) and small group of sarcomeres at very long lengths (filled bars). These very long lengths represent, presumably "popped" sarcomeres. (Data from: Talbot, J.A., Morgan, D.L. (1996). Quantitative analysis of sarcomere non-uniformities in active muscle following a stretch. *Journal of Muscle Research and Cell Motility, 17*, 261–268.)

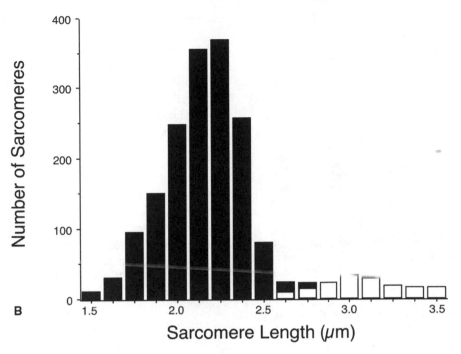

FIGURE 6-31. *(CONTINUED)*

require much more time. An attractive candidate for the proteolytic mechanism is the calcium activated protease, Calpain, which is present in skeletal muscle (Dayton, Goll, Zeece, Robson, & Reville, 1976) and for which desmin is a substrate (Belcastro, 1993). The mechanism of action of Calpain requires raised intracellular calcium ion $[Ca^{2+}]_i$) concentration.

CALPAIN-MEDIATED MECHANISM OF ECCENTRIC CONTRACTION-INDUCED MUSCLE INJURY

Although there is currently inconclusive evidence for such an increase in intracellular calcium (Balnave & Allen, 1995; Morgan & Allen, 1999), Duan et al. demonstrated an increase in the mitochondrial calcium concentration in muscles subjected to an exercise protocol biased toward eccentric contraction (Duan, Delp MD, Hayes, Delp PD, & Armstrong, 1990). Since mitochondrial calcium concentration indirectly reflects cytoplasmic $[Ca^{2+}]_i$, the results of Duan et al. might be construed as indirect evidence for increased $[Ca^{2+}]_i$. However, direct

measurement of $[Ca^{2+}]_i$ has provided less conclusive results (Morgan & Allen, 1999). The observations of rapid desmin loss in conjunction with our earlier demonstration that muscle fiber strain was the mechanical factor that most strongly influenced the magnitude of muscle injury (Lieber & Fridén, 1993) has led to the following hypothesis regarding the early mechanism of eccentric contraction induced muscle damage (Fig. 6-33):

1. Muscle fiber strain results in an increased $[Ca^{2+}]_i$. Such an increase may be due to calcium influx via strain-activated channels, by disruption of the intracellular stores of calcium in the sarcoplasmic reticulum (Guharay & Sachs, 1984), or by disruption of the T-system or sarcolemma (Fig. 6-33A). This could also result from the rapid "popping" of sarcomeres that was described above since each myofibril is surrounded by an extensive sarcoplasmic reticulum network that is full of calcium. Maybe this could also provide an explanation for the

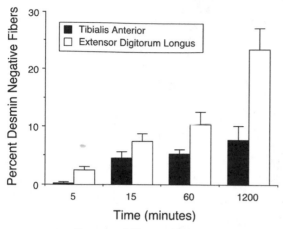

FIGURE 6-32. Percent of fibers which stain as desmin negative after various time periods of eccentric contraction and recovery. Note that a larger fraction of EDL (open bars) fibers are affected compared to TA (filled bars). The only change that is not statistically significant is the TA after 5 minutes. (Data combined from: Lieber, R.L., Schmitz, M.C., Mishra, D.K., Fridén, J. (1994). Contractile and cellular remodeling in rabbit skeletal muscle after cyclic eccentric contractions. *Journal of Applied Physiology, 77*, 1926–1934 and Lieber, R.L., Thornell L-E., Fridén, J. (1996). Muscle cytoskeletal disruption occurs within the first 15 minutes of cyclic eccentric contraction. *Journal of Applied Physiology, 80*, 278–284.)

observation that muscles composed primarily of fast fibers are more easily injured compared with muscles composed primarily of slow muscle fibers.

2. After $[Ca^{2+}]_i$ increases, Calpain activation results in selective hydrolysis or disruption of the intermediate filament network (Fig. 6-33B). It has been demonstrated that desmin is a substrate for Calpain while actin and myosin are not (Reddy, Etlinger, Robinowitz, Fischman, & Zak, 1975). This could explain the loss of desmin in sections that still demonstrate regular arrangements of contractile and metabolic proteins.

3. Finally, after the intermediate filament network has been altered due to proteolysis or conformational changes, the myofibrillar apparatus is disrupted on repeated muscle activation and unable to develop normal

tension (Fig. 6-33C). Of course, numerous variations to this scheme could be proposed. For example, mechanical events could alter intermediate filament structure, which would then render them vulnerable to mediated-mediated digestion or sarcolemmal integrity loss could trigger the entire sequence.

An alternate mechanism for desmin disruption could be that the primary injury occurs to the sarcolemma and results in the sequence of events presented above. Experimental evidence for primary sarcolemmal injury has been presented in rat skeletal muscle subjected to 90 minutes of eccentric exercise by downhill running (McNeil & Khakee, 1992). These authors used immunohistochemical identification of the circulating protein serum albumin within the myofibers as evidence for transient disruption of the sarcolemma. They found that, after 90 minutes of downhill running, a significant number of muscle fibers were labeled, indicating membrane disruption. Therefore, it is possible that transient change in sarcolemmal permeability represents a normal but heretofore unappreciated mechanism by which muscles meet the requirements for increasing mechanical performance or release intracellular growth factors to the extracellular matrix. Alternatively, perhaps the intermediate filament system depolymerizes after exposure to eccentric contractions much as occurs during mitosis in embryonic cardiac cells (Kuruc & Franke, 1988). Obviously, a lot of work needs to be done in this area.

MUSCLE INJURY IN A DESMIN KNOCKOUT MODEL

Based on the putative central role of desmin in mediating muscle injury, eccentric contractions were performed on a "knockout" model developed by Dr. Yassemi Capetanaki, a developmental biologist. This model was created in the mouse in which the desmin gene had been deleted by homologous recombination and thus, had no desmin intermediate filaments interconnecting the myofibrils within the muscle cell. Capetanaki and her colleagues had previously shown that desmin could play an important role in muscle development (Li et al., 1994; Weitzer, Milner, Kim, Bradley, & Carpetanaki, 1995) and they were interested in how the muscle would develop in the absence of desmin. They used modern genetic engineering to replace the desmin gene with a desmin "null" gene (a gene in which the DNA coding for desmin had been removed) and found that the mice, while living (which was itself somewhat of a surprise) had heart muscles that demonstrated abnormalities reminiscent of many heart muscle diseases (Milner et al., 1996, 2000). It was hypothesized that, in the absence of the intermediate filament

network, that the muscle would be much more mechanically fragile, analogous to the experiments performed by applying eccentric contractions to *mdx* mice (Petrof et al., 1993).

The experiments were performed on a muscle of the mouse extensor digitorum longus. This is a very fast muscle (>98% fast fibers) and has a small size that made it convenient for this experiment. The muscle belly was placed in a custom muscle chamber filled with physiological solution and secured to high-speed motor that could impose rapid length changes on the muscle belly. Approximately 30 minutes after the muscle was mounted in the chamber, passive and active "baseline" mechanical properties were measured. Each muscle then under-

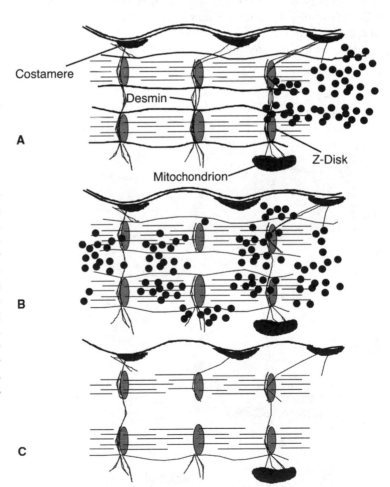

FIGURE 6-33. Schematic depiction of a possible mechanism of eccentric contraction-induced muscle damage. Calcium ions are represented as filled dots. **(A)** Muscle fiber strain results in an increased $[Ca^{2+}]_i$ from either extracellular or intracellular sources. **(B)** Increased $[Ca^{2+}]_i$ leads to mediated activation and selective hydrolysis or disruption of the intermediate filament network. **(C)** After intermediate filament network damage, the myofibrillar apparatus is disrupted on repeated muscle activation. (Used by permission from: Lieber, R.L., Thornell L-E., Fridén, J. (1996). Muscle cytoskeletal disruption occurs within the first 15 minutes of cyclic eccentric contraction. *Journal of Applied Physiology, 80,* 278–284.)

went a series of 10 eccentric contractions (ECs), one every 3 minutes. Note that this number is much smaller than used in many of the studies described above. This is because, as more and more data were reported suggesting that the initial injury was more mechanical in nature, experimental protocols were modified to minimize the influence of fatigue on muscle injury. For each EC, the muscle was first activated isometrically until tension stabilized (~200 ms), then a 15% fiber change was imposed resulting in a rapid tension rise (Fig. 6-34). This protocol was used in order to have a "contraction-by-contraction" estimate of the force generating ability of each muscle. During the first 200 ms, when the muscle is activated isometrically, this represents an estimate of the muscle's ability to generate tension in the absence of complicating factors of muscle lengthening. During the lengthening phase, as shown

before, tension increased in two phases, a reflection of the muscle short-range stiffness. Muscle length was held fixed during which tension declined due to active stress relaxation. Stimulation was then ceased and muscle length was returned to its starting value.

Measurement of the initial muscle properties, prior to any EC revealed that the knockout muscles generated lower isometric stress compared with the normal wild type muscles (Fig. 6-35). However, the most surprising result was that, after 10 ECs, the wild type muscles had dropped in isometric stress capability by ~25% whereas the knockouts had only dropped by ~9% (Fig. 6-35). In other words, the muscle that was *missing* its intermediate filaments was injured less compared with wild type muscle that contained desmin. There is experimental evidence supporting the idea that stress can be a major cause of muscle

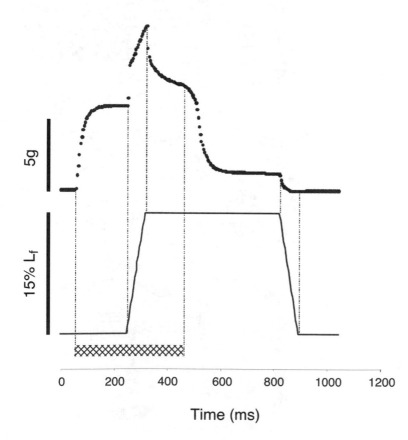

FIGURE 6-34. Sample eccentric contraction from the 5th toe of the mouse EDL muscle. Upper panel: muscle force; Lower Panel: muscle length. Hatched bar at bottom of figure represents period during which muscle is electrically stimulated. Vertical dotted lines represent corresponding times in force, length and muscle stimulation. Abbreviation: L_f, fiber length. (Modified from: Sam, M., Fridén, J., Shah, S., Milner, D.J., Capetanaki, Y., Lieber, R.L. (2000). Desmin knockout muscles generate lower stress and are less vulnerable to injury compared to wild type muscles. *American Journal of Physiology, 279,* C1116–C1122.)

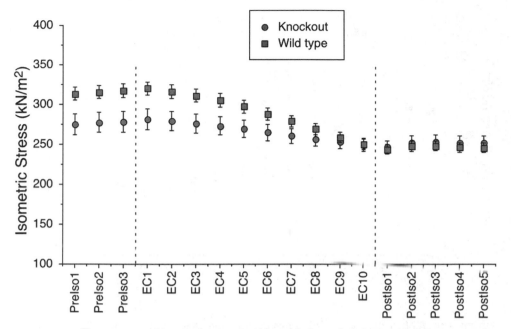

FIGURE 6-35. Time course of isometric stress achieved before, during, and after the eccentric contraction protocol. Note that the relative decrease in isometric stress of knockout animals is lower than the drop in muscles of the wild type animals. (■) wild type animals, (●) knockout animals. Abbreviations: Pre-Iso, Isometric testing prior to eccentric contraction protocol; EC, eccentric contractions; IC, isometric contractions; Post-Iso, Isometric testing after eccentric contraction protocol. Each symbol represents the mean±SEM of 6-7 experimental subjects per group. (Modified from: Sam, M., Fridén, J., Shah, S., Milner, D.J., Capetanaki, Y., Lieber, R.L. (2000). Desmin knockout muscles generate lower stress and are less vulnerable to injury compared to wild type muscles. *American Journal of Physiology, 279,* C1116–C1122.)

injury (Warren et al., 1993b) so perhaps the knockouts were injured less because they bore less stress. This is an excellent criticism and, at the time of the experiment, also caused great concern because it represented a confounding interpretation of these data. This issue was addressed directly by altering the stress-generating capability of the wild type and knockout mice. Based on what was already discussed, imagine how you might alter the stress-generating capability of a muscle? A relatively straight forward method is simply to age the animals because, as shown, active muscle stress decreases with age. After aging the mice ~40 weeks, isometric stress between the young knockouts and old wild type muscles was almost exactly the same (Fig. 6-36). This

fortuitous result permitted us to compare directly the "stress" effect to the "knockout" effect. All four data sets obtained by this experiment are shown in Figure 6-36 and provide a fairly clear result. Note that, independent of the presence or absence of desmin, the aged animals generate lower isometric stress compared with their younger counterparts. Also notice that, independent of age, the desmin knockout animals generate lower stress compared with their wild type counterparts. Finally, notice that, after the EC protocol, the stress generated by the knockout and wild type animals of the same age are, essentially, identical. This appears to provide direct mechanical evidence for the role that desmin plays in normal muscle force generation and, with EC,

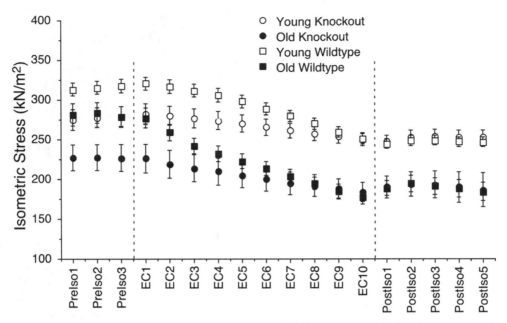

FIGURE 6-36. All four data sets used to demonstrate the time course of "injury" to young and old, wild type, and desmin-knockout muscles. Note that the relative decrease in isometric stress of knockout animals is lower than the drop in muscles of the age-matched animals. (□) Wild type young animals, (■) wild type mature animals, (○) knockout young animals, (●) knockout mature animals. Abbreviations as in Fig. 6-35. (Data from: Sam, M., Fridén, J., Shah, S., Milner, D.J., Capetanaki, Y., Lieber, R.L. (2000). Desmin knockout muscles generate lower stress and are less vulnerable to injury compared to wild type muscles. *American Journal of Physiology, 279,* C1116–C1122.)

for the fact that loss of desmin (in wild type muscles) is part of the reason why force declines over time.

Of course, the key question is, "Why should a desmin knockout muscle generate lower stress and be injured to a lesser extent compared with a wild type muscle?" The answer is not currently known but the following has been hypothesized: Intermediate filaments provide the normal interconnections between sarcomeres along and across the muscle fiber permitting efficient transfer of mechanical stress from the myofibril to the fiber exterior (Patel & Lieber, 1997). In the absence of desmin the intermyofibrillar connections may be more compliant permitting a greater degree of internal sarcomere shortening and motion, thereby decreasing the efficiency of force transfer across and along the fiber and decreasing stress generation. Similarly, based on the lack of these con-

nections, the opposite situation, where strain is transmitted from the fiber exterior to the myofibrils could also be less efficient. The result would be a decreased sarcomere strain during a fixed degree of lengthening in knockout compared with wild type muscles and thus, less injury in spite of the fact that the energy delivered to the desmin knockout muscle is identical.

There is some preliminary support for such a hypothesis. First, morphological analysis of the wild type and knockout muscles demonstrated many more cytoskeletal ultrastructural abnormalities in wild type compared with knockout muscles. One abnormality that was particularly striking was the percentage of "slanted" Z-disks seen after eccentric injury. In the wild type muscles, a significantly greater proportion of Z-disks were slanted greater than 30° in wild type ($10.4\pm1.5\%$) compared with knockout muscles ($5.8\pm0.9\%$) which support the concept of greater "strained" connection between adjacent myofibrils in wild type compared with knockout muscles. In addition, we recently measured, using numerous longitudinal electron micrographs of muscle from normal and desmin knockout animals, the "sliding" of myofibrils adjacent to one another as a muscle was stretched (Shah et al., 2002). This was quantified by measuring the horizontal displacement of adjacent Z-disks (Δx) as a function of sarcomere length (Fig. 6-37). Note that, in the wild type muscles, Δx was relatively constant as a function of sarcomere length, suggesting some type of mechanical tether that prevents excessive sliding. However, in the knockout Δx continued to get larger with sarcomere length, suggesting a greater ability for displacement of adjacent myofibrils. These

questions are currently being pursued on single muscle fibers with greater resolution.

Inflammation in Muscle Damage

The previous discussion on muscle injury focused primarily on mechanical events associated with muscle injury. There is a tremendous interest in the biological response of muscle to injury and repair. One aspect of muscle injury that has tremendous clinical implications is the inflammatory response mounted by a muscle in response to injury. Recall that the inflammatory response is the body's first line of defense to avoid prolonged disability. Several recent studies have showed that inflammation itself (*i.e.*, the infiltration of inflammatory cells such as neutrophils and macrophages) can injure muscle tissue. Thus, while mechanical injury may

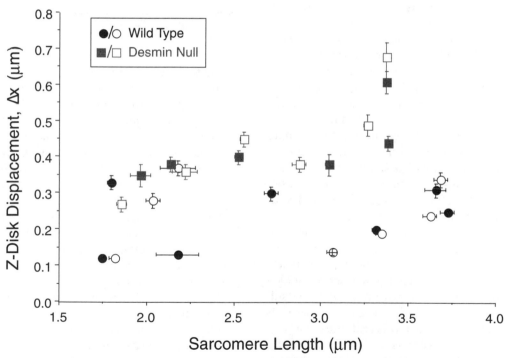

FIGURE 6-37. Relative displacement of Z-disks (Δx) from adjacent myofibrils in wild type (open circles) and desmin knockout (filled circles) mouse EDL muscles. Note that, in the knockout animals, a greater degree of sliding between adjacent myofibrils is permitted suggesting lack of physical tether normally provided by desmin. (Data from: Shah, S., Fridén, J., Su F-C, Milner, D.J., Capetanaki, Y., Lieber, R.L. (2002). Evidence for increased mobility of myofibrils in desmin null skeletal muscles. *Journal of Experimental Biology, 205,* 321–325.)

cause the initial injury, further injury may result from subsequent tissue inflammation. This hypothesis implies that the inflammatory process that can be used to repair tissue, may also cause further damage.

This hypothesis was directly tested by Dr. Joe Cannon working in Dr. Bill Evan's laboratory (Cannon et al., 1990, 1991). These investigators measured plasma CK levels in the same way as that described in the study reported in Figure 6-15. However, they performed these experiments on "young" (<30 years old) and "old" (>55 years old) human subjects. To study the effect of inflammation superimposed upon muscle injury, they also treated both groups with large doses of Vitamin E, a substance that stabilizes cell membranes and protects them against oxidative damage such as occurs during inflammation. The results were surprising. Cannon and colleagues observed the typical transient CK response in young individuals, whether or not they had received Vitamin E treatment. They also observed an increase in circulating levels of inflammatory cells in all young subjects. However, the elderly subjects demonstrated a much different response. The group that did not receive Vitamin E had a smaller CK transient response, similar to that previously described for training (filled circles, Figure 6-15). That is, the older, unprotected muscle demonstrated a smaller CK response. Since older muscle is known to be more vulnerable to exercise-induced injury, the simplest interpretation of these data is that CK levels clearly do not provide a reliable measure of muscle damage. This was confirmed by inspection of the CK data from the older subjects who received Vitamin E. Their CK response looked more like that seen for young, untrained subjects (open circles, Figure 6-15). What can be concluded about CK levels and muscle injury? The definitive answer is not yet available, but one must acknowledge that, as seen above in the animal studies, while increased CK levels are associated with muscle injury, they are not necessarily the direct result of the injury. Perhaps increased CK levels represent muscle remodeling which must occur following injury.

Box 6-8 Why Can Nonsteroidal Antiinflammatory Drugs (NSAIDs) Be Bad for Muscle?

Inflammation that occurs after muscle injury does cause tissue damage and is painful. Therefore, many people use NSAIDs to prevent these effects. This is essentially using the NSAID as an analgesic (pain reliever) rather than an antiinflammatory medication. Studies in animal models and young and old human and associated events appear to be necessary for proper muscle remodeling after injury as well as ultimate muscle strengthening. In an animal model, NSAIDs given after muscle injury actually resulted in weaker muscles in the long run. The take-home message is, "be careful when interfering with Nature's response to injury!"

Therapist's Comments

For the clinician, understanding the timing and the events of the inflammatory response help determine the type and intensity of the rehabilitation exercises. The time course of inflammation and repair after muscle injury suggests that myotubes are present and contractile ability is returning to normal within 1 week after the injury (although, complete regeneration and repair of the muscle takes many weeks). In the case of eccentric exercise-induced muscle injury, the pain subsides within 4 days after the injury, but the muscle is still swollen, strength is still decreased, and repair of the muscle is in the early stages. Therefore, even though the patient may have little pain a few days after the injury, the clinician should be cautious when beginning rehabilitation exercises understanding that the repair process is continuing. They should also educate the patient in this regard so that compliance with rehabilitative prescriptions is assured.

In terms of circulating inflammatory cells, the older subjects again demonstrated an unexpected response: the group that did not receive Vitamin E demonstrated an attenuated level of circulating neutrophils which was "increased to normal" by pretreatment with Vitamin E. Experiments such as these will have profound effects on our strategies for treating skeletal muscle injuries. It goes without saying that a rational basis for the prevention of muscle inflammation via the use of anti-inflammatory agents is not yet available.

Another direct demonstration of the ability of inflammatory cells to cause muscle injury was provided by Dr. James Tidball, who studied an injury model that results when animals who had been subjected to 10 days of hindlimb unloading (Chapter 5, pages 249 to 256) are then permitted normal weight bearing (Pizza, Hernandez, & Tidball, 1998). During this weight bearing period, muscle injury is observed. Tidball and colleagues demonstrated that, after permitting weight bearing, a steady invasion of neutrophils occurred for at least 24 hours (Fig.

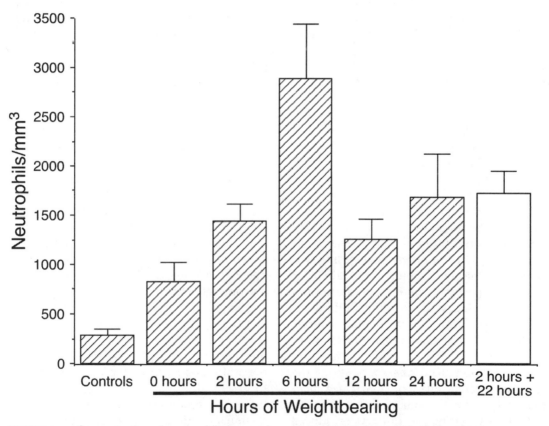

FIGURE 6-38. Concentration of neutrophils in muscle subjected to 10 days of hindlimb unloading followed by 2–24 hours of weightbearing (hatched bars). Note progressive invasion of these inflammatory cells. A separate group was subjected to 10 days of hindlimb unloading followed by 2 hours of weightbearing followed by 22 hours of resuspension (2 hours + 22 hours, open bar). The fact that the 24 hour data and 2 hour + 22 hour are the same supports the idea that inflammatory cells, not further loading, were responsible for the continued injury observed in the muscle (Data from: Tidball, J.G., Berchenko, E., Frenette, J. (1999). Macrophage invasion does not contribute to muscle membrane injury during inflammation. *Journal of Leukocyte Biology, 65,* 492–498.)

6-38, hatched bars), which could cause muscle injury (Tidball, Berchenko, & Frenette, 1999). To test whether the mechanical loading associated with weight bearing that permitted the neutrophil invasion, they permitted another group of animals to weight bear for 2 hours and then re-suspended them for 22 hours (Fig. 6-38, open bar). The magnitude of the muscle injury observed in this so-called 2+22 group was just as severe as the injury observed in the group that experienced 24 hours of continuous loading. Their interpretation of these data was that the presence and continued infiltration of these inflammatory cells themselves did not require continuous mechanical insult to the tissue and was the cause of the injury observed.

NSAIDs Provide a Short-Term Benefit but Long-Term Loss in Muscle Function

The process of inflammation and repair raises a potential conflict regarding the use of antiinflammatory medications after muscle injury. Since the inflammation process (which includes proteolysis by infiltrating neutrophils and macrophages) can itself cause damage in excess of that originally experienced by the tissue, it could be argued that prevention of inflammation would improve muscle status following injury. On the other hand, a "normal" inflammatory response might be required for the muscle to properly remodel after injury. Resolving this conflict would be difficult if experiments were performed using human subjects since the analgesic effect of nonsteroidal antiinflammatory drugs (NSAIDs) could itself permit improved performance, thus confounding the issue. Therefore, the effect of NSAID treatment was quantified on the rabbit skeletal muscle model following eccentric contraction-induced muscle injury. Six groups of animal subjects were subjected to an eccentric exercise and their contractile properties measured 3, 7, or 28 days after the exercise bout. After muscle injury due to eccentric contraction, three of the groups of animals were treated with flurbiprofen at a dosage of approximately 9 mg/day.

The remaining animals were permitted normal cage activity as untreated controls. The duration of drug treatment was 3 days for the 3-day group, and 7 days for the 7-day group and 7 days of treatment for the 28-day group. The NSAID-treated group demonstrated remarkable recovery compared with nontreated, eccentrically exercised muscles after only 3 days and 7 days, but then showed a significant decline in torque generation after 28 days (Fig. 6-39) (Mishra, Fridén, Schmitz, & Lieber, 1995). This was obvious in the torque records and the force records of both the EDL and TA. This represents a short-term benefit but long-term detriment of NSAID treatment. Thus, flurbiprofen-treated muscles demonstrated increased muscle strength at the early time periods but depressed strength after 28 days. Whether such a result is generally applicable to all forms of exercise-induced injury is not known. However, these results may cause one to rethink the relatively cavalier and widespread use of antiinflammatory medications which is often observed in the sports medicine community.

Another interesting by-product of this study was a detailed investigation of the morphology of these muscles after injury (Fridén & Lieber, 1998). Significant segmental lesions along the length of the muscle fiber were seen that resulted in "hypercontraction" of various muscle fiber regions (Fig. 6-40). Interestingly, these hypercontracted fibers also get very large in cross-section (does Fig. 6-40A look something like Fig. 6-24?) due to the fact that, as sarcomeres contract their volume stays constant. If the large fibers are viewed in longitudinal section, note the profound presence of infiltrating inflammatory cells near the lesion (Fig. 6-40B). Here then, is at least an association between inflammation and morphological changes in the muscle fibers within the tissue. The dramatic inflammatory response seen in these sections highlights the tremendous vascularity of muscle and thus the proximity to the circulatory system for the therapeutic use of medications or the use of muscles as a producer of substances using gene therapy.

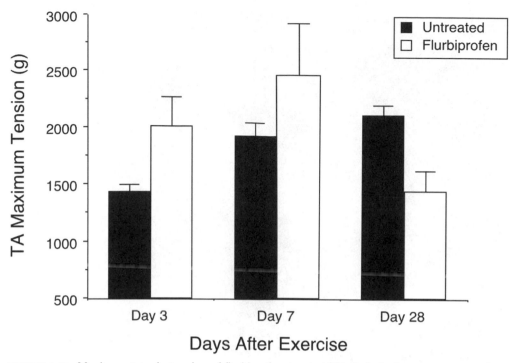

FIGURE 6-39. Maximum tetanic tension of flurbiprofen-treated (filled circles) versus untreated TA muscles. Tetanic tension mirrors the results obtained by measurement of dorsiflexion torque in that flurbiprofen-treated animals generate higher muscle forces early in the treatment and lower muscle forces later in the treatment. (Data from: Mishra, D.K., Fridén, J., Schmitz, M.C., Lieber, R.L. (1995). Antiinflammatory medication after muscle injury. A treatment resulting in short-term improvement but subsequent loss of muscle function. *Journal of Bone and Joint Surgery (American), 77,* 1510–1519.)

Excitation-Contraction Coupling and Muscle Injury

Up until now, primarily structural and biological changes within the contractile apparatus have been considered to provide the underlying mechanism for the loss of force in skeletal muscle after eccentric contraction. However, to date, there is still the unsatisfactory situation that no one has provided a structural basis for the large muscle force decline observed in either animal or human experimental models. This incongruity provided the motivation for a series of interesting experiments by physiologists Drs. Robert Armstrong and Gordon Warren and colleagues in which they suggested that it wasn't the structural damage to muscle that caused the force loss, rather it was the muscle's inability to activate the contractile apparatus that caused the force loss. In other words, their explanation for much of the muscle's force loss was an interruption in the normal process of excitation-contraction coupling.

To test this idea, they exploited the use of the "skinned muscle" preparation in which the membrane systems are rendered permeable by the use of mild detergents so that the contractile apparatus can be directly activated by exogenous applied calcium solutions. Thus, they eccentrically exercised mouse muscles and then measured the normal post-exercise maximum tetanic tension (Warren, Hayes, Lowe, & Armstrong, 1993b). Then, after skinning the muscles, they again measured maximum tetanic tension and found substantial increases

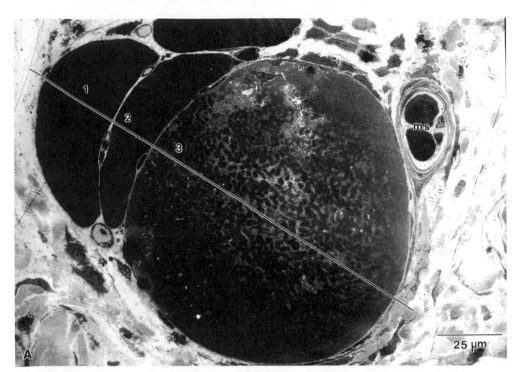

FIGURE 6-40. (A) Cross-section of muscle fibers showing enlarged fiber (#3) and two normal fibers (1 and 2). **(B)** Longitudinal section of muscle along plane shown in (A) revealing the inflammatory process that leads to the enlarged fiber type and size variation observed (c.f. Fig. 6-24). Thus, enlarged fibers represent "supercontracted" cells, which are being digested by inflammatory cells a short distance away. Calibration bar = 25 μm (Used with permission from: Fridén, J., Lieber, R.L. (1998). Segmental muscle fiber lesions after repetitive eccentric contractions. *Cell and Tissue Research, 293*, 165–171.)

(Fig. 6-41). What is the interpretation of these data? The most obvious interpretation is that force increase with direct calcium activation suggested that, after eccentric exercise, the normal magnitude of calcium release was diminished due to some breakdown in the excitation-contraction coupling scheme. Recall from Chapter 2 and the discussion of fatigue, that it is possible to interrupt this pathway at a number of sites. Warren et al. have pursued this line of experimentation since their first publication and have provided further evidence that the loss of excitation-contraction coupling can be detected using joint torque measurements and electromyography in intact animals. They argue that, because EMG does not decrease to the same extent as torque, this implicates loss of E-C coupling at some point distal to the muscle action potential (Ingalls, Warren, Williams, Ward, & Armstrong, 1998; Warren, Ingalls, Shah, & Armstrong, 1999).

Closing Thoughts on Muscle Injury
After having presented so many mechanical, biological, and structural theories of muscle injury, the student might be overwhelmed by the "lack" of consensus. It is encouraged that you view this field as a "work in progress" and learn to critically evaluate the literature on a

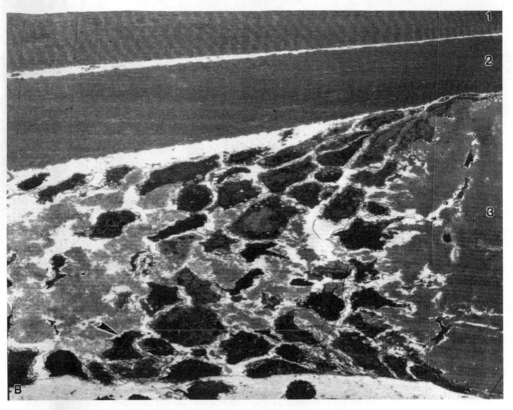

FIGURE 6-40. *(CONTINUED)*

study-by-study basis as well as in light of the historical and surrounding literature. Clearly there is much to learn about muscle injury and strengthening using eccentric exercise protocols. With so many excellent laboratories studying this phenomenon, answers will certainly emerge. No single laboratory has a "corner on the market" on truth in this area. Probably, the "real truth" represents some combination of many of these ideas. That is how the science will progress—experimentation, data analysis, interpretation, integration, and theorization.

Hopefully you have learned from this text how to think more critically, especially in the muscle realm. We are depending on you, the future laboratory directors in this area, to carry on this rich tradition of investigation and edu-cation. As a result, our patients, our colleagues and certainly, our society will benefit tremendously.

■ Chapter Summary

In this chapter, you saw the dramatic, dynamic, and impressive response of skeletal muscle fibers to traumatic injury. Skeletal muscle tissue regenerates vigorously following injury. The main "player" in the regenerative response is the satellite cell, which under cellular control, proliferates, fuses, and synthesizes proteins to restore fiber function to "normal." Such regeneration may someday be exploited in the therapeutic application of myogenic cells to myopathic tissue. Muscle injury during exercise is

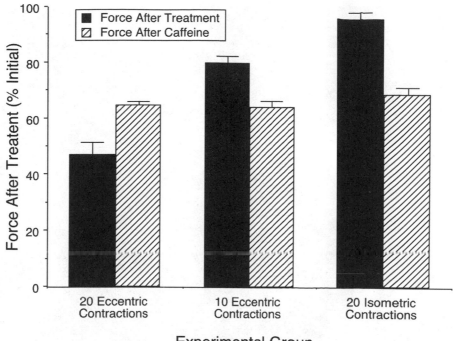

FIGURE 6-41. Maximum tetanic tension elicited electrically immediately after "treatment" (filled bars) and then, in the presence of 50 mM caffeine (hatched bars), which is known to augment calcium release by the sarcoplasmic reticulum. Muscles received treatment of 10 or 20 eccentric contractions compared to 20 isometric contractions that served as controls. The fact that force with caffeine-augmented contractions were no different than the force observed after isometric treatment was interpreted as indicating that eccentric contraction interrupted the excitation-contraction coupling process at some stage. (Data from: Warren, G.L., Lowe, D.A., Hayes, D.A., Karwoski, C.J., Prior, B.M., Armstrong, R.B. (1993). Excitation failure in eccentric contraction-induced injury of mouse soleus muscle. *Journal of Physiology (London), 468*, 487–499.)

selectively associated with eccentric contractions. Although high tensions are clearly required for muscle damage, the evidence to date suggests that a disruption of the muscle cell's ability to buffer calcium may provide the cellular signal to degenerate and regenerate a new fiber. The mechanical events associated with eccentric exercise are unique and have provided insights into normal muscle function. Finally, the inflammation that occurs after muscle injury appears to be necessary for proper remodeling, even strengthening, and the widespread use of anti-inflammatory medication may require rethinking.

REFERENCES

Allen, R.E., Sheehan, S.M., Taylor, R.G., Kendall, T.L., Rice, G.M. (1995). Hepatocyte growth factor activates quiescent skeletal muscle satellite cells in vitro. *Journal of Cell Physiology, 165,* 307–312.

Balnave, C.D., Allen, D.G. (1995). Intracellular calcium and force in single mouse muscle fibres following repeated contractions with stretch. *Journal of Physiology (London), 488,* 25–36.

Belcastro, A. (1993). Skeletal muscle calcium-activated neutral protease (Calpain) with exercise. *Journal of Applied Physiology, 74*, 1381–1386.

Bischoff, R. (1986). Proliferation of muscle satellite cells on intact myofibers in culture. *Developmental Biology, 115*, 129–139.

Bischoff, R. (1986). A satellite cell mitogen from crushed adult muscle. *Developmental Biology, 115*, 140–147.

Bischoff, R. (1990). Interaction between satellite cells and skeletal muscle fibers. *Development, 109*, 943–952.

Blau, H.M., Springer, M.L. (1995). Muscle-mediated gene therapy. *New England Journal of Medicine, 333*, 1554–1556.

Brown, S.C., Lucy, J.A. (1997). *Dystrophin: Gene, protein, and cell biology.* Cambridge, U.K.: Cambridge University Press

Byrnes, W.C., Clarkson, P.M., White, J.S., Hseih, S.S., Frykman, P.N., Maughan, R.J. (1985). Delayed onset muscle soreness following repeated bouts of downhill running. *Journal of Applied Physiology, 59*, 710–715.

Campbell, K.P. (1995). Three muscular dystrophies: loss of cytoskeletal-extracellular matrix linkage. *Cell, 80*, 675–679.

Cannon, J.G., Meydani, S.N., Fielding, R.A., Fiatarone, M.A., Meydani, M., Farhangmehr, M., Orencole, S.F., Blumberg, J.B., Evans, W.J. (1991). Acute phase response in exercise. II. Associations between Vitamin E, cytokines, and muscle proteolysis. *American Journal of Physiology, 260*, R1235–R1240.

Cannon, J.G., Orencole, S.F., Fielding, R.A., Meydani, M., Meydani, S.N., Fiatarone, M.A., Blumberg, J.B., Evans, W.J. (1990). Acute phase response in exercise: interaction of age and Vitamin E on neutrophils and muscle enzyme release. *American Journal of Physiology, 259*, R1214–R1219.

Carlson, B. (1973). The regeneration of skeletal muscle: a review. *American Journal of Anatomy, 137*, 119–150.

Carlson, B.M., Faulkner, J.A. (1989). Muscle transplantation between young and old rats: age of host determines recovery. *American Journal of Physiology, 256*, C1262–C1266.

Carlson, B.M., Faulkner, J.A. (1998). Muscle regeneration in young and old rats: effects of motor nerve transection with and without marcaine treatment. *Journal of Gerontology, 53*, B52–B57

Carpenter, S., Karpati, G. (1984). *Pathology of skeletal muscle.* New York, NY: Churchill Livingstone.

Dalakas, M.C., Park, K.Y., Semino-Mora, C., Lee, H.S., Sivakumar, K., Goldfarb, L.G. (2000). Desmin myopathy, a skeletal myopathy with cardiomyopathy caused by mutations in the desmin gene. *New England Journal of Medicine, 342*, 770–780.

Dayton, W.R., Goll, D.E., Zeece, M.G., Robson, R.M., Reville, W.J. (1976). A Ca^{2+}-activated protease possibly involved in myofibrillar protein turnover purification from porcine muscle. *Biochemistry, 15*, 2150–2158.

Donovan, C.M., Faulkner, J. (1987). Plasticity of skeletal muscle: regenerating fibers adapt more rapidly than surviving fibers. *Journal of Applied Physiology, 62*, 2507–2511.

Duan, C., Delp, M.D., Hayes, D.A., Delp, P.D., Armstrong, R.B. (1990). Rat skeletal muscle mitochondrial (Ca^{2+}) and injury from downhill walking. *Journal of Applied Physiology, 68*, 1241–1251.

Evans, W.J., Meredith, C.N., Cannon, J.G., Dinarello, C.A., Frontera, W.R., Hughes, V.A., Jones, B.H., Knuttgen, H.G. (1986). Metabolic changes following eccentric exercise in trained and untrained men. *Journal of Applied Physiology, 61*, 1864–1868.

Faulkner, J.A., Niemeyer, J.H., Maxwell, C., White, T.P. (1980). Contractile properties of transplanted extensor digitorum longus muscles of cats. *American Journal of Physiology, 238*, C120–C126.

Fridén, J., Lieber, R.L. (1998). Segmental muscle fiber lesions after repetitive eccentric contractions. *Cell and Tissue Research, 293*, 165–171.

Fridén, J., Lieber, R.L. (2001). Serum creatine kinase level is a poor predictor of muscle function after injury. *Scandinavian Journal of Medicine Science in Sports, 11*, 126–127.

Fridén, J., Sjöström, M., Ekblom, B. (1981). A morphological study of delayed muscle soreness. *Experientia, 37*, 506–507.

Fridén, J., Sjöström, M., Ekblom, B. (1983). Myofibrillar damage following intense eccentric exercise in man. *International Journal of Sports Medicine, 4*, 170–176.

Guharay, F., Sachs, F. (1984). Stretch-activated single ion channel currents in tissue-cultured embryonic chick skeletal muscle. *Journal of Physiology (London), 352*, 685–701.

Gulati, A.K., Reddi, A.H., Zalewski, A.A. (1983).

Changes in the basement membrane zone components during skeletal muscle fiber degeneration and regeneration. *Journal of Cell Biology, 97,* 957–962.

Gussoni, E., Blau, H.M., Kunkel, L.M. (1997). The fate of individual myoblasts after transplantation into muscles of DMD patients. *Nature Medicine 3,* 970–977.

Harry, J.D., Ward, A.W., Heglund, N.C., Morgan, D.L., McMahon, T.A. (1990). Cross-bridge cycling theories cannot explain high-speed lengthening behavior in frog muscle. *Biophysical Journal, 57,* 201–208.

Hawke, T.J., Garry, D.J. (2001). Myogenic satellite cells: physiology to molecular biology. *Journal of Applied Physiology, 91,* 534–551.

Hoffman, E.P., Brown, R.H., Kunkel, L.M. (1987a). Conservation of the Duchenne muscular dystrophy gene in mice and humans. *Science, 238,* 347–350.

Hoffman, E.P., Brown, R.H., Kunkel, L.M. (1987b). Dystrophin: the protein product of the Duchenne muscular dystrophy locus. *Cell, 51,* 919–928.

Huard, J., Fu, F.H. (2000). Gene therapy and tissue engineering in orthopaedic and sports medicine. In: *Methods in Bioengineering.* Vol 16. (pp. 286). Boston: Birkhäuser.

Huard, J., Labrecque, C., Dansereau, G., Robitaille, L., Tremblay, J.P. (1991). Dystrophin expression in myotubes formed by the fusion of normal and dystrophic myoblasts. *Muscle Nerve, 14,* 178–182.

Ingalls, C.P., Warren, G.L., Williams, J.H., Ward, C.W., Armstrong, R.B. (1998). E-C coupling failure in mouse EDL muscle after in vivo eccentric contractions. *Journal of Applied Physiology, 85,* 58–67.

Jaffe, A.S. (2001). New standard for the diagnosis of acute myocardial infarction. *Cardiology Review, 9,* 318–322.

Jennische, E., Ekberg, S., Matejka, G.L. (1993). Expression of hepatocyte growth factor in growing and regenerating rat skeletal muscle. *American Journal of Physiology, 265,* C122–C128.

Johnson, S.E., Allen, R.E. (1993). Proliferating cell nuclear antigen (PCNA) is expressed in activated rat skeletal muscle satellite cells. *Journal of Cell Physiology, 154,* 39–43.

Johnson, S.E., Allen, R.E. (1995). Activation of skeletal muscle satellite cells and the role of fibroblast growth factor receptors. *Experimental Cell Research, 219,* 449–453.

Karpati, G., Pouliot, Y., Stirling, C., Holland, P. (1989). *Implantation of nondystrophic allogenic myoblasts into dystrophic muscles of mdx mice produces "mosaic" fibers of normal microscopic phenotype* (pp. 973–985). New York: Alan R Liss.

Kuruc, N., Franke, W.W. (1988). Transient coexpression of desmin and cytokeratins 8 and 18 in developing myocardial cells of some vertebrate species. *Differentiation, 38,* 177–193.

Kyrolainen, H., Takala, T.E., Komi, P.V. (1998). Muscle damage induced by stretch-shortening cycle exercise. *Medicine and Science in Sports and Exercise, 30,* 415–420.

Lazarides, E. (1980). Intermediate filaments as mechanical integrators of cellular space. *Nature, 283,* 249–256.

Lazarides, E. (1982). Intermediate filaments: a chemically heterogeneous, developmentally regulated class of proteins. *Annual Review of Biochemistry, 51,* 219–250.

Li, H., Choudhary, S.K., Milner, D.J., Munir, M.I., Kuisk, I.R., Capetanaki, Y. (1994). Inhibition of desmin expression blocks myoblasts fusion and interferes with the myogenic regulators myoD and myogenin. *Journal of Cell Biology, 124,* 827–841.

Lieber, R.L., Fridén, J. (1988). Selective damage of fast glycolytic muscle fibers with eccentric contraction of the rabbit tibialis anterior. *Acta Physiologica Scandinavica, 133,* 587–588.

Lieber, R.L., Fridén, J. (1993). Muscle damage is not a function of muscle force but active muscle strain. *Journal of Applied Physiology, 74,* 520–526.

Lieber, R.L., McKee-Woodburn, T., Fridén, J. (1991). Muscle damage induced by eccentric contractions of 25% strain. *Journal of Applied Physiology, 70,* 2498–2507.

Lieber, R.L., Schmitz, M.C., Mishra, D.K., Fridén, J. (1994). Contractile and cellular remodeling in rabbit skeletal muscle after cyclic eccentric contractions. *Journal of Applied Physiology, 77,* 1926–1934.

Lieber, R.L., Thornell, L-E., Fridén, J. (1996). Muscle cytoskeletal disruption occurs within the first 15 minutes of cyclic eccentric contraction. *Journal of Applied Physiology, 80,* 278–284.

Lynn, R., Morgan, D.L. (1994). Decline running produces more sarcomeres in rat vastus intermedius muscle fibers than does incline running. *Journal of Applied Physiology, 77,* 1439–1444.

Mauro, A. (1970). *Regeneration of striated muscle and myogenesis.* Amsterdam: Excerpta Medica.

Mauro, A.J. (1961). Satellite cell of skeletal muscle fibers. *Journal of Biophysical and Biochemical Cytology, 9*, 493–495.

McCully, K.K., Faulkner, J.A. (1985). Injury to skeletal muscle fibers of mice following lengthening contractions. *Journal of Applied Physiology, 59*, 119–126.

McHugh, M.P., Connolly, D.A., Eston, R.G., Kremenic, I.J., Nicholas, S.J., Gleim, G.W. (1999). The role of passive muscle stiffness in symptoms of exercise-induced muscle damage. *American Journal of Sports Medicine, 27*, 594–599.

McNeil, P.L., Khakee, R. (1992). Disruptions of muscle fiber plasma membranes. *American Journal of Pathology, 140*, 1097–1109.

Megeney, L.A., Kablar, B., Garrett, K., Anderson, J.E., Rudnicki, M.A. (1996). MyoD is required for myogenic stem cell function in adult skeletal muscle. *Genes and Development, 10*, 1173–1183.

Milner, D.J., Mavroidis, M., Weisleder, N., Capetanaki, Y. (2000). Desmin cytoskeleton linked to muscle mitochondrial distribution and respiratory function. *Journal of Cell Biology, 150*, 1283–1298.

Milner, D.J., Weitzer, G., Tran, D., Bradley, A., Capetanaki, Y. (1996). Disruption of muscle architecture and myocardial degeneration in mice lacking desmin. *Journal of Cell Biology, 134*, 1255–1270.

Mishra, D.K., Fridén, J., Schmitz, M.C., Lieber, R.L. (1995). Antiinflammatory medication after muscle injury. A treatment resulting in short-term improvement but subsequent loss of muscle function. *Journal of Bone and Joint Surgery, 77*, 1510–1519.

Morgan, D.L. (1990). New insights into the behavior of muscle during active lengthening. *Biophysical Journal, 57*, 209–221.

Morgan, D.L., Allen, D.G. (1999). Early events in stretch-induced muscle damage. *Journal of Applied Physiology, 87*, 2007–2015.

Newham, D.J. (1988). The consequences of eccentric contractions and their relationship to delayed onset muscle pain. *European Journal of Applied Physiology, 57*, 353–359.

Newham, D.J., Jones, D.A., Clarkson, P.M. (1987). Repeated high-force eccentric exercise: effects on muscle pain and damage. *Journal of Applied Physiology, 63*, 1381–1386.

Niklason, L.E. (1999). Techview: medical technology. Replacement arteries made to order. *Science, 286*, 1493–1494.

Niklason, L.E., Gao, J., Abbott, W.M., Hirschi, K.K., Houser, S., Marini, R., Langer, R. (1999). Functional arteries grown in vitro. *Science, 284*, 489–493.

Ohlendieck, K., Ervasti, J.M., Snook, J.B., Campbell, K.P. (1991). Dystrophin-glycoprotein complex is highly enriched in isolated skeletal muscle sarcolemma. *Journal of Cell Biology, 112*, 135–148.

Partridge, T.A., Morgan, J.E., Coulton, G.R., Hoffman, E.P., Kunkel, L.M. (1989). Conversion of mdx myofibres from dystrophin-negative to -positive by injection of normal myoblasts. *Nature, 337*, 176–179.

Patel, T., Cuizon, D., Mathieu-Costello, O., Fridén, J., Lieber, R.L. (1998). Increased oxidative capacity does not protect skeletal muscle from eccentric contraction-induced muscle injury. *American Journal of Physiology, 274*, R1300–R1308.

Patel, T.J., Fridén, J., Lutz, G.J., Lieber, R.L. (2002). Active sarcomere strain causes injury and differential cytoskeletal damage to frog skeletal muscle fiber bundles. (submitted) 2002.

Patel, T.J., Lieber, R.L. (1997). Force transmission in skeletal muscle: from actomyosin to external tendons. *Exercise and Sport Sciences Reviews, 25*, 321–363.

Petrof, B.J., Shrager, J.B., Stedman, H.H., Kelly, A.M., Sweeney, H.L. (1993). Dystrophin protects the sarcolemma from stresses developed during muscle contraction. *Proceedings of the National Academy of Sciences of the United States of America, 90*, 3710–3714.

Pizza, F.X., Hernandez, I.J., Tidball, J.G. (1998). Nitric oxide synthase inhibition reduces muscle inflammation and necrosis in modified muscle use. *Journal of Leukocyte Biology, 64*, 427–433.

Rack, P.M.H., Westbury, D.R. (1974). The short range stiffness of active mammalian muscle and its effects on mechanical properties. *Journal of Physiology (London), 240*, 331–350.

Rando, T.A., Blau, H.M. (1994). Primary mouse myoblast purification, characterization, and transplantation for cell-mediated gene therapy. *Journal of Cell Biology, 125*, 1275–1287.

Reddy, M.K., Etlinger, J.D., Rabinowitz, M., Fischman, D.A., Zak, R. (1975). Removal of Z-lines and α-actinin from isolated myofibrils by a calcium-activated neutral protease. *Journal of Biological Chemistry, 250*, 4278–4284.

Sam, M., Fridén, J., Shah, S., Milner, D.J., Capetanaki, Y., Lieber, R.L. (2000). Desmin knockout muscles generate lower stress and are less vulnerable to injury compared to wild type muscles. *American Journal of Physiology, 279,* C1116–C1122.

Shah, S., Fridén, J., Su, F-C., Milner, D.J., Capetanaki, Y., Lieber, R.L. (2002). Evidence for increased mobility of myofibrils in desmin null skeletal muscles. *Journal of Experimental Biology, 205,* 321–325.

Shansky, J., Del Tatto, M., Chromiak, J., Vandenburgh, H. (1997). A simplified method for tissue engineering skeletal muscle organoids in vitro. *In Vitro Cell and Developmental Biology in Animals, 33,* 659–661.

Snow, M.H. (1976). Myogenic cell formation in regenerating rat skeletal muscle injured by mincing. *Anatomical Record, 188,* 201–217.

Talbot, J.A., Morgan, D.L. (1996). Quantitative analysis of sarcomere non-uniformities in active muscle following a stretch. *Journal of Muscle Research and Cell Motility, 17,* 261–268.

Tatsumi, R., Anderson, J.E., Nevoret, C.J., Halevy, O., Allen, R.E. (1998). HGF/SF is present in normal adult skeletal muscle and is capable of activating satellite cells. *Developmental Biology, 194,* 114–128.

Tidball, J.G., Berchenko, E., Frenette, J. (1999). Macrophage invasion does not contribute to muscle membrane injury during inflammation. *Journal of Leukocyte Biology, 65,* 492–498.

Vandenburgh, H.H. (1982). Dynamic mechanical orientation of skeletal myofibers in vitro. *Developmental Biology, 93,* 438–443.

Vandenburgh, H., Del Tatto, M., Shansky, J., Lemaire, J., Chang, A., Payumo, F., Lee, P., Goodyear, A., Raven, L. (1996). Tissue-engineered skeletal muscle organoids for reversible gene therapy. *Human Gene Therapy, 17,* 2195–2200.

Vandenburgh, H.H., Hatefaludy, S., Karlisch, P., Shansky, J. (1991a). Mechanically induced alterations in cultured skeletal muscle growth. *Journal of Biomechanics, 24,* 91–99.

Vandenburgh, H.H., Swasdison, S., Karlisch, P. (1991b). Computer-aided mechanogenesis of skeletal muscle organs from single cells in vitro. *FASEB Journal, 5,* 2860–2867.

Warren, G.L., Ingalls, C.P., Shah, S.J., Armstrong, R.B. (1999). Uncoupling of in vivo torque production from EMG in mouse muscles injured by eccentric contractions. *Journal of Physiology (London), 515,* 609–619.

Warren, G.L., Lowe, D.A., Hayes, D.A., Karwoski, C.J., Prior, B.M., Armstrong, R.B. (1993a). Excitation failure in eccentric contraction-induced injury of mouse soleus muscle. *Journal of Physiology (London), 468,* 487–499.

Warren, G.W., Hayes, D., Lowe, D.A., Armstrong, R.B. (1993b). Mechanical factors in the initiation of eccentric contraction-induced injury in rat soleus muscle. *Journal of Physiology (London), 464,* 457–475.

Weitzer, G., Milner, D.J., Kim, J-U., Bradley, A., Capetanaki, Y. (1995). Cytoskeletal control of myogenesis: a desmin null mutation blocks the myogenic pathway during embryonic stem cell differentiation. *Developmental Biology, 172,* 422–439.

Index

Page numbers in italic denote figures; those followed by a t denote tables; those followed by a b denote boxes.